Imaging of the Phar and the Esophagus

Often neglected or wrongfully discarded as obsolete, barium swallows are still a staple of the daily routine of radiology departments worldwide, serving as an important tool to support the clinical and endoscopic diagnosis of the upper gastrointestinal tract. Like other imaging methods, barium radiography and fluoroscopy have also undergone radical technological changes and upgrades. This book constitutes a seminal volume on the subject, easily accessible to junior graduate students and specialists, showcasing that before being a diagnostic tool of utmost importance, it is a form of art worth preserving and passing on to future generations. Covering sections such as oral and pharyngeal anatomy and an overview of clinical disorders, the basics of pharyngoesophageal endoscopy, CT, and MR imaging, as well as the art of interpreting the images, this book provides an extensive and well-illustrated guide to the morphodynamic imaging of the pharynx and esophagus.

Key Features

- Underscores the value of the barium swallow study in the evaluation of the upper gastrointestinal tract in both routine and complex diagnostic scenarios

- Illustrates the technological advancements in imaging, such as radiographic and fluoroscopic techniques supplemented by digital imaging and improved contrast media

- Caters to both early career learners and experienced clinicians and offers a structured exploration of anatomy, pathology, and radiologic techniques

Imaging of the Pharynx and the Esophagus

Giovanni Fontanella MD FRSA MBSImPc

CRC Press
Taylor & Francis Group
Boca Raton London New York

CRC Press is an imprint of the
Taylor & Francis Group, an **informa** business

Designed cover image: Giovanni Fontanella

First edition published 2026
by CRC Press
2385 NW Executive Center Drive, Suite 320, Boca Raton, FL 33431

and by CRC Press
4 Park Square, Milton Park, Abingdon, Oxon, OX14 4RN

CRC Press is an imprint of Taylor & Francis Group, LLC

© 2026 Giovanni Fontanella

ISBN: 978-1-032-83166-4 (hbk)
ISBN: 978-1-032-79178-4 (pbk)
ISBN: 978-1-003-50811-3 (ebk)

DOI: 10.1201/9781003508113

Typeset in Palatino
by Deanta Global Publishing Services, Chennai, India

"La vita non finisce, è come il sonno;
la nascita è come il risveglio.

...

Torneremo ancora, ancora, e ancora."

F. Battiato

A mio padre Eugenio, ora in una dimensione senza dolore
A mia madre Mirella, esempio di vita e di coraggio
A Simona, futura moglie, che condivide con me ogni giorno pane e sogni
Ad Ivana, figlia mia, che mi mantiene bambino come lei

"Life does not end, it is like sleep;
birth is like awakening.

...

We will return again, and again, and again."

F. Battiato

To my father Eugenio, now in a dimension free from pain.
To my mother Mirella, a true example of life and courage.
To Simona, my future wife, who shares her daily bread and dreams with me.
To Ivana, my daughter, who keeps my inner child alive, a child like her.

Contents

Foreword by Bonnie Martin-Harris

The modified barium swallow study (MBSS) stands as one of the most enduring, informative tools in the evaluation of swallowing physiology. With its origins in structural imaging, the procedure has evolved to capture dynamic events at the intersection of anatomy, physiology, and functional health. Through decades of refinement, the MBSS has become not only a diagnostic procedure but a platform for interdisciplinary understanding, linking image-based impairment with clinical management, patient goals, and outcome prediction.

This volume by Dr. Giovanni Fontanella is a timely and vital contribution to that evolution. It reflects the discipline, clinical empathy, and integrative thinking that high-fidelity fluoroscopic evaluation demands. It is not enough to capture images in shades of black, white, and gray. True clinical impact requires interpreting those images within the context of the patient, bringing together their physiology, their symptoms, their environment, and their care team. That synthesis is at the heart of this book.

Dr. Fontanella's work is particularly meaningful at a time when radiology trainees are often distanced from the functional implications of what they image. This book bridges that divide. It offers detailed anatomic and physiologic exposition while grounding those details in real clinical relevance. It trains the eye to see impairment not in isolation but as part of a complex, dynamic system. It elevates the role of the radiologist to that of a full participant in the management of dysphagia, highlighting the neural underpinnings of function and the translational value of imaging findings.

This book exemplifies an integrative approach to fluoroscopic imaging, one that emphasizes standardized protocols, physiologic detail, and clinical interpretation grounded in reproducibility and relevance. It advances a broader ethos: that methodological rigor is not an academic exercise but a foundation for responsible, impactful patient care. Excellence in this field demands more than image acquisition; it requires the ability to interpret findings with precision, to communicate across disciplines with clarity, and to act with shared purpose.

Comprehensive in scope and thoughtful in execution, this text offers essential insight for the full team of clinicians engaged in the management of oropharyngeal and esophageal swallowing disorders. Its strength lies in its clarity, its clinical applicability, and its insistence on seeing patients, rather than images, as the central focus of practice.

Dr. Fontanella has crafted more than a procedural guide; he has created a teaching companion and a clinical reference. It belongs in the hands of every resident, fellow, and practicing clinician committed to pursuing this work with fidelity, transparency, and compassion.

Bonnie Martin-Harris, PhD, CCC-SLP, BCS-S

Foreword by Francesco Giuseppe Biondo

Every significant scientific work is born from a question, a conflict, an act of resistance.

This book was conceived in precisely this way—as a response to the hasty tendency to dismiss fluoroscopy as an "outdated" technique, in an era where technological innovation has profoundly transformed the diagnostic and therapeutic approach to pharyngeal and esophageal diseases.

This volume, beyond offering exceptional clinical and scientific value, powerfully reaffirms that fluoroscopy is far from obsolete; rather, it remains a modern clinical frontier, maintaining its diagnostic dignity—and even a humanistic dimension.

Dr. Giovanni Fontanella, whom I had the pleasure of knowing and appreciating during our clinical and scientific collaboration when I served as Director of the Department of General and Specialist Surgery at the "Sacro Cuore di Gesù—Fatebenefratelli" Hospital in Benevento, Italy, presents a work that goes well beyond describing the morphology, pathophysiology, and dynamic imaging of the pharyngoesophageal tract. It highlights, with rigor and depth, the irreplaceable role of the radiologist in the multidisciplinary management of patients with functional and organic pharyngoesophageal disorders.

Such an approach restores to the patient a precise, dynamic, and integrated diagnostic language—where technique becomes a tool for connection, understanding, and ultimately, care.

The clinical acumen and human sensitivity that permeate each page of the book reflect the author's mature approach, shaped by extensive field experience and deep reflection on the very meaning of our profession.

This is not merely a technical manual. It is an act of awareness—of the history of medicine, and of attentive listening to patients and to the human body, which speaks beyond words.

In my 40 years of experience as a surgeon of the esophagus and pharynx—at the University of Naples, the "Moscati" Hospital of Avellino, and the "Sacro Cuore di Gesù—Fatebenefratelli" Hospital in Benevento—I have witnessed tools and methodologies evolve. Yet, the value of clinical interpretation and observation—guided by sensitivity, scientific curiosity, interpretative skill, and technical precision—has never diminished.

The author invites us to "speak with patients" before, during, and after the examination.

A simple phrase—yet profoundly revolutionary in a medical context increasingly at risk of becoming procedural and depersonalized. I fully share this vision.

Like surgery, fluoroscopy is not merely technique: it is presence, it is language, it is relationship.

Imaging of the Pharynx and the Esophagus is a complete, scholarly yet accessible volume, intended not only for radiologists, surgeons, and gastroenterologists, but for all those who recognize dysphagia as not only a clinical, but also an existential concern.

I therefore consider this volume an important reference—not only to be studied and consulted, but also to be lived, as knowledge lives when it meets experience. It is a book that informs, guides, and inspires.

Francesco Giuseppe Biondo, MD
Specialist in General and Thoracic Surgery
Professor of Thoracic Surgery
Head of the General Surgery Unit
Avellino, Italy

Acknowledgments

This book would not be here without the help of many people, especially Professor Bonnie Martin-Harris and her group, who provided images, guidance, expertise, and a brilliant foreword.

This is true for Dr. Paul Hellerhoff, too, who kindly gave me permission to use his extensive collection of clinical images on the matter.

Special thanks go to Dr. Francesco Giuseppe Biondo, who also contributed a foreword to this text-book and has always supported me, even when I was much younger and inexperienced—his words surely come from the heart, too, but he captured the essence of my fluoroscopic practice.

I am truly grateful to Dr. Emilio Parente, a fatherly figure who dispenses daily pearls of wisdom and has always shown me respect and trust, both on and off duty—a true maestro in his surgical craft.

To my soon-to-be wife Simona, thank you for a couple of excellent drawings that feature in this book and for supporting me daily with true love and dedication.

I wish to thank all the Imaging and Surgery staff at the Sacro Cuore di Gesù—Fatebenefratelli Hospital in Benevento, Italy, which has been my home for eight years.

ACKNOWLEDGMENT LIST

Bonnie Martin-Harris	Ferdinando Giorgione
Kate Davidson	Giovanni Fuggi
Paul Hellerhoff	Saverio Mazzeo
Simona Borrelli	Gianfranco Micco
Francesco Giuseppe Biondo	Giuliano Fabrizio
Emilio Parente	Carlo Nazzaro
Maurizio Russo	Marco Russo
Fabio Pacifico	Maurizio Orso
Luciano Onofrio	Vincenza De Lucia
Federica Mastella	Diego De Stasio
Michele Schettino	Luigi Di Cerbo
Gianluca Rossetti	Annamaria Carbone
Giuseppe Fuggi	Sonia Lanzilli
Francesca Russo	Roberta De Luca
Nicola Forte	Paola Covino
Silvio De Lucia	Antonietta Cardone
Andrea Festa	Adriana Insogna
Felice De Rosa	Giacomo Sica

Author

Giovanni Fontanella, MD FRSA MBSImPc, is an Abdominal and Gastrointestinal Consultant Radiologist based in Benevento, Italy, at the Sacro Cuore di Gesù—Fatebenefratelli Hospital. His alma mater is the historical Vanvitelli University in Naples, Italy, one of the most important schools for gastrointestinal imaging in Italy. His interest in gastrointestinal (GI) and abdominal imaging was consolidated at the prestigious St. Mark's Hospital in London, United Kingdom, a competitive and top-level environment. In Benevento, he conducts both clinical activities and research, with a focus on constant testing, innovation, and optimization of all imaging techniques to meet the needs of clinical practice. He is currently working on further developments of gel-enhanced MR fistulography, which was entirely developed and used in clinical routine for the first time at the Fatebenefratelli Hospital, morphodynamic imaging techniques in pharyngoesophageal motility diseases, and virtual colonoscopy. His academic record stands, at the time of writing, at over 40 top-level publications, most of them in the field of GI imaging, including the seminal book *Morphodynamic Imaging in Achalasia*, with several occasions as a speaker at international radiology meetings, such as the European Congress of Radiology (ECR 2019, 2020, 2021, 2024), Congress of the European Society of Gastrointestinal and Abdominal Imaging (ESGAR 2019, 2020), and the Annual Radiology Meeting in Dubai (2020, 2021). He works as a regular reviewer for several radiology journals, including the *European Journal of Radiology* and *Clinical Case Reports* to name a few. Dr. Fontanella is a member of several radiology societies worldwide, such as the European Society of Radiology, European Society of Gastrointestinal and Abdominal Imaging, British Society of Gastrointestinal and Abdominal Imaging, Radiological Society of North America, and the Korean Society of Radiology. He regularly hosts GI-themed seminars for the Radiological Society of the Emirates. In 2021, Dr. Fontanella was nominated Fellow of the Royal Society of Arts in London, while in 2023 he was recognized as a registered clinician for the Modified Barium Swallow Impairment Profile.

Introduction

I still remember the day this book was conceptually born, more than ten years ago. That day, while working on my daily barium swallow routine, a risky game of trial and error at the time, one of my senior tutors approached me and, out of the blue, bluntly said that gastrointestinal imaging was done with and should have been disposed of, subtly implying that my efforts were, in the best of cases, useless. I had, up until that day, always listened to my teachers, tutors, and professors, almost always convinced they were talking and teaching in the light of a superior collective well-being. That day, curiously enough, my last patient on the list, well into the afternoon, was a man I had met years before as a child, the father of a schoolmate. I struggled to recognize him, on a wheelchair, due to amyotrophic lateral sclerosis and a devastating weight loss. In my daily practice, I have never seen anyone as happy as he was when meeting me in a medical context. Needless to say, it was an extremely difficult and even somewhat perilous examination to carry out for many reasons. But we all—patient, radiologist, speech therapist—made it. If this was something to be disposed of, how would I have helped that man retain even a grain of his quality of life? That was the day this book was born, not only a mere collection of X-rays but a series of different life paths colliding with mine, each one of them leaving a trace. Moreover, that was the day in which I recognized that teachers will be teachers, but not always are their teachings to be read positively. I started going back to the roots of upper gastrointestinal fluoroscopy, to the classics, especially Marcel Brombart and, nearer to our time, Olle Ekberg and Bonnie Martin-Harris. My aim was to produce something that would be comprehensive and explicative enough to be both a reference and a self-help guide for junior radiologists—something I would want a still unborn son of mine to read. What I ended up learning, because yes, compiling a book is an extensive learning process, is that the best teachers in the field of fluoroscopy are patients themselves; of course, you have to be very well versed in anatomy, pathophysiology, and technique, but the actual learning, the experience-growing process happens while with the patients. Talk to them before, during, and after the examinations: even when the barium swallow comes out negative, you will at least learn something about yourselves. In the end, fluoroscopy stands on the border between the physical and the metaphysical. The people we help, basically, struggle with swallowing, and often eating, drinking, and even breathing capabilities are severely impaired—often overlooked pleasures of life, gone. The observation and interpretation of fluoroscopy should not and cannot be, then, a mere repetitive, mechanical job. It requires discipline in technique, method in interpretation, but more importantly, profound respect, empathy, and a mindful knowledge of self. And I'm sure, if you approach fluoroscopy this way, you will experience everything differently: a cool glass of water, your dog quietly snoring on the carpet, and, especially, daily routine at work and the impact on the patients. Because, of course, we are not done with gastrointestinal imaging and most probably never will be.

Porticcio, Corse-du-Sud, France

1 Oral, Pharyngeal, and Esophageal Anatomy

1.1 INTRODUCTION

The radiographic assessment of a bolus's transit from the mouth through the pharynx and into the esophagus is dependent on the recognition of particular anatomical landmarks and the coordinated movement executed by the pharyngeal and oral muscles during swallowing. Transporting liquids and hard food from the mouth into the esophagus is a complex physiological activity that requires the coordinated action of 26 muscles and 6 cranial nerves. Understanding its morphology, neuro-vascular supply, musculature, surgical consequences, and clinical relevance can help us appreciate its significance; moreover, a profound knowledge of pharyngeal anatomy is therefore mandatory for those approaching the radiographic evaluation [1].

1.2 EMBRYOLOGICAL OVERVIEW

The formation of the adult bony skull is a result of intricate embryological processes involving various tissue precursors [2]. Typically, the skeletal bones of mammals may be classified into two distinct histologic-level origins: those that are produced in cartilage, known as endochondral bone, and those that undergo direct ossification from mesenchyme, referred to as membranous bone. The majority of postcranial bones exhibit endochondral ossification, but a significant number of bones in the head and neck area are characterized by membranous ossification. The vault of the skull is composed of membranous bones, such as the parietal, temporal, and frontal bones, and some parts of the occipital bones. These bones are believed to have originated from the skeletal armor found in primitive fish. Direct ossification is responsible for the formation of the maxilla, mandible, and some parts of the palate and zygomatic bone. The endochondral bones of the cranium have diverse origins in terms of the cartilaginous templates. The cranial base bones, which provide a foundation for the brain, may be traced back to the chondrocranium, a cartilaginous structure that encased the brain in early vertebrates. In human beings, the aforementioned tissues originally exist as a collection of capsules, including the olfactory, optic, and otic capsules, which subsequently fuse with a group of embryonic midline cartilaginous structures, including the prechordal cartilage, hypophyseal cartilage, and parachordal cartilage. Collectively, these structures comprise the ethmoid bone, the main body, the smaller and larger wings of the sphenoid bone, the dense component of the temporal bone, and the lower part of the occipital bone. The bones that originate from cartilage are derived from the pharyngeal arches, which are intricate structures that have evolved from the supportive and protective structures that housed the gills in early vertebrates. This collection of five sequential structures, commonly referred to as the branchial arches, extends in a cranial-to-caudal direction. The formation of these structures commences on day 22 of human embryonic development, namely during the onset of the fourth week, inside the craniofacial area. However, it is important to note that these structures are present in embryos of all mammalian species. Every arch is comprised of an outside layer of ectodermal tissue, a central core of mesodermal tissue that will give rise to nerve, muscle, and cartilage, and an inner layer of endoderm. The arch-derived cartilage contributes to the development of several oropharyngeal structures, including the ossicles of the middle ear, the styloid process, the hyoid bone, and the laryngeal cartilages. The tissue present in each of the arches undergoes differentiation into muscle, nerve, and blood vessels. Typically, the first arch develops into the jaws, the second arch contributes to facial and ear structures, the third arch is connected with the hyoid and upper pharynx, and the fourth and sixth arches (with the disappearance of the fifth arch) give rise to structures related to the larynx and lower pharynx (Table 1.1).

The development of the face, palate, and superior components of the oral cavity is contingent upon the intricate processes involved in the development of the first arch. The first arch undergoes an early division, resulting in two distinct components: a mandibular segment and a maxillary segment. At the conclusion of the fourth week of embryonic development, a series of five discrete protuberances emerges, namely two maxillary swellings, two mandibular swellings, and a superior, centrally located protuberance known as the frontonasal process. The tissues in question are infiltrated by a population of cells known as neural crest cells, which play a pivotal role in the development and expansion of these protuberances. Ultimately, the amalgamation of these protuberances culminates in the formation of the outer visage. The formation of the oral cavity involves the development of a narrow opening, while the ectodermal midline undergoes thickening, leading to the formation of depressions that will subsequently develop into nasal openings. The development of these tissues also gives rise to the formation of the palate. The mucosa of the tongue is formed by tissue originating from the pharyngeal arches. The intricate arrangements

Table 1.1 Branchial Arches

Arch No.	Adult Skeletal Elements	Muscles	Blood Vessels	Cranial Nerves
1	Incus (maxillary portion) malleus (mandibular portion)	Muscles of mastication, mylohyoid, ant. digastric, tensor tympani, tensor veli palatini	Terminal branch of maxillary	V1 (maxillary portion) V2 (mandibular portion)
2	Stapes, styloid process, stylohyoid ligament, lesser horn, and upper rim of hyoid	Muscles of facial expression	Stapedial/ corticotympanic	VII (facial)
3	Greater horn and lower rim of hyoid	Stylopharyngeus	Common carotid, root of internal carotid	IX (glossopharyngeal)
4	Laryngeal cartilages	Constrictors of the pharynx, cricothyroid, levator veli palatini	Arch of aorta, right subclavian	Superior laryngeal (branch of X)
6	Laryngeal cartilages	Intrinsic muscles of larynx	Ductus arteriosis (embryonic), pulmonary	Recurrent laryngeal (branch of X)

of both general and particular sensory perception inside the tongue are indicative of its intricate developmental processes. The mesoderm originating from the first arch is responsible for the development of the front two-thirds of the tongue, extending to the foramen cecum. On the other hand, the mesoderm derived from the third and fourth arches contributes to the formation of the posterior third of the tongue. The tongue musculature receives contributions from additional tissue originating from the occipital somites. The tissue in question, which was initially located behind the pharyngeal arches, receives its blood supply from the hypoglossal nerve, also known as cranial nerve XII. The interstitial gaps seen outwardly between the arches are commonly referred to as clefts, while internally they are known as pouches. The construction of the external acoustic meatus is facilitated by the presence of the outer cleft between the first two arches, whereas the remaining clefts undergo absorption during the developmental process. The inner pouch located between the initial two arches undergoes differentiation to form the tympanic cavity, sometimes known as the auditory or Eustachian tube. The remaining pouches aid the development of glandular tissue in the region of the head and neck. The structures derived from the pharyngeal pouches consist of the palatine tonsils originating from pouch two, the inferior parathyroid glands and thymus originating from pouch three, the superior parathyroid glands originating from pouch four, and the ultimobranchial body originating from the most inferior part of pouch four. Following their creation, these tissues undergo migration to their respective adult regions as part of the normal developmental process. The embryologic linkages, as well as the adult anatomy, appear to exhibit relatively minimal patterns. The cranial nerves, despite being assigned numerical designations ranging from I to XII, exhibit overlapping regions of innervation, rather than adhering strictly to a hierarchical superior-to-inferior or anterior-to-posterior arrangement. In organisms exhibiting a less advanced anatomical structure, such as early chordates and certain fish, amphibians, and reptiles, the adult anatomical features are arranged in a sequential manner that precisely corresponds to the embryological sequence of the arches. Consequently, structures innervated by cranial nerve II consistently appear anterior to those innervated by cranial nerve III. The head and neck regions undergo substantial evolutionary remodeling, leading to a mammalian pattern that deviates from a linear and orderly arrangement. The evolutionary processes that gave rise to these alterations are of great interest. There are two separate forces at play in this context: constraint and adaptability. The process of evolution rarely produces morphological structures that are optimally designed for their respective functions. In order to effectively address the demands posed by a dynamic environment and the presence of competing species, the process of selection acts upon the diversity created by mutation, and often minor genetic modifications can yield substantial alterations in an organism's developmental program. Hence, the structures already present, such as the branchial or pharyngeal arches, impose a limitation. Nevertheless, as creatures undergo adaptations to new settings, such as transitioning from aquatic to terrestrial habitats and developing the ability to breathe air, they undergo structural modifications to accommodate these novel capabilities. The current morphology underwent significant modifications as a result of subsequent adaptations for endothermy, which refers to the ability to generate and maintain body heat, as well as the increased energy consumption associated with it. Additionally, changes were made to separate the processes of swallowing (deglutition) and breathing (respiration). However, it is valuable to acknowledge the evolutionary connection that is evident in the embryonic development of humans. There is a multitude of clinical disorders that seem to exert an impact on various structures. However, the structures that are impacted are connected by their shared embryological origin (Table 1.1). The aforementioned conditions, often known as syndromes of the first and second arches, include Goldenhar syndrome, mandibulofacial dysostoses such as Treacher–Collins or Hallermann–Streiff and DiGeorge syndromes.

1.2.1 Branchial Origin of Oral Cavity and Pharynx

The branchial or visceral arches and pharyngeal pouches are anatomical structures that are of significant importance in developmental biology and embryology. The front portion of the foregut has five pharyngeal pouches, which are situated in the lateral walls (Figure 1.1). The upper four pouches extend into both a dorsal and a ventral diverticulum. The ectoderm undergoes invaginations, resulting in the formation of branchial or outer pharyngeal grooves. The mesoderm that is present in between is displaced, allowing the ectoderm to temporarily make contact with the entodermal lining of the foregut. Consequently, the two layers merge along the grooves' lower surfaces, resulting in the formation of delicate closure membranes that separate the foregut from the external environment. Subsequently, the mesoderm once again undergoes penetration, positioning itself between the entoderm and the ectoderm. In organisms possessing gills, the occlusion of sealing membranes ceases, leading to the transformation of grooves into fully formed clefts known as gill clefts. These clefts open from the throat to the external environment. It is worth noting that perforation of gill clefts does not take place in avian or mammalian species. The grooves serve to demarcate a sequence of curved bars or arches, known as the branchial or visceral arches, whereby there is a localized thickening of the mesoderm (as seen in Figures 1.2 and 1.3). The posterior portions of these arches are affixed to the lateral aspects of the cranium, while the anterior ends finally converge along the median plane of the cervical region. A total of six arches are present; however, only the initial four are outwardly observable. The initial arch is referred to as the mandibular arch, while the next one is known as the hyoid arch; the other arches lack specific designations. Within each arch, a cartilaginous bar is formed, including bilateral components, and accompanying each of these bars is one of the original aortic arches. The mandibular arch is situated in the anatomical region between the first branchial groove and the stomodeum. It serves as the developmental foundation for several structures including the lower lip, the jaw, the muscles responsible for mastication, and the front portion of the tongue. The formation of its cartilaginous bar is

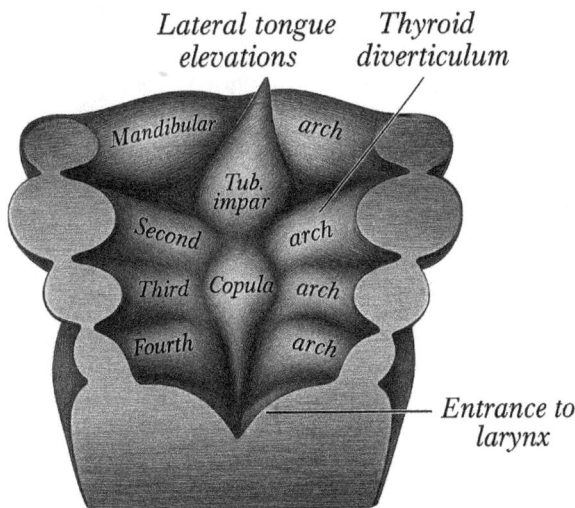

Figure 1.1 Scheme of the floor of the pharynx of an embryo.

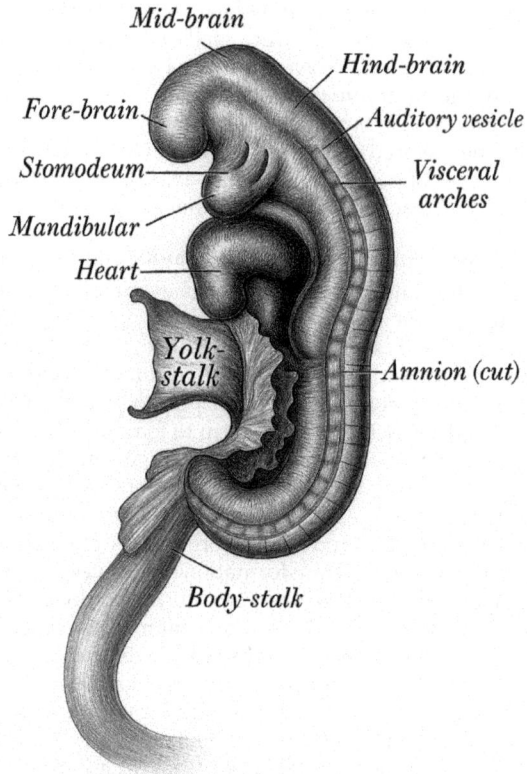

Figure 1.2   Embryo between days 18 and 21.

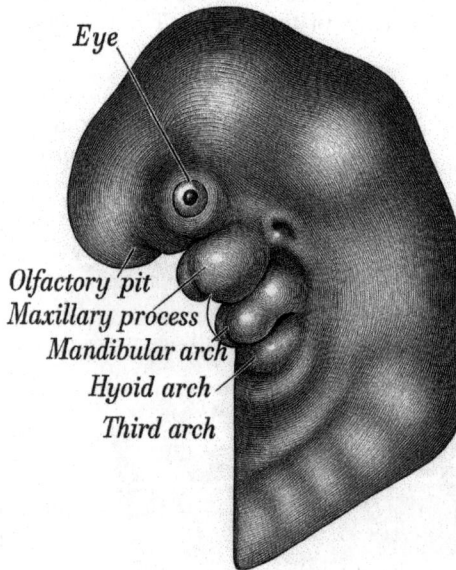

Figure 1.3   Head end of a human embryo, about the end of the fourth week.

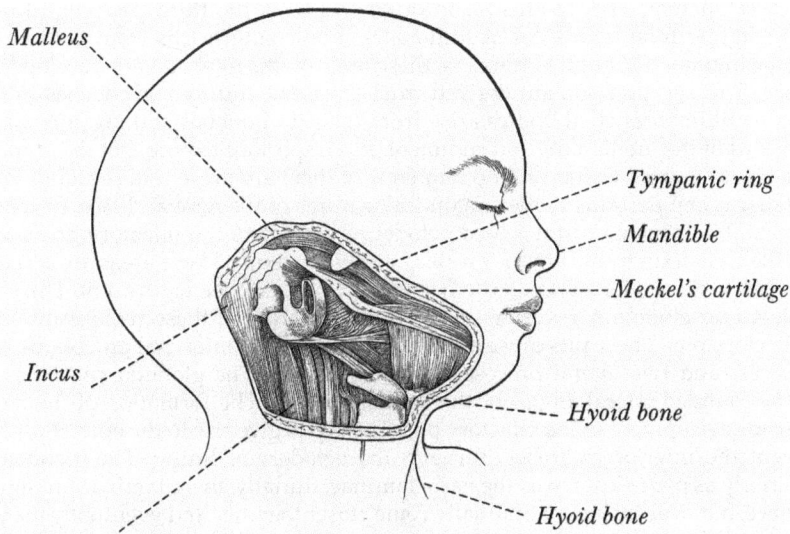

Figure 1.4 Head and neck of a human embryo 18 weeks old, with Meckel's cartilage and hyoid bar exposed.

attributed to Meckel's cartilages, namely the right and left ones, as seen in Figure 1.4. Positioned above this structure, the incus undergoes development. The dorsal extremity of each cartilage is anatomically linked to the ear capsule and undergoes ossification to give rise to the malleus. The ventral extremities converge in the area of the symphysis menti and are commonly considered to undergo ossification, forming the section of the mandible that houses the incisor teeth. The intervening section of the cartilage becomes indiscernible, with the area directly opposite to the malleus being substituted by a fibrous membrane known as the spheno-mandibular ligament. Meanwhile, the majority of the mandible is ossified from the connective tissue that covers the remaining piece of the cartilage. The maxillary process emerges from the dorsal ends of the mandibular arch, extending forward on both sides to shape the cheek and lateral region of the upper lip. The second, or hyoid, arch contributes to the development of the lateral and anterior aspects of the neck. The styloid process, stylohyoid ligament, and smaller cornu of the hyoid bone are derived from its cartilage. The phases are likely to emerge in the top portion of this arch. The hyoid bone's larger cornu originates from the cartilage of the third arch. The ventral terminations of the second and third arches conjoin with their counterparts on the other side, resulting in the formation of a horizontal strip. This strip serves as the foundation for the development of the body of the hyoid bone and the posterior region of the tongue. The ventral components of the cartilages originating from the fourth and fifth arches combine to create the thyroid cartilage. The cartilages derived from the sixth arch give rise to the cricoid and arytenoid cartilages, as well as the cartilages found in the trachea. The mandibular and hyoid arches have a higher rate of growth compared to the posterior arches, leading to a partial overlapping of the latter within the former. Consequently, the formation of a profound depression, known as the sinus cervicalis, occurs bilaterally in the neck region. The sinus in question is delimited anteriorly by the hyoid arch and posteriorly by the thoracic wall. Eventually, its walls undergo fusion, resulting in its complete obliteration. The concha auriculae and external auditory meatus are derived from the first branchial groove. Additionally, a series of protuberances emerges on the mandibular and hyoid arches around the groove, contributing to the formation of the auricula or pinna. The first pharyngeal pouch extends dorsally to give rise to both the auditory canal and the tympanic cavity. Additionally, the membrane that separates the mandibular and hyoid arches is infiltrated by the mesoderm, ultimately developing into the tympanic membrane. There is no evidence of the persistence of the second, third, and fourth branchial grooves. The anatomical structure located within the second pharyngeal pouch is referred to as the sinus tonsillaris. This region is responsible for the development of the tonsil, with a remnant of the sinus remaining as the supratonsillar fossa. The fossa of Rosenmüller, also known as the lateral recess of the pharynx, is considered by certain individuals to be a permanent component of the second pharyngeal pouch. However, it is more likely that this structure is formed as a subsequent development. The thymus gland originates from the third pharyngeal pouch as an endodermal outgrowth on both sides. Additionally, minor outgrowths from the fourth pouches merge with the thymus, although in humans, these outgrowths likely do not develop into genuine thymus tissue. The parathyroids are derived from the third and fourth pouches in the form of diverticula. The ultimobranchial bodies arise from the fifth pouches and are surrounded by the lateral extensions of the median thyroid rudiment. It is important to note that these entities do not develop into actual thyroid tissue, and no remnants of them are present in the adult human body. The topic of discussion pertains to the anatomical features of the nose and face. In the third week of development, two regions of thickened ectoderm, known as the olfactory areas, emerge just underneath the fore-brain in the anterior wall of the stomodeum. These areas are situated on each side of a specific region referred to as the frontonasal process (see Figure 1.5). The surrounding regions undergo development, resulting in the transformation of these regions into depressions known as olfactory pits. These pits cause an indentation in the frontonasal process, dividing it into a medial process and two lateral processes (see Figure 1.6). The globular processes of His are formed by the rounded lateral angles of the medial process. The formation of the nasal cavities begins with the development of the olfactory pits. These pits give rise to the epithelium of the nasal cavities, except the inferior meatuses, through the ectodermal lining. The globular processes extend posteriorly as plates known as the nasal laminae. Initially, these laminae are separated by a certain distance, but over time they gradually come closer together and eventually merge to create the nasal septum. The processes themselves converge at the midline, giving rise to the premaxillae and the philtrum, which is the central portion of the upper lip (see Figure 1.7). The inferior portion of the nasal septum, also known as the columella, is situated between the globular processes of the medial nasal process. Above this region, there is a noticeable angle that will develop into the future apex of the nose (as seen in Figure 1.6). Further, superiorly, there is a flat surface referred to as the future bridge of the nose. The alae of the nose are formed by the lateral nasal processes. The maxillary process is a triangular process that extends forward from the cephalic border of the mandibular arch. It is continuous with the dorsal end of the mandibular arch. The ventral extremity of the maxillary process is separated from the mandibular arch by a notch in the shape of the letter "V" (see Figure 1.5). The maxillary process is responsible for the development of the lateral wall and floor of the orbit. Within this process, the zygomatic bone and a significant portion of the maxilla undergo ossification. Initially, the maxillary process is distinct from the lateral nasal process, but they eventually come into contact. A groove called the naso-optic furrow separates these two processes temporarily. This furrow extends from the groove encircling the eyeball to the olfactory pit.

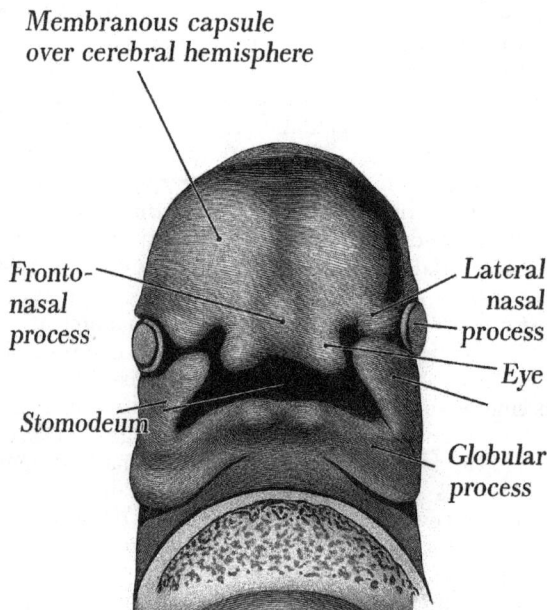

Figure 1.5 Undersurface of the head of a human embryo at about 29 days old.

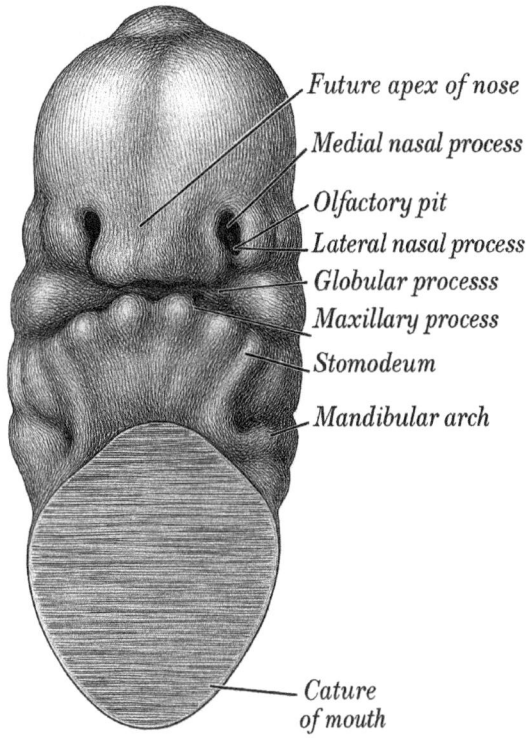

Future apex of nose

Medial nasal process

Olfactory pit

Lateral nasal process

Globular processs

Maxillary process

Stomodeum

Mandibular arch

Cature
of mouth

Figure 1.6   Head end of a human embryo at about 30–31 days old.

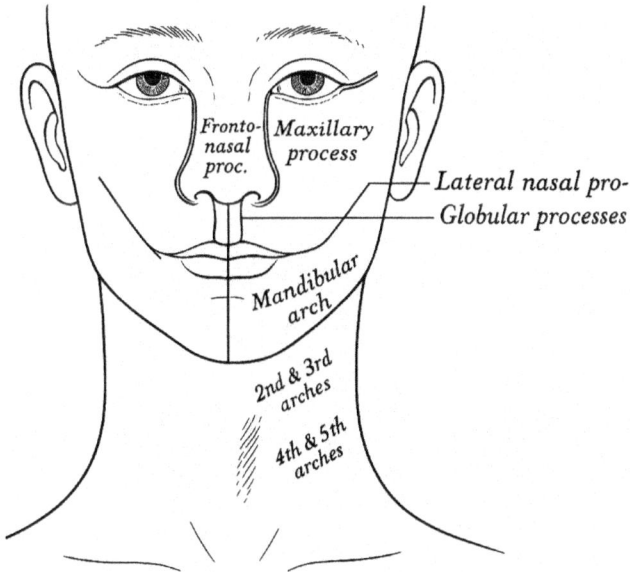

Fronto-
nasal
proc.

Maxillary
process

Lateral nasal pro-

Globular processes

Mandibular
arch

2nd & 3rd
arches

4th & 5th
arches

Figure 1.7   Diagram showing the regions of the adult face and neck related to the frontonasal process and the branchial arches.

The fusion of the maxillary processes with the lateral nasal and globular processes results in the formation of the lateral portions of the upper lip and the posterior limits of the nare. During the period spanning from the third to the fifth month, the nasal passages become obstructed by accumulation of epithelial tissue. The subsequent breakdown and disappearance of these tissue masses lead to the formation of the permanent nasal apertures. The maxillary process is responsible for the development of the inferior segment of the lateral wall of the nasal cavity. The development of the roof of the nose and other components of the lateral wall, including as the ethmoidal labyrinth, inferior nasal concha, lateral cartilage, and lateral crus of the alar cartilage, occurs inside the lateral nasal process. The primitive palate is created by the union of the maxillary and nasal processes in the roof of the stomodeum. Additionally, the olfactory pits extend posteriorly above the primitive palate. The bucco-nasal membrane, an epithelial membrane, is created by the nasal and stomodeal epithelium and serves to shut the posterior end of each pit. The establishment of the primordial choanae, or apertures between the olfactory pits and the stomodeum, occurs through the rupture of these membranes. The formation of the floor of the nasal cavity is accomplished through the growth of palatine processes, resembling shelves, which project medially from the maxillary processes. These processes merge with each other at the midline, forming the entirety of the palate, with the exception of a small anterior portion that is constructed by the premaxillary bones. There are two persistent holes that exist temporarily between the palatine processes and the premaxillae. These apertures serve as the permanent channels found in lower animals that connect the nose and mouth. The fusion of the constituent components that constitute the palate starts anteriorly, with the premaxillary and palatine processes conjoining during the eighth week of embryonic development. Subsequently, the formation of the hard palate area is finalized by the ninth week, followed by the completion of the soft palate region by the eleventh week. Upon the culmination of the development of the palate, the permanent choanae are established and are positioned at a significant distance posterior to the primitive choanae. The condition referred to as cleft palate arises due to a lack of fusion between the palatine processes, whereas harelip occurs due to a lack of fusion between the maxillary and globular processes. The nasal cavity undergoes division through the presence of a vertical septum. This septum extends in a downward and backward direction from the medial nasal process and nasal laminae, ultimately joining with the palatine processes below. A plate of cartilage extends from the inferior side of the ethmoid plate of the chondrocranium into this septum. The front segment of this cartilaginous structure remains as the septal cartilage of the nose and the medial crus of the alar cartilage, while the posterior and higher segments are substituted by the vomer and perpendicular plate of the ethmoid bone. The ectoderm undergoes invagination on both sides of the nasal septum, namely in its lower and anterior region. This invagination results in the formation of a blind pouch or diverticulum, which spreads in a posterior and superior direction within the nasal septum. This structure is further reinforced by a curved cartilaginous plate. The aforementioned pouches serve as the initial stages of the Jacobson's vomero-nasal organs, situated in close proximity to the intersection of the premaxillary and maxillary bones, and positioned below the lateral nasal processes (Figures 1.5–1.7).

1.3 ORAL CAVITY

The oral cavity, sometimes referred to as the buccal cavity or mouth, is the initial part of the digestive system [3]. It is composed of many physically distinct features that cooperate to carry out multiple tasks in an effective and efficient manner. The palate, teeth, lips, and tongue are some of these features. The mouth cavity, despite its modest size, is a unique and intricate structure that contains a variety of nerves and blood vessels. This complex network is essential to its distinct and varied function in human existence. The oral cavity is situated at the beginning of the gastrointestinal tract (Figure 1.10). It is an approximately oval-shaped cavity comprised of two distinct sections: a smaller outside piece known as the vestibule and a larger interior region referred to as the oral cavity proper. The vestibule, also known as the vestibulum oris, is a narrow region that is visually enclosed by the lips and cheeks and internally by the gums and teeth. The means of communication between the body's surface and the external environment occurs through the rima or aperture of the mouth. The upper and lower boundaries of this area are determined by the reflection of the mucous membrane from the lips and cheeks onto the gum, which covers the upper and lower alveolar arches, respectively. The glandular secretion from the parotid salivary glands is received by it. When the jaws are closed, it establishes communication with the oral cavity through an aperture located on both sides, posterior to the wisdom teeth, as well as through thin gaps between opposing teeth. The mouth cavity proper, also known as cavum oris proprium, is delimited on the sides and anteriorly by the alveolar arches containing the teeth. Posteriorly, it connects

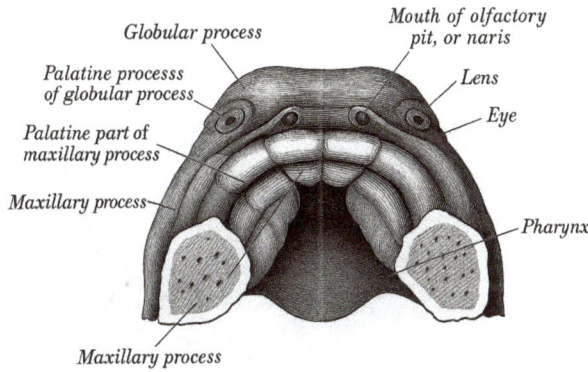

Figure 1.8 The roof of the mouth of a human embryo, aged about 2.5 months, showing the mode of formation of the palate.

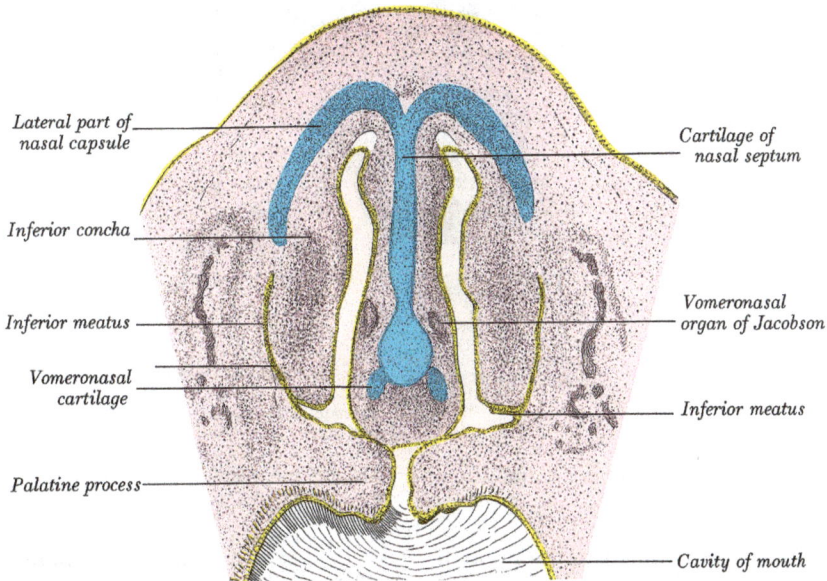

Figure 1.9 Frontal section of nasal cavities in a human embryo 28 mm long.

with the pharynx by a narrow opening called the isthmus faucium. The oral cavity is enclosed by the hard and soft palates, with the majority of the floor being comprised of the tongue. The remaining portion of the floor is created by the mucous membrane, which extends from the sides and underside of the tongue to the gums lining the inner aspect of the jaw. The secretion from the submaxillary and sublingual salivary glands is received by it. The structure of the subject matter is comprised of three main components. The mucous membrane that lines the oral cavity maintains a continuous connection with the integument at the unfettered edge of the lips, as well as with the mucous lining of the pharynx posteriorly. This membrane has a rosy-pink hue when alive and is notably thick where it covers the bony structures that enclose the oral cavity. The surface is lined by stratified squamous epithelium. The lips, also known as labia oris, refer to the pair of fleshy folds that encircle the rima or opening of the mouth. These structures consist of an external layer of integument and an internal layer of mucous membrane. Within this anatomical arrangement, one can find the orbicularis oris muscle, labial vessels, various nerves, areolar tissue, adipose tissue, and numerous small labial glands. The mucous membrane forms a fold known as the frenulum, which connects the inner surface of each lip to the corresponding gum. It is worth noting that the upper frenulum is greater in size. The labial glands, also known as

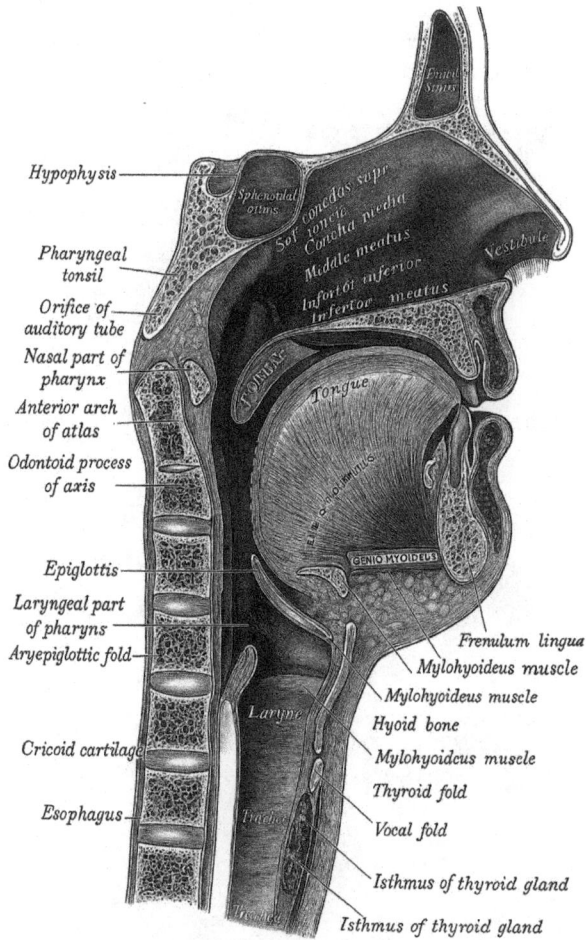

Figure 1.10 Sagittal section of nose, mouth, pharynx, and larynx.

glanduloe labiales, are located in the perioral region between the mucosal membrane and the orbicularis oris muscle, encircling the oral opening. The objects in question have a circular morphology and possess dimensions akin to those of small peas. Their ducts are characterized by minute apertures that facilitate their connection to the mucosal membrane. In terms of their anatomical composition, they have a resemblance to the salivary glands. The buccae, commonly referred to as the cheeks, constitute the lateral aspects of the face and maintain a contiguous relationship with the front portion of the lips. The surface composition of these structures consists of integument, while the interior composition is comprised of mucous membrane. Additionally, there exists a muscle layer between the integument and mucous membrane, accompanied by a substantial amount of adipose tissue, areolar tissue, blood vessels, nerves, and buccal glands. The mucous membrane that lines the cheek is mirrored both above and below onto the gums, and it maintains continuity with the lining membrane of the soft palate posteriorly. Located across from the second maxillary molar tooth is a papilla, which contains the opening of the parotid duct at its apex. The primary muscle responsible for the structure and function of the cheek is known as the buccinator. However, it is important to note that other muscles also contribute to its construction, such as the zygomaticus, risorius, and platysma. The buccal glands are situated within the buccinator muscle, positioned between the mucous membrane and the muscle itself. These glands have a comparable structural composition to the labial glands, however on a smaller scale. Approximately five glands, which are somewhat bigger compared to the others, are positioned in the vicinity of the distal end of the parotid duct, specifically between the masseter and buccinator muscles. These particular glands have ducts that open in the oral cavity, precisely opposite to the final molar tooth. The anatomical structures in question are commonly referred to as molar glands. The gingivae, also known as the gums, are comprised of thick fibrous tissue that is strongly associated with the periosteum of the alveolar processes. They encircle the cervical regions of the teeth. The surface of these structures is lined by a smooth and vascular mucous membrane, characterized by its relatively low sensitivity. The membrane surrounding the teeth exhibits several delicate papillae along the necks of the teeth. It is also reflected into the alveoli, where it maintains continuity with the periosteal membrane that lines these cavities. The anatomical structure known as the palate, or palatum, is situated in the upper part of the oral cavity and serves as the roof of the mouth. It is composed of two distinct regions: the front area referred to as the hard palate, and the posterior half known as the soft palate. The hard palate, also known as palatum durum (Figure 1.11), is anatomically delimited anteriorly and laterally by the alveolar arches and gums. Posteriorly, it maintains continuity with the soft palate. The oral cavity is encompassed by a compact arrangement, comprised of the periosteum and mucous membrane, which exhibit a close and intimate adherence. A linear ridge may be observed along the central axis, terminating anteriorly in a tiny elevation that corresponds with the incisive canal. The mucous membrane surrounding the raphé exhibits distinct characteristics depending on its location. On both sides and in the anterior region, it appears thick, pale, and exhibits a corrugated texture. Conversely, in the posterior region, it appears thin, smooth, and possesses a deeper coloration. This mucous membrane is lined with stratified squamous epithelium and contains numerous palatal glands situated between the mucous membrane and the underlying bone surface. The soft palate, also known as palatum molle, is a dynamic fold that is suspended from the posterior

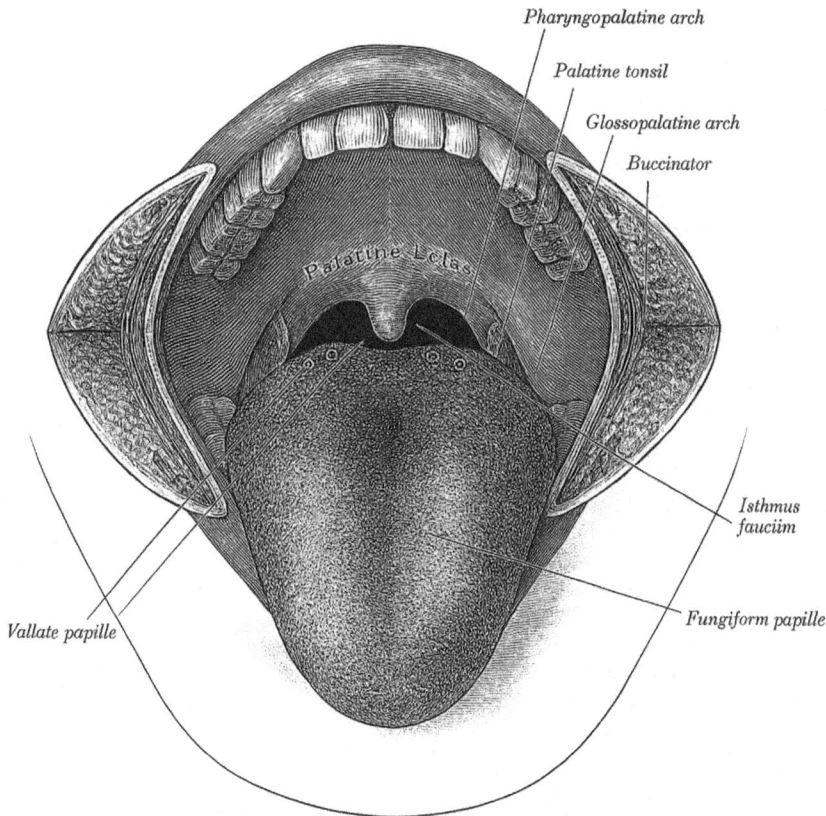

Figure 1.11 The hard and soft palate.

edge of the hard palate. It serves as an imperfect partition, separating the oral cavity from the pharynx. The structure comprises a mucous membrane fold that encloses muscle fibers, an aponeurosis, blood vessels, nerves, adenoid tissue, and mucous glands. When in its typical state, namely when it is relaxed and hanging down, the tongue's front surface is concave and seamlessly connected to the roof of the mouth. It is also distinguished by a central ridge known as the median raphé. The posterior aspect of the structure exhibits convexity and maintains a seamless connection with the mucous membrane that envelops the lower region of the nasal cavities. The superior boundary of the structure is connected to the posterior edge of the hard palate, while its lateral aspects are integrated with the pharynx. The bottom boundary is unobstructed. The anatomical structure referred to as the palatine velum is located in the lower region, serving as a curtain-like partition between the oral cavity and the throat. A tiny, conical, pendulous structure known as the palatine uvula is suspended from the middle of the lower border. Additionally, on either side of the base of the uvula, there are two curved folds of mucous membrane that contain muscle fibers. These folds are referred to as the arches or pillars of the fauces, and they arch laterally and downward. Humans are equipped with two distinct sets of teeth that emerge at various stages of development. The initial group of teeth emerges during early stages of development and is commonly referred to as deciduous or milk teeth. The individuals belonging to the second category, who also manifest during the first stages, have the potential to persist until advanced age, and are referred to as permanent. There are a total of 20 deciduous teeth, comprising four incisors, two canines, and four molars, in each jaw. There are a total of 32 permanent teeth, consisting of four incisors, two canines, four premolars, and six molars, located in each jaw.

1.3.1 The Tongue

The tongue serves as the primary sensory organ for taste perception and plays a significant role in speech production. Additionally, it aids in the process of chewing and swallowing food. The location of the structure is within the oral cavity, specifically in the sublingual region, which is positioned under the mandibular body. The root, also known as the radix linguae (Figure 1.11) exhibits a posterior orientation and is anatomically linked to the hyoid bone through the hyoglossi and genioglossi muscles as well as the hyoglossal membrane. Additionally, it establishes connections with the epiglottis through three folds of mucous membrane known as the glosso-epiglottic folds. Furthermore, it is associated with the soft palate via the glossopalatine arches, and with the pharynx through the constrictores pharyngis superiores muscles and the mucous membrane. The apex of the tongue, specifically the apex linguae tip, is slender and elongated, positioned in an anterior direction toward the lingual surfaces of the lower incisor teeth. The inferior surface, also known as the facies inferior linguae under surface, is anatomically linked to the mandible through the genioglossi muscle. The mucous membrane extends from this surface to cover the lingual surface of the gum and continues onto the floor of the mouth. In the midline of the floor of the mouth, the mucous membrane forms a prominent vertical fold known as the frenulum linguae. Adjacent to the frenulum, there exists a little crease of the mucous membrane known as the plica fimbriata. Occasionally, the unattached edge of this crease may display a sequence of fringe-like structures. The tip of the tongue, together with the inferior surface, sides, and dorsum, exhibits freedom of movement. The dorsum of the tongue, also known as the dorsum linguae, exhibits a convex shape and is characterized by a central groove that divides it into two symmetrical halves. This groove terminates posteriorly, approximately 2.5 cm from the base of the tongue, forming a depression called the foramen cecum. From this point, a shallow groove known as the sulcus terminalis extends laterally and anteriorly on both sides, reaching the edge of the tongue. The front portion of the dorsum of the tongue, which constitutes approximately two-thirds of its surface, is characterized by an upward orientation and a rough texture due to the presence of papillae. In contrast, the posterior third of the dorsum faces backward, exhibiting a smoother surface and housing a considerable number of muciparous glands and lymph follicles, sometimes referred to as the lingual tonsil. The foramen cecum is the residual structure of the superior segment of the thyroglossal duct or diverticulum, which serves as the developmental origin of the thyroid gland. The presence of the pyramidal lobe of the thyroid gland serves as an anatomical marker for the location of the inferior segment of the duct. The papillae of the tongue are protrusions originating from the corium. The structures are densely dispersed throughout the anterior two-thirds of its dorsum, resulting in the distinctive rough texture observed on this surface. The several types of papillae encountered include the vallate papillae, fungiform papillae, filiform papillae, and simple papillae. The tongue is anatomically bisected into lateral halves

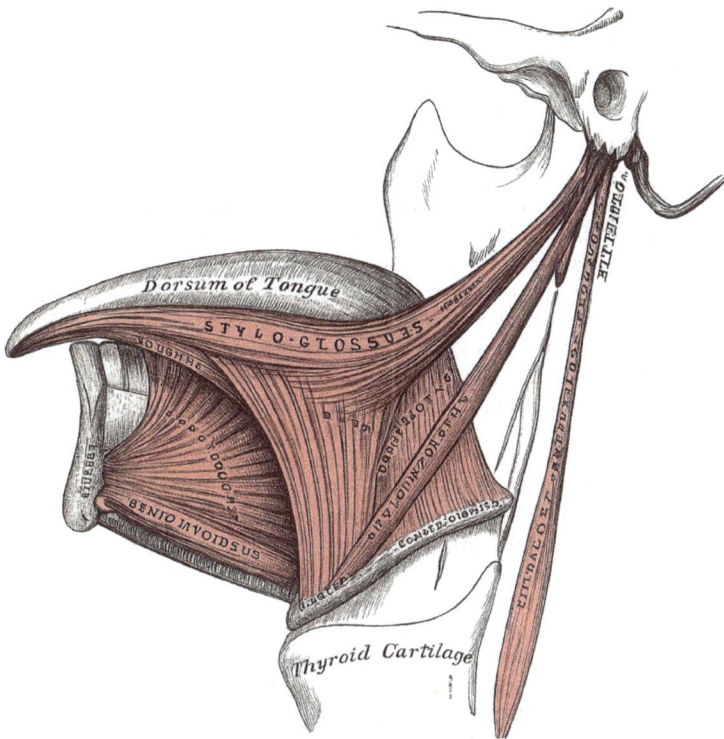

Figure 1.12 Extrinsic muscles of the tongue. Left side.

by a centrally located fibrous septum that spans the whole length of the tongue and is anchored inferiorly to the hyoid bone. Within each half of the tongue, there are two distinct sets of muscles, namely extrinsic and intrinsic muscles. The extrinsic muscles originate from outside the tongue, while the intrinsic muscles are fully contained within its structure. The extrinsic muscles, as seen in Figure 1.12, include the genioglossus and hyoglossus. The genioglossus (geniohyoglossus) is a planar triangle muscle located in close proximity to and aligned with the median plane. Its apex corresponds to its origin from the jaw, while its base corresponds to its insertion into both the tongue and hyoid bone. The muscle in question originates from the superior mental spine located on the inner surface of the symphysis menti, positioned just above the geniohyoideus muscle. It then extends outward in a fan-shaped manner. The inferior fibers descend and attach via a thin aponeurosis to the upper portion of the body of the hyoid bone. Some of these fibers pass between the hyoglossus and chondroglossus muscles to merge with the constrictores pharyngis muscles. The middle fibers extend posteriorly, while the superior fibers extend upward and forward, spanning the entire undersurface of the tongue from its base to its tip. The muscles on opposing sides are anatomically divided by the median fibrous septum of the tongue. Toward the front, these muscles are partially fused due to the crossing of bundles in the central plane. The hyoglossus muscle, characterized by its slender and quadrilateral shape, originates from the lateral aspect of the body and extends along the whole length of the larger cornu of the hyoid bone. It ascends almost vertically and inserts into the lateral aspect of the tongue, positioned between the styloglossus and longitudinalis inferior muscles. The fibers originating from the corpus of the hyoid bone exhibit a degree of overlap with those originating from the larger cornu. The chondroglossus muscle has been occasionally characterized as a component of the hyoglossus muscle. However, it is distinguished from the hyoglossus by the presence of fibers from the genioglossus muscle, which traverse laterally to the pharynx. The length of the structure in question measures approximately 2 cm. It originates from the medial side and base of the lesser cornu, as well as the neighboring section of the body of the hyoid bone. From there, it ascends straight and merges with the intrinsic muscular fibers of the tongue, situated between the hyoglossus and genioglossus muscles. Occasionally, a little occurrence of muscular fibers can be observed, originating from the cartilago triticea within the lateral hyothyroid ligament and extending into the tongue across the posterior fibers of the hyoglossus muscle. The styloglossus muscle, which is the most diminutive and briefest of the trio of styloid muscles, originates from the anterior and lateral aspects of the styloid process in close proximity to its peak, as well as from the stylomandibular ligament. The lingual artery descends and advances from the internal to the external carotid arteries. It then bifurcates on the lateral aspect of the tongue, in close association with the dorsal surface. At this point, it merges with the fibers of the inferior longitudinal muscle, which is located anterior to the hyoglossus muscle. Additionally, another branch of the lingual artery, known as the oblique branch, overlaps the hyoglossus muscle and crosses over its fibers. The sensory nerves responsible for the perception of taste and general sensation in the tongue can be categorized as follows: (1) the lingual branch of the mandibular nerve, which is distributed to the papillae located at the front and sides of the tongue, and serves as the primary nerve for general sensation in the anterior two-thirds of the tongue; (2) the chorda tympani branch of the facial nerve, which travels within the lingual sheath and is commonly recognized as the primary taste nerve for the anterior two-thirds of the tongue; this nerve is a continuation of the sensory root of the facial nerve (known as the nervus intermedius); (3) the lingual branch of the glossopharyngeal nerve, which is distributed to the mucous membrane at the base and sides of the tongue, as well as the vallate papillae, providing both gustatory filaments and general sensory fibers to this region; and (4) the superior laryngeal nerve, which sends small branches to the root of the tongue near the epiglottis.

1.3.2 The Fauces

The anatomical term used to describe the opening connecting the mouth and the pharynx is known as the isthmus faucium. The structure in question is delimited superiorly by the soft palate, inferiorly by the dorsum of the tongue, and laterally by the glossopalatine arch. The structure known as the glossopalatine arch, also referred to as the arcus glossopalatinus or anterior pillar of fauces, extends in a downward, lateral, and forward direction toward the base of the tongue. This arch is produced by the protrusion of the glossopalatinus, along with its accompanying mucous membrane. The pharyngopalatine arch, also known as the arcus pharyngopalatinus or posterior pillar of fauces, exhibits greater size and extends more prominently toward the midline compared to the anterior arch. It descends, moves laterally, and extends posteriorly toward the side of the pharynx. This arch is formed by the projection of the pharyngopalatinus, which is covered by a layer of mucous membrane. The two arches on either side are distinctly divided by a triangular space, inside which the palatine tonsil is situated. The palatine tonsils, also known as tonsillae palatinae, are bilateral structures located between the glossopalatine and pharyngopalatine arches. The tonsils are composed mostly of a cluster of lymphoid tissue located under the mucous membrane situated between the palatine arches. The lymphoid mass does not entirely occupy the space between the two arches, resulting in the presence of a small concavity known as the supratonsillar fossa in the top portion of the gap. Moreover, the tonsil protrudes to varying lengths beneath the protection of the glossopalatine arch, and in this region, it is enveloped by a duplicated layer of mucous membrane. The upper portion of this fold extends over the supratonsillar fossa, positioned between the two arches, resembling a delicate fold referred to as the plica semilunaris. The remaining section of the fold is known as the plica triangularis. The area located between the plica triangularis and the outer layer of the tonsil is referred to as the tonsillar sinus. It is worth noting that in several instances, this sinus is rendered nonexistent due to the walls of the sinus fusing together. Based on this description, it becomes evident that a segment of the tonsil is situated below the level of the adjacent mucous membrane, indicating its embedded nature, and the remaining piece protrudes as the observable tonsil. In pediatric individuals, the size of the tonsils is comparatively greater, and often much larger, than that of adults. Additionally, approximately one-third of the tonsil is embedded. Following the onset of puberty, the embedded section of the tonsil undergoes a significant reduction in size, causing the tonsil to adopt a flattened, disk-like shape. It is important to note that the shape and size of the tonsil can vary substantially among different individuals.

1.3.3 Muscles of the Palate and Mouth

The muscles of the palate include the levator veli palatini, glossopalatinus, tensor veli palatini, pharyngopalatinus, and musculus uvulae (see Figure 1.13). The levator veli palatini, also known as the levator palati, is a robust and rounded muscle located in a lateral position relative to the choanae. The origin of this structure may be found at the lower surface of the apex of the petrous portion of the temporal bone, as well as from the medial lamina of the auditory tube's cartilage. Upon

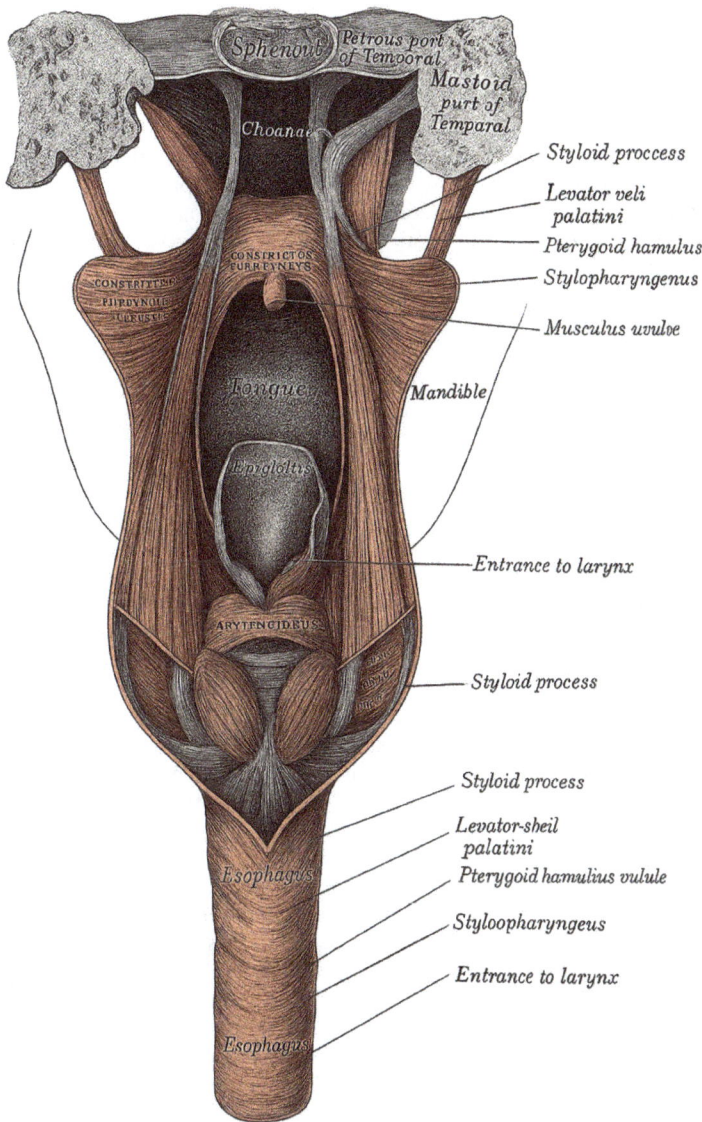

Figure 1.13 Dissection of the muscles of the palate from behind.

surpassing the top concave boundary of the constrictor pharyngis superior, it expands within the palatine velum, with its fibers reaching diagonally downward and toward the midline, where they merge with the fibers of the contralateral side. The tensor veli palatini, also known as the tensor palati, is a wide and thin muscle located laterally to the levator veli palatini. The structure in question originates from the scaphoid fossa located at the base of the medial pterygoid plate, as well as from the spina angularis of the sphenoid bone and the lateral wall of the cartilage of the auditory tube. The structure descends in a vertical manner, positioned between the medial pterygoid plate and the pterygoideus internus. It terminates as a tendon that wraps around the pterygoid hamulus, remaining in place due to the presence of some fibers originating from the pterygoideus internus. A tiny bursa is located between the tendon and the hamulus. Subsequently, the tendon traverses in a medial direction and becomes affixed to the palatine aponeurosis, as well as the region situated posterior to the transverse ridge on the horizontal segment of the palatine bone. The musculus uvulae, also known as the azygos uvulae, originates from the posterior nasal spine of the palatine bones and the palatine aponeurosis. It then descends to its insertion point in the uvula. The glossopalatinus, also known as palatoglossus, is a compact fasciculus that exhibits a smaller width in its central region compared to its ends. It combines with the mucous membrane that envelops its exterior to produce the glossopalatine arch. The muscle in question originates from the front surface of the soft palate, where it maintains a continuous connection with the muscle on the opposite side. It then proceeds downward, forward, and laterally, positioning itself in front of the palatine tonsil. Finally, it inserts into the side of the tongue, with certain fibers extending over the upper surface of the tongue, while others penetrate deeply into the tissue of the tongue to intermingle with the transversus linguae muscle. The pharyngopalatinus, also known as the palatopharyngeus, is a lengthy and fleshy bundle of fibers that is smaller in its central region compared to its ends. It combines with the mucous membrane that envelops it to create the pharyngopalatine arch. The glossopalatinus is anatomically distinct from the palatine tonsil, with an angular interval between the two structures. The uvula originates from the soft palate and is anatomically separated into two fasciculi by the levator veli palatini and musculus uvulae. The posterior fasciculus is situated in close proximity to the mucous membrane and connects with the contralateral muscle in the median plane. The anterior fasciculus, which is thicker, is located in the soft palate between the levator and tensor muscles, and also connects with the equivalent portion of the contralateral muscle in the median plane. The pharyngopalatinus muscle traverses in a lateral and downward direction behind the palatine tonsil. It converges with the stylopharyngeus muscle, and together they are inserted into the posterior border of the thyroid cartilage. Some of the fibers of the pharyngopalatinus muscle are dispersed on the side of the pharynx, while others cross over the midline posteriorly to intersect with the muscle of the contralateral side.

The muscles responsible for the movement and control of the mouth include the quadratus labii superioris, quadratus labii inferioris, caninus, triangularis, zygomaticus, buccinator, mentalis, orbicularis oris, and risorius (Figure 1.14). The quadratus labii superioris is a wide muscular structure that originates from the lateral aspect of the nose and extends toward the zygomatic bone. The medial fibers of the structure give rise to the angular head, which emerges from the top portion of the frontal process of the maxilla with a pointed end. It then proceeds in a diagonal downward and lateral direction, ultimately dividing into two separate sections. One of these structures is inserted into the larger alar cartilage and skin of the nose, while the other extends into the lateral portion of the upper lip, merging with the infraorbital head and the orbicularis oris (Figure 1.15). The infraorbital head, which is situated in the intermediate region, originates from the lower boundary of the orbit just above the infraorbital foramen. It is characterized by its fibers being connected to both the maxilla and the zygomatic bone. The fibers of the muscle come together and are placed into the muscular tissue of the upper lip, namely between the angular head and the caninus. The zygomatic head is composed of lateral fibers that originate from the malar surface of the zygomatic bone, located just below the zygomaticomaxillary suture. These fibers then descend in a medial direction toward the upper lip. The caninus muscle, also known as levator anguli oris, originates from the canine fossa located just below the infraorbital foramen. Its fibers are then inserted into the corner of the mouth, where they intertwine with the fibers of the zygomaticus, triangularis, and orbicularis oris muscles. The zygomaticus major muscle originates from the zygomatic bone, specifically in front of the zygomaticotemporal suture. It descends obliquely with a medial inclination and inserts into the angle of the mouth. At this point, it merges with the fibers of the caninus, orbicularis oris, and triangularis muscles. The facial nerve innervates this particular set of muscles. The action of the mentalis muscle involves the elevation and projection of the lower lip, concomitant with the formation of wrinkles on the chin, conveying a sense of skepticism or contempt. The quadratus labii inferioris muscle is responsible for the downward and somewhat lateral movement of the lower lip, commonly observed during the expression of irony. The triangularis muscle functions as a depressor of the mouth angle, opposing the actions of the caninus and zygomaticus muscles. When working in conjunction with the caninus muscle, it causes the mouth angle to move toward the midline. The platysma muscle, which is responsible for the retraction and depression of the angle of the mouth, is classified under this particular category. The buccinator muscle, as seen in Figure 1.14, is a slender quadrilateral muscle located in the facial region between the maxilla and the mandible. The origin of this structure is located on the outer surfaces of the alveolar processes of the maxilla and mandible, specifically aligned with the three molar teeth. Posteriorly, it originates from the anterior border of the pterygomandibular raphé, which serves as a demarcation from the constrictor pharyngis superior. The fibers of the muscle converge toward the angle of the mouth, where the central fibers intersect each other. The fibers originating from below are connected to the upper segment of the orbicularis oris, while those originating from above are connected to the lower segment. The upper and lower fibers extend forward into their respective lips without crossing over.

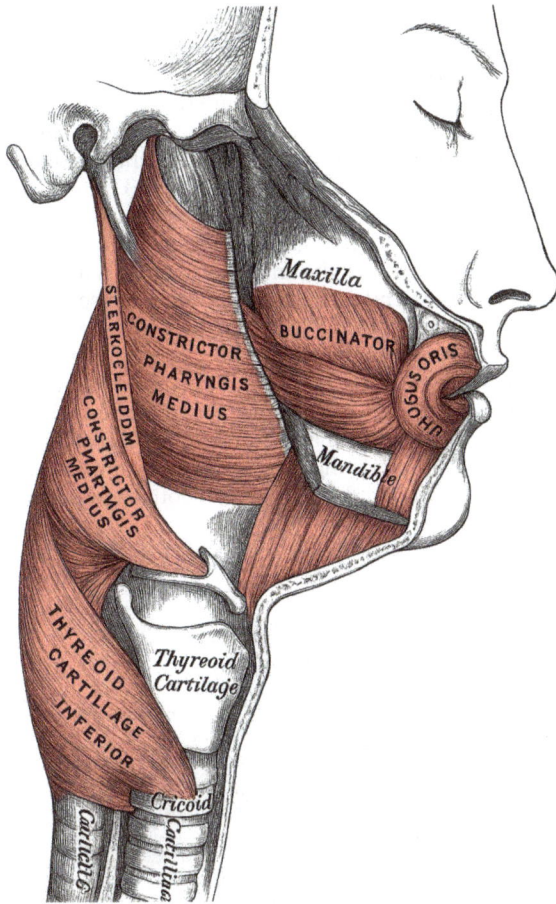

Figure 1.14 Muscles of the pharynx and cheek.

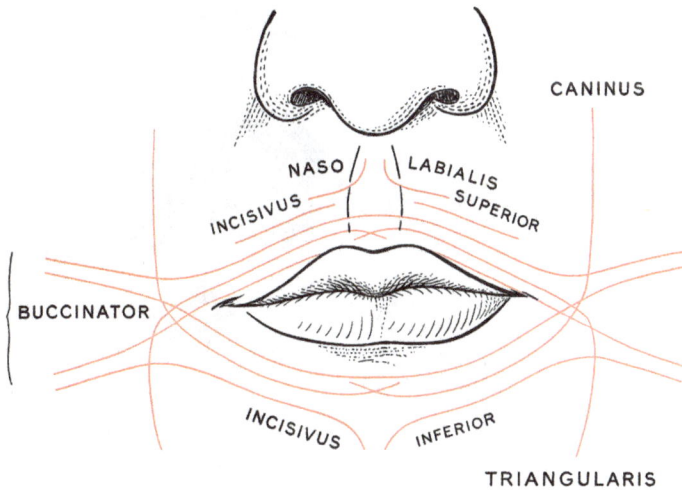

Figure 1.15 Scheme showing arrangement of fibers of the orbicularis oris.

1.3.4 Muscles of Mastication

The primary muscles responsible for the process of mastication include the masseter, pterygoideus externus, temporalis, and pterygoideus internus [4].

The masseter muscle is enveloped by a robust fascial layer known as the masseteric fascia, with which it is firmly interconnected. This fascial layer originates from the deep cervical fascia. The fascia mentioned above is connected to the inferior edge of the zygomatic arch, and posteriorly, it envelops the parotid gland. The masseter muscle, as seen in Figure 1.16, is a robust and slightly quadrilateral muscle that has two distinct sections: the superficial portion and the deep portion. The superficial portion, which is larger in size, originates from a thick, tendinous aponeurosis located at the zygomatic process of the maxilla and the anterior two-thirds of the lower border of the zygomatic arch. Its fibers descend and extend posteriorly, ultimately inserting into the angle and lower half of the lateral surface of the ramus of the mandible. The inferior component is comparatively diminutive and exhibits a denser muscular composition. It originates from the posterior segment of the inferior margin and encompasses the entirety of the medial aspect of the zygomatic arch. Its fibers descend in a forward trajectory, ultimately inserting into the upper portion of the ramus and the lateral facade of the coronoid process of the mandible. The buried nature of the deep component of the muscle is due, in part, to its positioning anteriorly to the superficial portion, while its posterior aspect is covered by the parotid gland. The fibers of both segments exhibit continuity at their

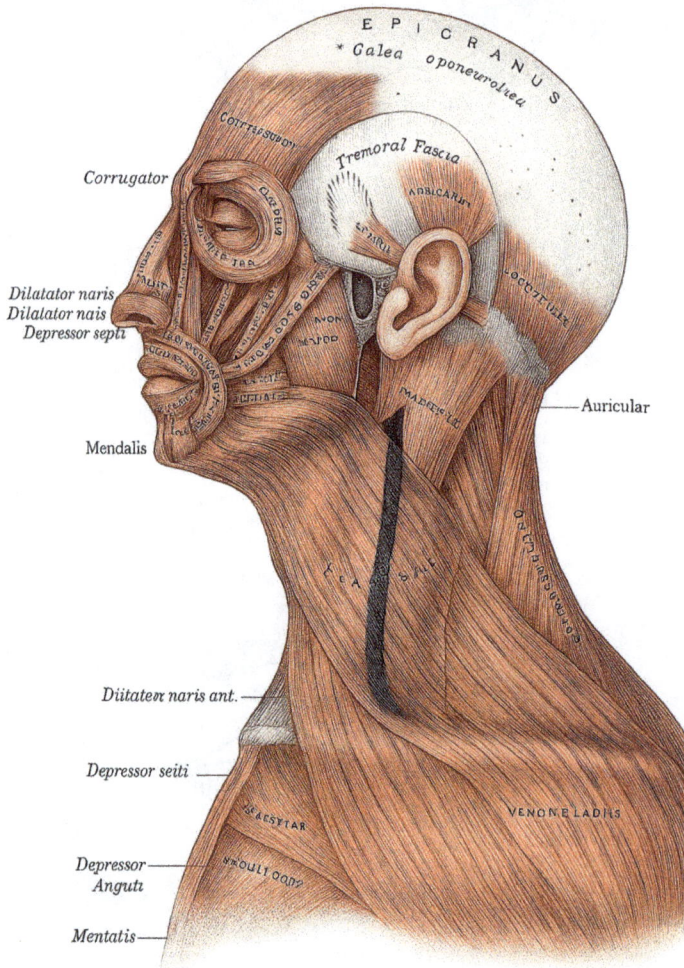

Figure **1.16** The masseter is one of the muscles of the head, face, and neck.

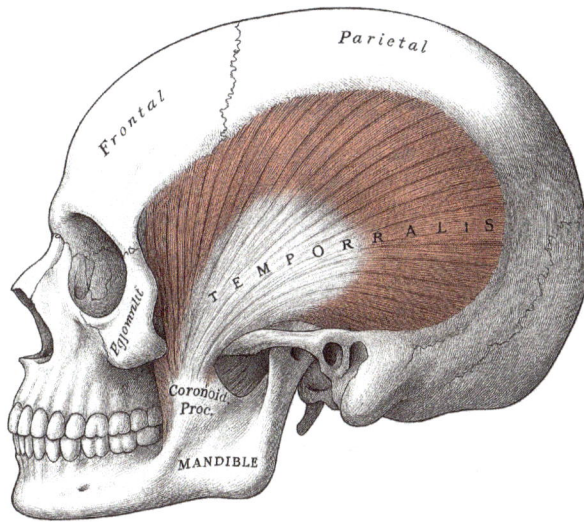

Figure 1.17 The temporalis, zygomatic arch, and masseter have been removed.

point of insertion. The temporal fascia envelops the temporalis muscle. The structure in question is a robust and resilient anatomical entity, enveloped on its sides by the auricularis anterior and superior muscles, on its top by the galea aponeurotica, and partially by the orbicularis oculi muscle. The superficial temporal arteries and the auriculotemporal nerve traverse the area in a caudal to cranial direction. The structure mentioned above is a singular layer that is connected to the full length of the superior temporal line. However, below this point, where it is anchored to the zygomatic arch, it comprises two layers. One of these layers is inserted into the lateral border of the arch, while the other is inserted into the medial border. Between these two layers, there exists a small amount of adipose tissue, the orbital branch of the superficial temporal artery, and a filament originating from the zygomatic branch of the maxillary nerve. The deep surface of the structure allows for attachment to the superficial fibers of the temporalis muscle.

The temporalis (Figure 1.17), also known as the temporal muscle, is a wide and diverging muscle located on the lateral aspect of the cranium. The origin of this structure encompasses the entirety of the temporal fossa, except for the section produced by the zygomatic bone, as well as the deep surface of the temporal fascia. The fibers of the muscle converge in a downward direction and terminate in a tendon. This tendon passes beneath the zygomatic arch and attaches to the medial surface, apex, and anterior border of the coronoid process, as well as the anterior border of the ramus of the mandible, extending almost as far forward as the final molar tooth. The external pterygoid muscle, also known as the pterygoideus externus, is a compact, robust muscle that has a conical shape. It spans horizontally from the infratemporal fossa to the mandibular condyle. The origin of this structure can be attributed to two sources: an upper origin from the lower portion of the lateral surface of the great wing of the sphenoid bone and the infratemporal crest, and a lower origin from the lateral surface of the lateral pterygoid plate. The fibers of this structure traverse in a horizontal direction, extending posteriorly and laterally, ultimately attaching to a concave area located anterior to the neck of the condyle of the jaw. Additionally, they enter the anterior border of the articular disk of the temporomandibular joint. The internal pterygoid muscle, also known as the pterygoideus internus, is a muscular structure that has a quadrilateral shape (see Figure 1.18). The muscle in question originates from the medial surface of the lateral pterygoid plate and the grooved surface of the pyramidal process of the palatine bone. Additionally, it has another point of origin from the lateral surfaces of the pyramidal process of the palatine bone and the tuberosity of the maxilla. The fibers of this structure descend, move to the side, and move toward the rear. They are then attached to the lower and posterior region of the inner surface of the mandible's ramus and angle, extending up to the mandibular foramen, through a robust tendinous lamina.

The mandibular nerve is responsible for innervating the muscles of mastication. The muscles known as the temporalis, masseter, and pterygoideus internus exert significant power to elevate the mandible in opposition to the maxillae. The primary function of the pterygoideus externus muscle is to aid in the process of mouth opening. However, its principal action involves the advancement

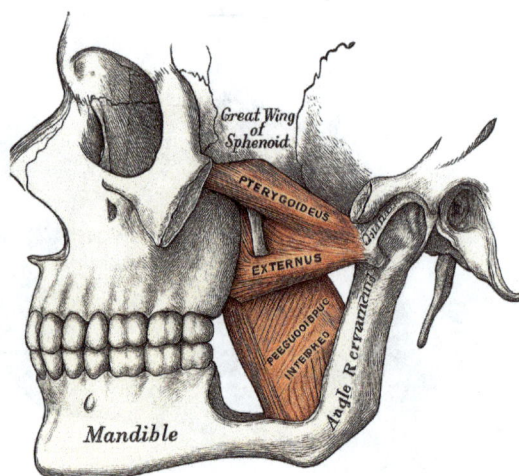

Figure 1.18 The pterygoidei, the zygomatic arch, and a portion of the ramus of the mandible have been removed.

of the condyle and articular disk, resulting in the protrusion of the mandible and the projection of the inferior incisors in front of the upper incisors. The pterygoideus internus muscle provides assistance in this particular activity. The retraction of the jaw is facilitated by the posterior fibers of the temporalis muscle. When the pterygoideus internus and externus muscles on one side are activated, the mandible on the corresponding side is brought forward, while the opposing condyle remains relatively stable, allowing for lateral motions.

1.4 THE PHARYNX

The pharynx is a component of the gastrointestinal tract that is situated posteriorly to the nasal cavities, oral cavity, and larynx [5]. The structure in question may be described as a tubular formation composed of muscle and membrane. It has a conical shape, with the wider end oriented upward and the narrower end pointing downward. This tubular structure extends from the lower surface of the skull to the level of the cricoid cartilage in the anterior region and to the sixth cervical vertebra in the posterior region. The length of the pharynx cavity measures around 12.5 cm, and it exhibits a greater width in the transverse dimension compared to the anteroposterior dimension. The maximum width of the structure is located just under the cranial base, where it extends bilaterally, posterior to the pharyngeal opening of the auditory tube, forming the pharyngeal recess (also known as the fossa of Rosenmüller). The narrowest point of the structure is at its end, where it connects to the esophagus. The pharynx is anatomically bounded by the body of the sphenoid and the basilar part of the occipital bone above, and it is continuous with the esophagus below. Posteriorly, it is connected to the cervical portion of the vertebral column through loose areolar tissue and the prevertebral fascia that covers the longus colli and longus capitis muscles. Anteriorly, it is incomplete and sequentially attached to the medial pterygoid plate, pterygomandibular raphé, mandible, tongue, hyoid bone, and thyroid and cricoid cartilages. Laterally, it is connected to the styloid processes and their associated muscles, and it is in contact with the common and internal carotid arteries; internal jugular veins; glossopharyngeal, vagus, and hypoglossal nerves; sympathetic trunks; and small portions of the pterygoidei interni above. There are a total of seven interconnected cavities with which it communicates. These are the two nasal cavities, the two tympanic cavities, the mouth, the larynx, and the esophagus. The pharynx may be split into three segments, namely nasal, oral, and laryngeal, when considering its cavity. This division is seen in Figure 1.10. The nasal part of the pharynx, also known as the pars nasalis pharyngis or nasopharynx, is situated posterior to the nasal cavity and superior to the soft palate. It is distinguished from the oral and laryngeal portions of the pharynx by its consistent openness. The lateral wall of the structure contains the pharyngeal ostium of the auditory tube, which has a slightly triangular shape. This ostium is bordered posteriorly by a prominent and hard structure known as the torus or cushion. The torus is formed by the medial portion of the cartilage of the auditory tube, which causes an elevation of the surrounding mucous membrane. The salpingopharyngeal fold, which is a vertical fold of mucous membrane, extends from the bottom portion of the torus and encompasses the salpingopharyngeus muscle. A secondary and rather diminutive fold, known as the salpingopalatine fold, extends from the superior region of the torus to the palate. The pharyngeal recess, also known as the fossa of Rosenmüller, is located posterior to the ostium of the auditory canal. The pharyngeal tonsil, sometimes referred to as a mass of lymphoid tissue, is located on the posterior wall. It is most prominent throughout childhood. The mucous membrane located above the pharyngeal tonsil has an irregular flask-shaped depression in the midline. Occasionally, this depression continues upward to the basilar process of the occipital bone. This anatomical feature is referred to as the pharyngeal bursa. The segment of the pharynx known as the pars oralis pharyngis extends from the soft palate to the hyoid bone. The orifice of the structure is located in the front region, namely via the isthmus faucium, leading into the oral cavity. Positioned within the lateral wall, between the two palatine arches, is the palatine tonsil. The anatomical region known as the laryngeal part of the pharynx, or pars laryngea pharyngis, extends from the hyoid bone to the lower boundary of the cricoid cartilage. At this point, it seamlessly transitions into the esophagus. The front aspect of the larynx exhibits a triangular entry, with its base oriented toward the front. This entrance is comprised of the epiglottis, which forms the base, and the aryepiglottic folds, which represent the lateral limits. The laryngeal orifice is flanked by a recess known as the sinus piriformis. This recess is delimited medially by the aryepiglottic fold and laterally by the thyroid cartilage and hyothyroid membrane. There is a total of six muscles that comprise the pharynx, as seen in Figure 1.14. The muscles involved in the pharyngeal constrictor complex include the inferior constrictor, stylopharyngeus, middle constrictor, salpingopharyngeus, superior constrictor, and pharyngopalatinus (Figure 1.19). The inferior constrictor, also known as the constrictor pharyngis inferior, originates from the lateral aspects of the cricoid and thyroid cartilage. It is the thickest of the three constrictor muscles. The structure in question originates from the cricoid cartilage, specifically within the space located between the cricothyreoideus muscle anteriorly and the articular facet for the inferior cornu of the thyroid cartilage posteriorly. The origin of the muscle on the thyroid cartilage is located at the oblique line on the lateral aspect of the lamina, extending from the posterior border and reaching the surface behind it,

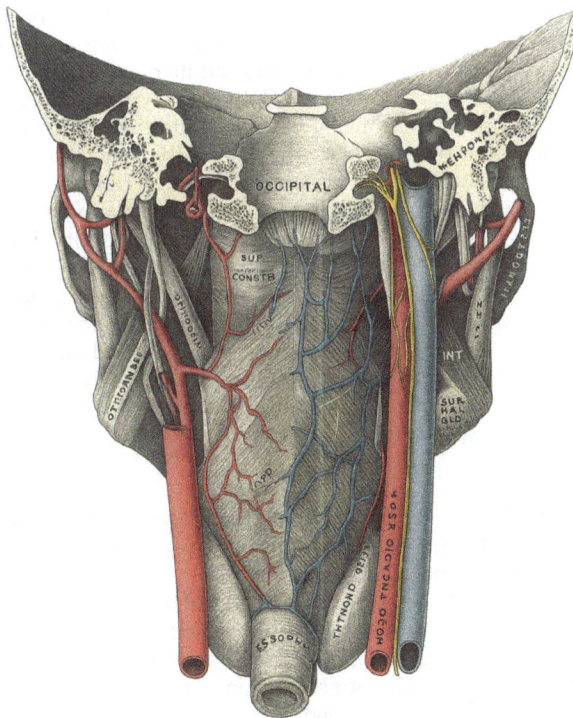

Figure 1.19 The pharyngeal muscles.

as well as from the inferior cornu. The fibers originating from these points extend in a posterior and medial direction, ultimately joining with the muscle on the other side to form a connection at the fibrous raphé located in the posterior median line of the pharynx. The horizontal inferior fibers of the esophagus are seamlessly connected to the circular fibers. The remaining fibers ascend in an oblique manner, gradually increasing in angle, and overlap the constrictor medius. The middle constrictor muscle, also known as the constrictor pharyngis medius, is a muscle that has a fan-like structure and is smaller than the muscle that comes before it. The origin of this structure is derived from the entire extent of the superior margin of the larger cornu of the hyoid bone, as well as from the smaller cornu and the stylohyoid ligament. The fibers exhibit a pattern of divergence from their point of origin. The lower fibers proceed downward, passing beneath the constrictor inferior. The intermediate fibers traverse horizontally, while the top fibers ascend and overlap with the constrictor superior. The structure is introduced into the posterior median fibrous raphé, where it merges along the central axis with the muscle on the contralateral side. The superior constrictor muscle, also known as the constrictor pharyngis superior, is a quadrilateral muscle that has a thinner and paler appearance compared to the other two muscles. The origin of this structure may be traced to the lower third of the posterior edge of the medial pterygoid plate and its hamulus, as well as the pterygomandibular raphé. Additionally, it originates from the alveolar process of the jaw above the posterior end of the mylohyoid line, and is supplemented by a small number of fibers from the side of the tongue. The fibers have a posterior curvature when they are placed into the median raphé. Additionally, they are extended by an aponeurosis toward the pharyngeal spine located on the basilar portion of the occipital bone. The more superior of the fibers arch below the levator veli palatini muscle and the auditory canal. The anatomical space located between the superior margin of the muscle and the cranial base is anatomically sealed by the pharyngeal aponeurosis, and is commonly referred to as the sinus of Morgagni. The stylopharyngeus muscle, as seen in Figure 1.12, is characterized by its elongated and thin structure, with a cylindrical shape above and a flattened shape below. The structure originates from the medial aspect of the base of the styloid process, descends next to the throat between the constrictores superior and medius muscles, and expands under the mucous membrane. A portion of the fibers of the muscle in question is anatomically integrated inside the constrictor muscles, whilst another portion of these fibers, upon convergence with the pharyngopalatinus, is affixed to the posterior edge of the thyroid cartilage. The glossopharyngeal nerve courses along the lateral aspect of this muscle, traversing it in order to innervate the tongue. The salpingopharyngeus muscle (Figure 1.12) originates from the lower region of the auditory tube in close proximity to its opening. It descends and merges with the posterior bundle of the pharyngopalatinus muscle. The constrictores and salpingopharyngeus muscles receive innervation from branches originating from the pharyngeal plexus. In addition, the constrictor inferior muscle is supplied by extra branches originating from the external laryngeal and recurrent nerves. The stylopharyngeus muscle, on the other hand, receives innervation from the glossopharyngeal nerve. During the initiation of deglutition, the pharynx undergoes elevation and expansion in various orientations, facilitating the reception of food pushed from the oral cavity. The stylopharyngei muscles exhibit a greater distance between their points of origin compared to their points of insertion. These muscles elevate and move the sides of the pharynx in an upward and lateral direction, thereby augmenting its transverse diameter. Additionally, the breadth of the pharynx in the anteroposterior direction is expanded as the larynx and tongue are propelled forward during their ascent. Upon the arrival of the food bolus in the pharynx, the elevator muscles undergo relaxation, causing the pharynx to drop. Simultaneously, the constrictores muscles contract around the bolus, facilitating its movement downward into the esophagus.

1.5 THE LARYNX

The larynx, often known as the vocal organ, is situated in the top portion of the respiratory tract [6]. The thyroid gland is located in the front region of the neck, positioned between the trachea and the base of the tongue. It prominently protrudes in the midline of the neck. The structure in question constitutes the inferior portion of the anterior pharyngeal wall and is posteriorly lined by the mucous membrane of said cavity. Adjacent to it are the major neck veins. The vertical extent of the structure aligns with the fourth, fifth, and sixth cervical vertebrae; however, it is positioned somewhat higher in females and children. The upper portion of the larynx has a wide structure resembling a flattened triangular box, with flattened surfaces at the posterior and lateral sides. It is delimited anteriorly by a distinct vertical ridge. The object in question has a slender and tubular shape. The structure consists of cartilages that are interconnected by ligaments and mobilized by a

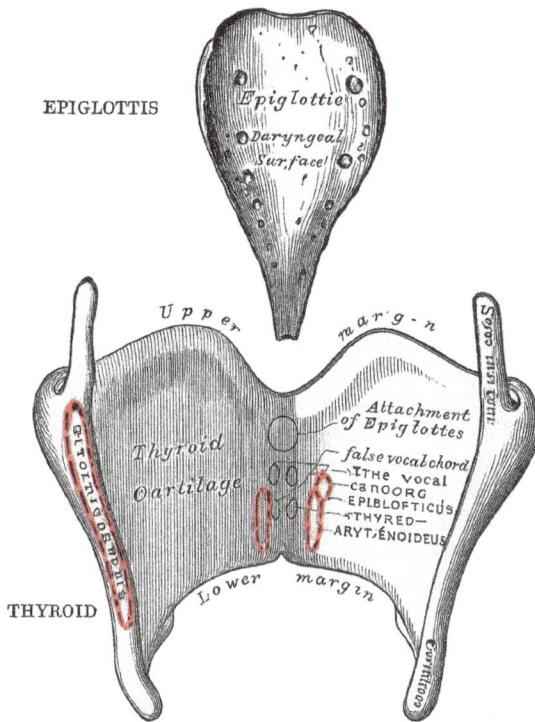

Figure 1.20 The laryngeal cartilages.

multitude of muscles. The structure in question is bordered by a mucous membrane that is uninterrupted in its connection to the pharynx above and the trachea below. The cartilages of the larynx, known as cartilagines laryngis, consist of a total of nine components (Figure 1.20). Among them, there are three single cartilages and three pairs of cartilages. The single cartilages include the thyroid cartilage, the cricoid cartilage, and the epiglottis. The paired cartilages consist of two corniculate cartilages, two cuneiform cartilages, and two arytenoid cartilages. The cartilago thyreoidea, commonly referred to as the thyroid cartilage, is the largest cartilage structure found within the larynx. The structure is composed of two laminae, with their anterior borders fused together at an acute angle along the midline of the neck. This fusion creates a subcutaneous projection known as the laryngeal prominence, also referred to as the pomum Adami. The aforementioned prominence exhibits its most notable characteristics in its upper region and displays a greater size disparity between males and females. Directly superior to it, the laminae are distinctly divided by a V-shaped indentation known as the superior thyroid notch. The laminae have an irregular quadrilateral form, with their posterior angles extending into structures known as the superior and inferior cornua. The superior thyroid tubercle, located at the root of the superior cornu, is connected to the inferior thyroid tubercle on the lower border by an oblique line that goes downward and forward on the outer surface of each lamina. This line provides connection to the sternothyreoideus, thyreohyoideus, and constrictor pharyngis inferior muscles. The inner surface of the object has a smooth texture, while its upper and posterior regions possess a small concavity and are enveloped by a layer of mucous membrane. Located in the anterior aspect, within the angle created by the convergence of the laminae, many anatomical structures are affixed, including the epiglottis stem, the ventricular and vocal ligaments, the thyreoarytaenoidei, thyreoepiglottici, and vocales muscles, as well as the thyroepiglottic ligament. The superior margin has a concave shape posteriorly and a convex shape anteriorly, serving as the point of attachment for the corresponding portion of the hyothyroid membrane. The inferior border has a concave shape posteriorly and a nearly straight configuration anteriorly, with the presence of the inferior thyroid tubercle serving as the demarcation between these two regions. The cricoid cartilage is attached to a portion of the midline, both within and in close proximity to it, through the middle cricothyroid ligament. The posterior border, which is characterized by its thickness and rounded shape, serves as the site of insertion for the stylopharyngeus and pharyngopalatinus muscles. The termination point of the structure is situated superiorly in the cornu and inferiorly in the cornu. The superior cornu is characterized by its elongated and slender shape, with an upward, backward, and medialward orientation. It terminates in a conical tip, serving as the point of attachment for the lateral hyothyroid ligament. The inferior cornu is characterized by its compact dimensions, exhibiting a shortened and robust structure. It is oriented in a downward direction, displaying a minor anterior and medial inclination. Additionally, it features a diminutive oval articular facet on its medial aspect, which facilitates articulation with the lateral surface of the cricoid cartilage. During infancy, the laminae of the thyroid cartilage are linked to each other by a narrow, lozenge-shaped strip, dubbed the intrathyroid cartilage. The aforementioned strip spans from the superior to the inferior boundary of the central cartilage and is characterized by its increased transparency and flexibility compared to the laminae. The cricoid cartilage, known as cartilago cricoidea in anatomical terminology, is smaller than the thyroid cartilage. However, it compensates for its reduced size by possessing greater thickness and strength. Functionally, it serves to constitute the lower and posterior regions of the larynx's wall. The structure is comprised of two distinct components: a posterior quadrate lamina and a rather slender anterior arch, which measures around one-fourth or one-fifth of the depth of the lamina. The posterior portion of the lamina cartilaginis cricoideae is characterized by its deep and broad structure, measuring approximately 2–3 cm in a superior-inferior direction. Positioned on its posterior surface, in the midline, is a vertical ridge. The lower part of this ridge serves as an attachment site for the longitudinal fibers of the esophagus. Additionally, on each side of this ridge, there is a wide depression specifically designed to accommodate the cricoarytenoideus posterior muscle. The front segment of the arch, known as the arcus cartilaginis cricoideae, is characterized by its thin and convex shape. It has a vertical measurement ranging from 5 to 7 mm. This arch provides external attachment points for the cricothyreiodei muscles at the front and sides, and at the back, it attaches to a piece of the constrictor pharyngis inferior muscle. Located near the intersection of the lamina and the arch, there exists a diminutive circular articular surface on both sides, which facilitates the articulation with the inferior cornu of the thyroid cartilage. The inferior margin of the cricoid cartilage is oriented horizontally and is anatomically linked to the uppermost ring of the trachea by the cricotracheal ligament. The superior boundary has an oblique upward and posterior trajectory, which can be attributed to the significant depth of the lamina. The structure in question exhibits anterior attachment to the middle cricothyroid ligament, lateral attachment to both the conus elasticus and the cricoarytaenoidei laterales, and posteriorly, it displays a central shallow notch. On either side of this notch, there are smooth, oval, convex surfaces that are oriented in an upward and lateral direction. These surfaces serve as points of articulation with the base of an arytenoid cartilage. The inner surface of the cricoid cartilage has a smooth texture and is covered by a layer of mucous membrane. The arytenoid cartilages, also known as cartilagines arytaenoideae, consist of a pair of structures located near the superior margin of the lamina of the cricoid cartilage, positioned posteriorly inside the larynx. Each object possesses a pyramidal structure, characterized by three distinct surfaces, a foundational base, and a singular apex. The posterior aspect of the structure has a triangle shape, displaying a smooth and concave morphology. This surface serves as the site for the attachment of the arytaenoidei obliquus and transversus muscles. The anterolateral surface exhibits a moderate convexity and a coarse texture. Located in close proximity to the apex of the cartilage, there exists a rounded prominence known as the colliculus. Extending from this colliculus is a ridge referred to as the crista arcuata, which first bends in a posterior direction before subsequently descending and then moving forward toward the vocal process. The inferior portion of this crest is situated between two concavities known as foveae, namely an upper triangular fovea and a lower oblong fovea. The latter fovea serves as the point of attachment for the vocalis muscle. The medial surface is characterized by its narrowness, smoothness, and flattened shape. It is covered by a layer of mucous membrane and serves as the lateral border of the intercartilaginous portion of the rima glottidis. The cartilage base has a wide structure, including a concave and sleek surface that facilitates articulation with the cricoid cartilage. The lateral angle of the structure is characterized by its short length, rounded shape, and notable prominence. It extends in a posterior and lateral direction, and is referred to as the muscular process. This particular region provides attachment points for the cricoarytenoid posterior muscle at its posterior aspect, and for the cricoarytenoid lateral muscle at its anterior aspect. The anterior angle, which is likewise notable but possesses a sharper tip, extends horizontally in a forward direction. It serves as the site of attachment for the vocal ligament and is referred to as the vocal process. The superior aspect of each cartilage has a pointed shape, with a posterior and medial curvature, and is topped with a little conical nodule composed of cartilage, known as the corniculate cartilage. The corniculate cartilages, also known as cartilagines corniculatae or cartilages of Santorini, are a pair of tiny conical nodules composed of elastic cartilage with a yellowish appearance. These cartilages interact with the tops of the arytenoid cartilages and function to extend them posteriorly and medially. The structures in question are located inside the posterior regions of the aryepiglottic folds of mucous membrane, and on occasion, they may be conjoined with the arytenoid cartilages. The cuneiform cartilages, also known as cartilagines cuneiformes or cartilages of Wrisberg, consist of two elongated structures composed of yellow elastic cartilage. These cartilages are situated bilaterally within the aryepiglottic fold, resulting in the formation of small whitish elevations on the mucous membrane's surface. These elevations are located anteriorly to the arytenoid cartilages.

The epiglottis, also known as the cartilago epiglottica, is a slender fibrocartilaginous structure with a leaf-like form. It is positioned at an oblique angle, extending upward beyond the base of the tongue and in front of the opening of the larynx. Its coloration is often yellowish in appearance. The distal end of the structure is characterized by a wide and rounded shape, while the proximal portion or stalk is elongated, slender, and linked to the juncture formed by the two plates of the thyroid cartilage by the thyroepiglottic ligament, situated a short distance under the superior thyroid notch. The hyoepiglottic ligament serves as a connecting structure between the top border of the body of the hyoid bone and the lower section of the anterior surface. The anterior or lingual surface has a pronounced curvature in the forward direction. This surface is overlaid by a layer of mucous membrane on its upper section, which extends onto the sides and base of the tongue. Consequently, a central glossoepiglottic fold and two lateral glossoepiglottic folds are formed. The lateral folds are partially connected to the pharyngeal wall. The anatomical structures referred to as the valleculae are the depressions located between the epiglottis and the root of the tongue, specifically situated on both sides of the median fold. The lower section of the anterior surface is beneath the hyoid bone, the hyothyroid membrane, and upper part of the thyroid cartilage, but is separated from these structures by a mass of fatty tissue. The surface located behind or on the larynx is characterized by its smoothness and concave shape from side to side, as well as its concavo-convex shape from top to bottom. Toward its lower portion, there is a protrusion known as the tubercle or cushion. Upon removal of the mucous membrane, the cartilage surface exhibits indentations characterized by many tiny pits that serve as housing for mucous glands. The aryepiglottic folds are connected to the lateral aspects.

The anatomical structure known as the larynx cavity, or cavum laryngis, spans from the entrance of the larynx to the lower boundary of the cricoid cartilage, where it seamlessly connects with the cavity of the trachea. The structure in question is anatomically separated into two distinct sections by the presence of the projection of the vocal folds. Positioned between these folds is a slender triangular opening referred to as the rima glottidis. The anatomical region located above the vocal folds within the larynx is referred to as the vestibule. This region has a broad and triangular morphology, with its anterior wall serving as its foundation. Notably, the tubercle of the epiglottis projects backward from the central area of this anterior wall. The structure in question encompasses the ventricular folds, and situated between these folds and the vocal folds are the ventricles of the larynx. The region situated underneath the vocal folds initially has an elliptical shape, but as it descends, it progressively widens and adopts a circular configuration, ultimately connecting seamlessly with the tracheal tube. The laryngeal entry, as seen in Figure 1.21, is a triangular aperture that exhibits a wider anterior aspect, a narrower posterior aspect, and an oblique downward and backward inclination. The structure in question is demarcated anteriorly by the epiglottis, posteriorly by the apices of the arytenoid cartilages, corniculate cartilages, and the interarytenoid notch, and laterally by a mucous membrane fold. This fold contains ligamentous and muscular fibers that extend between the side of the epiglottis and the apex of the arytenoid cartilage. Specifically, this fold is known as the aryepiglottic fold, and on the posterior portion of its margin, the cuneiform cartilage forms a discernible whitish prominence referred to as the cuneiform tubercle. The ventricular folds, also known as plicoe ventriculares or superior vocal cords, consist of two thick folds of mucous membrane. Each fold encloses a narrow band of fibrous tissue called the ventricular ligament. The ventricular ligament is attached at the front to the angle of the thyroid cartilage, just below the attachment of the epiglottis. At the back, it is connected to the anterolateral surface of the arytenoid cartilage, located a short distance above the vocal process. The inferior edge of this ligament, surrounded by a layer of mucous membrane, creates a curved and unrestricted barrier that serves as the upper limit of the laryngeal ventricle. The vocal folds, also known as plicoe vocales or lower vocal cords, play a crucial role in sound generation. They consist of two robust bands called the

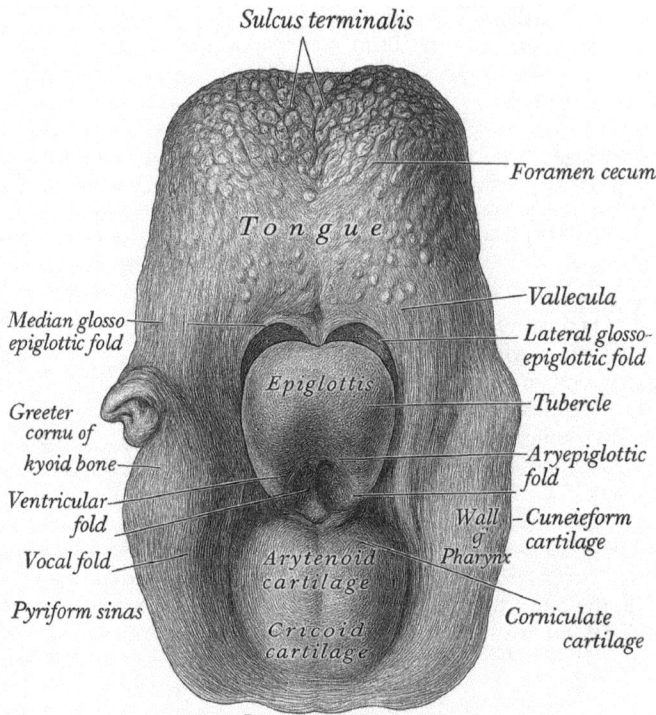

Figure 1.21 The entrance to the larynx, viewed from behind.

vocal ligaments, which are sometimes referred to as ligamenta vocales or inferior thyroarytenoid. Each ligament is composed of a yellow elastic tissue band that is connected anteriorly to the angle of the thyroid cartilage and posteriorly to the vocal process of the arytenoid. The inferior boundary of this structure exhibits continuity with the slender lateral component of the conus elasticus. The superior margin of this structure constitutes the inferior demarcation of the laryngeal ventricle. Horizontally, the vocalis muscle is positioned parallel to it. The structure in question is medially enveloped by a delicate mucous membrane that exhibits a very thin composition and adheres tightly to its surface. The anatomical structure known as the ventricle of the larynx, sometimes referred to as ventriculus laryngis (Morgagni) or laryngeal sinus, is a spindle-shaped depression located bilaterally between the ventricular and vocal folds. It spans a significant portion of the length of these folds. The fossa is delimited superiorly by the arched border of the ventricular fold, inferiorly by the straight margin of the vocal fold, and laterally by the mucous membrane that covers the corresponding thyreoarytenoideus muscle. The anterior region of the ventricle ascends through a tiny aperture into a cecal pouch composed of mucous membrane, which exhibits variability in terms of its dimensions, and is commonly referred to as the appendix. The anatomical structure known as the appendix of the laryngeal ventricle, also referred to as the appendix ventriculi laryngis or laryngeal saccule, is a sac-like membranous structure located between the ventricular fold and the inner surface of the thyroid cartilage. In some cases, it may extend up to the upper border of the thyroid cartilage or even beyond. The appendix of the laryngeal ventricle exhibits a conical shape and a slight posterior curvature. The mucous membrane of the subject in question contains openings for around 60–70 mucous glands, which are situated inside the submucous areolar tissue. The sac in question is contained within a fibrous capsule, which remains uninterrupted as it extends below to form the ventricular ligament. The medial surface of the structure is enveloped by a limited number of tiny muscle bundles, originating from the apex of the arytenoid cartilage and terminating within the aryepiglottic fold of mucous membrane. On its lateral side, it is distinctly separated from the thyroid cartilage by the thyreoepiglotticus. The aforementioned muscles exert pressure on the sac, facilitating the expulsion of its contained secretion onto the vocal folds, so providing lubrication to their surfaces. The rima glottidis, as seen in Figure 1.22, refers to the elongated fissure or narrow opening that exists between the vocal folds anteriorly, and the bases and vocal processes of the arytenoid cartilages posteriorly. Consequently, the structure may be separated into two distinct

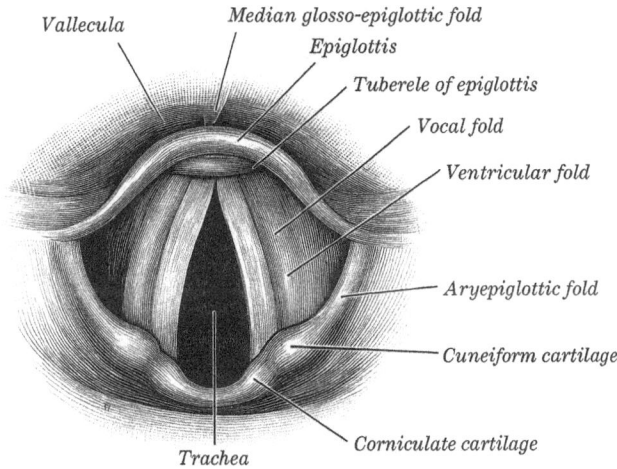

Figure 1.22 Laryngoscopic view of the interior of the larynx.

components: the larger anterior intramembranous section, known as the glottis vocalis, which occupies around 60% of the total aperture length, and the posterior intercartilaginous part, referred to as the glottis respiratoria. The posterior limitation is determined by the presence of the mucous membrane that traverses the arytenoid cartilages. The rima glottidis, which correlates with the bases of the arytenoid cartilages, is the most constricted region inside the laryngeal cavity. The length of the specimen in the male is around 23 mm, while in the female it ranges from 17 to 18 mm. The dimensions and configuration of the rima glottidis exhibit variability in response to the actions of the vocal folds and arytenoid cartilages during the processes of breathing and phonation. In a state of rest, specifically when these structures are unaffected by muscular activity, such as during calm respiration, the intramembranous portion assumes a triangular shape, with its apex positioned in front and its base located at the back. The base is represented by a line measuring approximately 8 mm in length, connecting the anterior ends of the vocal processes. Additionally, the medial surfaces of the arytenoids are parallel to each other, resulting in a rectangular shape for the intercartilaginous part. During the production of a high note, the vocal folds undergo extreme adduction. This causes the intramembranous part of the vocal folds to become a linear slit due to their apposition. Simultaneously, the intercartilaginous part of the vocal folds takes on a triangular shape, with its apex aligning with the anterior ends of the vocal processes of the arytenoids. This triangular shape is achieved through the medial rotation of the cartilages. On the other hand, in cases of severe abduction of the vocal folds, such as during forced inspiration, the arytenoids and their vocal processes undergo lateral rotation. This results in a triangular form of the intercartilaginous section, with its apex pointing toward the posterior region. In this particular state, the complete glottis exhibits a shape resembling a lozenge, with the sides of the intramembranous portion diverging in a front-to-back direction, and the sides of the intercartilaginous portion diverging in a back-to-front direction. The widest part of the opening aligns with the points where the vocal folds attach to the vocal processes.

1.6 THE ESOPHAGUS

The esophagus is a hollow muscular structure with two high-pressure zones, the upper and lower esophageal sphincters, that span 18–26 cm (Figure 1.23) [7]. It has a compressed oval shape in the axial plane, with the long axis extending laterally. The diameter is roughly 2 cm at rest and can reach up to 3 cm laterally when inflated with a meal bolus. Symptoms of dysphagia often appear when the lumen is constricted to less than 13 mm, improve when the lumen is more than 15 mm, and disappear completely when the lumen is greater than 18 mm. The esophagus, unlike the remainder of the gastrointestinal tract, lacks a genuine serosa. Mucosa, submucosa, muscularis propria, and adventitia are the four layers that make up the esophageal wall (Figure 1.24). A thin outer longitudinal layer and a broader inner circular layer split the muscularis propria. The esophagus is made up of striated muscle in the proximal third and smooth muscle in the distal third, with a moderate transition zone in between. On high-resolution esophageal manometry, this transition zone can be identified as a decrease or small break in peristalsis. The esophagus's motor activity is

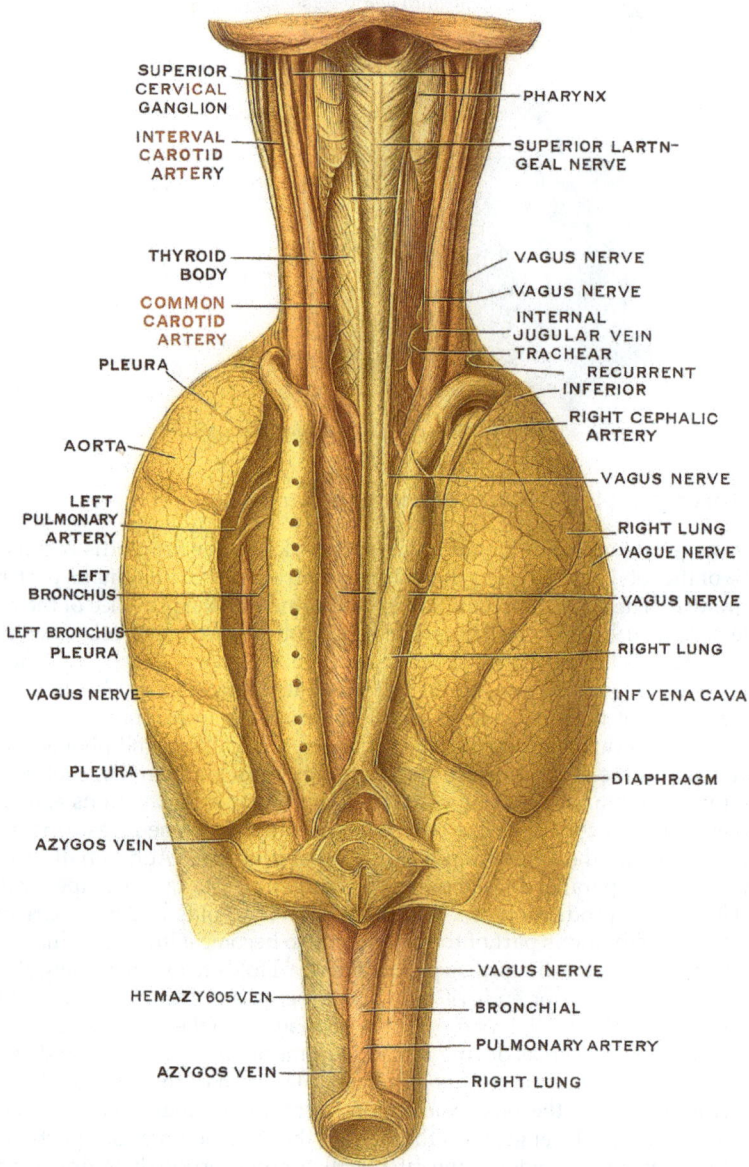

Figure 1.23 The esophagus within the thorax.

not rhythmic like that of the rest of the gastrointestinal tract, and it is controlled by extrinsic and intrinsic innervations. Peristalsis is principally controlled in the proximal striated muscle by direct sequential vagal stimulation originating in the nucleus ambiguous. The peripheral enteric nervous system and central impulses from the dorsal motor nucleus work together to control peristalsis in the distal smooth muscle. Two nerve plexuses make up the peripheral enteric nervous system. The distal peristalsis is primarily coordinated by the myenteric plexus (Auerbach's plexus), which is located between the two muscular layers. The submucosal plexus (Meissner's plexus) is scarce in the esophagus and is primarily responsible for transmitting sensory information to the brain via vagal afferent neurons. Mucosal chemoreceptors and muscular mechanoreceptors can also send pain signals back to the somatosensory cortex via these same afferent neurons. Because of its large circulatory network, esophageal ischemia is relatively unusual. The vascular supply is variable, although branches from the inferior thyroid artery in the proximal third, the thoracic aorta in the middle third, and the left stomach artery in the distal third are the most common. Small tributaries

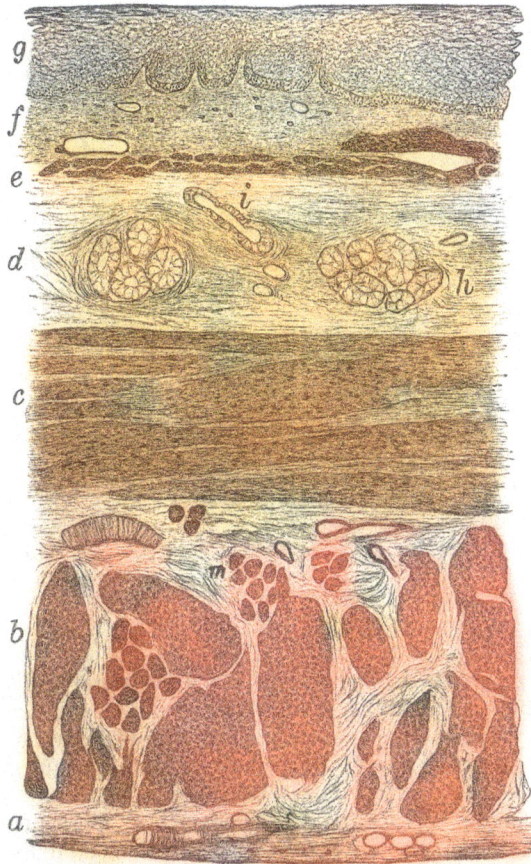

Figure 1.24 Histology of the esophageal wall.

discharge venous blood to the azygos and hemiazygos veins, which go to the superior vena cava in the thoracic cavity. The left gastric vein drains the distal esophagus. The development of distal esophageal varices is caused by retrograde flow through the left gastric vein in the presence of portal hypertension. Proximal esophageal varices, also known as downhill varices, occur infrequently and are mainly caused by obstruction of the superior vena cava. The esophagus is separated into three distinct segments based on topography: cervical, thoracic, and abdominal. The cervical esophagus begins where the inferior pharyngeal constrictor muscles join the cricopharyngeus muscle to form the upper esophageal sphincter (UES), a 1 cm high-pressure zone located at the level of C5–C6, and usually around 16 cm from the incisors. The UES is in a contracted position at rest to prevent air from entering and regurgitation from leaving the esophagus. Killian's triangle is a zone of scant musculature on the posterior wall immediately proximal to the UES. A Zenker's diverticulum might form in this location of relative muscular weakness. The most common cause of pharyngeal pressurization is poor UES opening due to cricopharyngeus muscle fibrosis, which results in a false diverticulum with only a mucosal and submucosal outpouching. The cervical esophagus is made entirely of striated muscle and extends about 5 cm along the cervical spine to the suprasternal notch. It is located between the carotid sheaths and the cervical vertebral bodies, posterior to the trachea and anterior to the trachea. Other common pathologies contributing to dysphagia can be observed in this area, including extrinsic compression from anterior cervical osteophytes and anterolateral outpouchings below the cricopharyngeus due to Killian–Jamieson diverticula, a congenital weakening of the esophagus wall. Rather than flowing straight down, the esophagus produces a modest reverse S shape when it enters the thoracic cavity, leaning to the left of the spinal column, then right, then left again. It creates several close relationships with the vasculature and airways as it descends, resulting in distinctive indentations that can be observed endoscopically. The aortic arch,

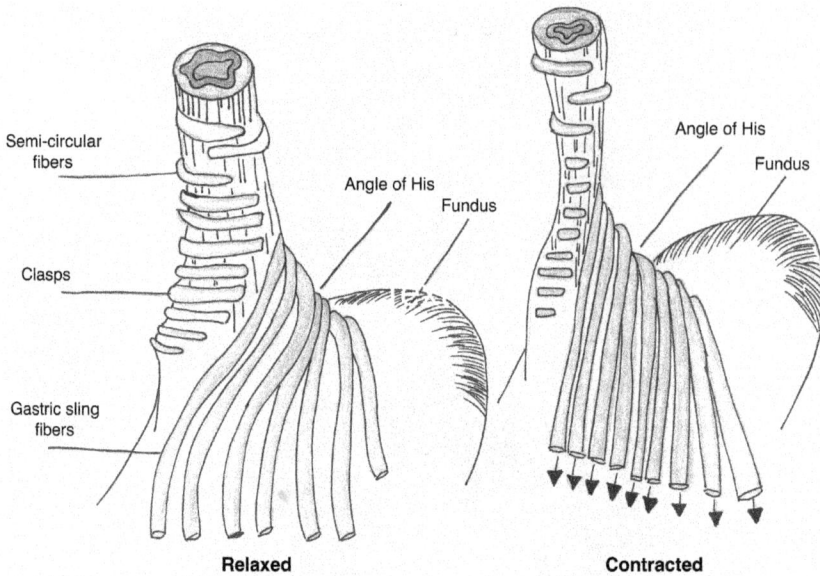

Figure 1.25 Clasp and sling fibers of the gastroesophageal junction.

which curves posteriorly and makes an impression on the left lateral wall of the esophagus, causes the initial indentation, which is around 23 cm from the incisors. Characteristic pulsations can often be seen on endoscopy to identify this. The left major bronchus passes anterior to the esophagus around 2 cm distal to this, causing a second depression. The esophagus lies below this, posterior to the left atrium of the heart, separated from it by a narrow pericardium. An enlarged left atrium might result in a third indentation, as seen here anteriorly. Any of these indentations, if accentuated, can cause dysphagia and are also places where pill esophagitis is more likely to occur. Dysphagia aortica is caused by the aorta compressing the esophagus, which usually occurs in the presence of a thoracic aortic aneurysm. Dysphagia lusoria is defined by a pencil-like indentation at T3–T4 above the aortic arch and is caused by an abnormal right subclavian artery, which affects 0.7% of the population. A short section of the esophagus (about 1 cm) reaches the abdomen as it departs the thoracic chamber through its own hiatus within the right crus of the diaphragm. The esophagus creates an indentation on the posterior surface of the liver's left lobe. A second high-pressure zone, the lower esophageal sphincter, marks the esophagus's distal end (LES). The LES is made up of an asymmetrically thickened circular smooth muscle that is 2–4 cm long on average. The proximal border of the LES is difficult to discern endoscopically; however, the presence of a proportionally thickened muscular band can help. This area of the LES is sometimes referred to as the phrenic ampulla or vestibule on an esophagram. The LES and the crural diaphragm are two structures that make up the high-pressure zone at the esophagogastric junction (EGJ). The LES is made up of two muscular fibers called sling and clasp fibers (Figure 1.25). At the EGJ, the clasp fibers form an incomplete muscular ring. They cover the esophagus from the front, on the lesser curve side, and from the back. Sling fibers originate on the anterior gastric body, travel cephalad around the EGJ's larger curve side, and terminate on the posterior gastric body. The squamocolumnar junction is 1.5 cm proximal and 2 cm distal to the high-pressure zone. The phrenoesophageal ligament, which inserts circumferentially into the esophageal musculature, holds these two independent components of the EGJ in place. They can maintain a competent anti-reflux barrier by working together to constantly counterbalance a variable pressure gradient between the stomach and the esophagus and prevent excessive esophageal acid exposure [8].

REFERENCES

1. Butler P. *Applied radiological anatomy*. Cambridge: Cambridge University Press; 1999.
2. Ryan S, McNicholas M, Eustace SJ. *Anatomy for diagnostic imaging*. 3rd ed. Edinburgh: Churchill Livingstone; 2011.

3. Noh H, Fishman E, Forastiere A, Bliss D, Calhoun P. CT of the esophagus: spectrum of disease with emphasis on esophageal carcinoma. *Radiographics*. 1995;15(5):1113–34. doi:10.1148/radiographics.15.5.7501854.
4. Schünke M, Schulte E, Schumacher U. *Thieme atlas of anatomy*. Stuttgart: Thieme; 2006.
5. Singh I. *Textbook of anatomy with colour atlas*. New Delhi: Jaypee Brothers Medical Publishers; 2008.
6. Federle MP, Jeffrey RB, Woodward PJ. *Diagnostic imaging*. Salt Lake City: Amirsys; 2010.
7. Sinnatamby CS. *Last's anatomy: regional and applied*. 12th ed. Edinburgh: Churchill Livingstone; 2011.
8. Woodland P, Sifrim D, Krarup A, et al. The neurophysiology of the esophagus. *Ann N Y Acad Sci*. 2013;1300(1):53–70. doi:10.1111/nyas.12238.

2 Physiology of Deglutition

2.1 INTRODUCTION

Swallowing is a systematic physiological process that conveys food and saliva from the mouth to the stomach. The process of swallowing often appears to be smooth and uncomplicated, but it actually involves a sophisticated neuromuscular machinery that carries out and coordinates the sequence of swallowing. Swallowing is typically seen as a deliberate action, as it may be initiated by conscious thought of "swallow" [1]. Many swallows, especially those that happen between meals, occur without deliberate input. Voluntary swallowing typically happens at a rate of around one per minute in those who are awake. The rapid pace of swallowing is triggered by salivation, which occurs at around 0.5 mL per minute and must be either ingested or expelled. During periods of alertness, there is a consistently high rate of swallowing. This results in around 1000 swallows per day or 3 to 4 million swallows every decade [2]. While most swallows happen automatically as a result of salivation, there are also voluntary swallows that occur. These voluntary swallows are actively triggered when eating and tend to occur in close succession. During the process of eating, swallowing is linked to heightened salivation, which aids in the commencement of swallowing and serves as a lubricant. During sleep, the production of saliva and the act of swallowing significantly decrease, but these activities quickly resume when a person wakes up from sleep. Swallowing may be categorized into four distinct phases for descriptive purposes: the preparation phase, oral phase, pharyngeal phase, and esophageal phase [3]. The preliminary phase entails the process of chewing a bolus and combining it with saliva. The bolus is prepared, with its size, shape, and position optimized for swallowing, and placed on the tongue. In the oral phase, the bolus is driven from the oral cavity into the pharynx [4]. The typical pharyngeal phase entails the movement of the food bolus from the oropharynx to the esophagus without any inhalation of foreign substances. In the esophageal phase, the bolus is driven along the whole length of the esophagus and into the stomach.

2.2 NEURAL CONTROL OF DEGLUTITION

It is mandatory to know the essential afferent and efferent impulses, their origin, their destination, and the functions that integrate this process, in order to comprehend how the nervous system regulates any biological process [5]. Swallowing is a motor function that has been the focus of numerous disagreements and a very challenging neurophysiological investigation. A significant portion of the established mechanisms for the brain control of swallowing could not be regarded as reliable hypotheses, as demonstrated by these data and the literature study. In this sense, the study of the brain regulation of swallowing is still open to fresh ideas. The mechanics behind the oral, pharyngeal, and esophageal phases that make up the swallowing process are hotly debated [6]. Observations of neurological diseases have led to significant advances, and there are numerous techniques for verifying theories that ultimately remain theories [7]. Even if they are merely theories, there are a number of novel morphological and functional concepts that are at least more organized than the empirical ones that have been employed up to this point to describe the swallowing mechanisms. It was previously thought that the whole swallowing process, including the automatic and semiautomatic actions of chewing and swallowing, was involuntary by genesis and regulation, and that the swallowing control center was solely found in the brainstem [8]. The role of the cerebral cortex in the swallowing control mechanism has been identified and thoroughly investigated based on observations of patients with cortical dysphagia. According to the embryology of the nervous system, the brainstem and cerebellum originated from a rhombencephalic center that was created when the third primordial vesicle (the hindbrain) joined with the second one (the mesencephalon or midbrain). Through pre-existing receptors on the palate, palatoglossal and palatopharyngeal pillars, the base of the tongue, and the pharyngeal walls, particularly the posterior one, the rhombencephalic center would receive stimuli produced by the food bolus passage, initiating an involuntary and coordinated process that would define the pharyngeal phase of swallowing. It was thought that under physiological conditions, this phase would be regulated by a framework that was constantly altered by peripheral afferent stimuli [9]. This framework would specifically affect muscle function, modifying contraction time and strength in response to the size of the bolus that was swallowed. Soft palate elevation and reflex contraction of the upper pharyngeal constrictor would result from the bolus admission in the oropharynx. The bolus entrance would also start a peristaltic wave that would spread to the other muscles, closing the pharynx to protect the airways. However, the cricopharyngeal muscle would relax, allowing the pharyngeal content to flow through to the esophagus. The coordination mentioned is complemented by a center in the brainstem that consists of sensory and motor nuclei connected by a network of interneurons. A novel method takes into account the

DOI: 10.1201/9781003508113-2

oral and pharyngeal phases of swallowing as the components of the oropharynx's functional activity. Muscle contraction would generate this functional activity, which would be regulated by the central pattern generator (CPG) for swallowing, a control center located in the brainstem [10].

Under normal circumstances, the bilateral contraction of the pharyngeal and oral muscles would be coordinated and organized by this pattern-generating center, which would be made up of two hemicenters, one on each side of the brainstem [11]. With swallowing-linked neurons in the dorsal and ventral parts of the brainstem, their nerve fibers would connect the two halves of the implicated production centers by crossing the brainstem's midline. It has been acknowledged that information from the cerebral cortex and peripheral impulses caused by the swallowing stimulus would converge to the solitary tract nucleus in this pattern-generating area. The induction of voluntary swallowing would be the main function of this convergence of inputs to the solitary tract nucleus. The oropharyngeal cavity (oral and pharyngeal cavities) is thought to be the site of the initial "swallowing reflex" event. Here, the bolus would generate a sensory afferent stimulation that would alert the brainstem and cortex. The solitary tract nucleus would receive the initial cerebral command during nutritive swallowing. Therefore, the cerebral cortex could consciously initiate or facilitate consecutive eating and drinking through the brainstem's neural network (CPG) [12]. It was also thought that the primary function of swallowing-related cortical and subcortical regions in voluntary deglutition would be to initiate and regulate the swallowing motor sequence, particularly the oral phase. It has previously been described that the dorsal (sensory) and ventral (motor) regions represented on both sides of the brainstem would be able to independently coordinate the pharyngeal and esophageal phases of swallowing on each side, which is in opposition to the bilateral integration of the brainstem acknowledged in the pattern-generating center conception. The pharyngeal and oral swallowing phases differ from one another in terms of structure, innervation, and brain regulation, despite the fact that the two cavities are anatomically adjacent and work sequentially [13]. The pharyngeal phase is reflexive, while the oral phase is elective. While very uncommon, it is insufficient to classify the oral and pharyngeal stages as oropharyngeal or buccopharyngeal [14]. The functional role of the oral and pharyngeal phases of swallowing is not defined by the oropharynx, which is the anatomical intermediary segment that connects the oral and pharyngeal chambers and receives the contents conveyed during swallowing. Oropharyngeal dysphagia is a common definition of high dysphagia. Although impairment of both stages may result in high dysphagia, it is impossible to rule out the potential of injury that is solely oral or pharyngeal [15]. The commitment of the sequence, not of both phases, is emphasized by the fact that damage to one adjacent phase affects the dynamics of the other. With questionable therapeutic efficacy, the oropharyngeal classification for this type of dysphagia shifts the clinical and treatment focus, which ought to be on the truly impaired phase. Due to the classification of oropharyngeal dysphagia, we incorrectly classified esophageal dysphagia as a conduction dysphagia and the dysphagia affecting the oral and pharyngeal phases as transference dysphagia. Conduction is appropriate for the pharyngeal and esophageal phases, and transference is appropriate for the oral phase [16]. Conduction takes place in the reflex pharyngeal and esophageal stages, while transference is a voluntary process that takes place in the voluntary oral phase. It is true that studying neurological dysphagia has taught us a lot. Furthermore, there are a number of different approaches to studying swallowing and related difficulties nowadays, which help us better understand the physiology of swallowing but also show how many contradictory ideas are still in use [17]. In order to give the theories used to explain the swallowing mechanics and, by extension, the brain regulation of swallowing a stronger foundation, this work aims to provide new conceptual alternatives based on personal research and the literature.

2.2.1 Chewing

The chewing muscles, innervated by the trigeminal pair (V), the tongue muscles, innervated by the hypoglossal pair (XII), and, with less obvious involvement, the expression muscles, particularly the buccinators and lips' orbicular, which are innervated by the facial pair (VII), are all part of mastication, which is essentially voluntary. Axons from the trigeminal lemniscus travel to the thalamus, from where they travel to the postcentral gyrus (somatosensory cortex) in the parietal region of the cerebral cortex. Trigeminal afferent fibers arrive at the dorsal region of the brainstem, the primary sensory nucleus of the V. Through the nuclear cortical route (pyramidal-voluntary), the postcentral gyrus transmits information to the precentral gyrus (somatomotor cortex) in the frontal region, producing a motor efferent response that travels to the ventral region of the brainstem, where the trigeminal motor nucleus is situated on either side. The chewing muscles are activated by the trigeminal nerve's motor pathway from this nucleus. The hypoglossal motor nucleus in the brainstem provides the tongue with dynamics while chewing by activating the cortex-nuclear connection. By modifying the tension of the cavity walls, afferent and efferent facial nerve pathways work together to accommodate the bolus and control the pressure of the oral cavity. This process is particularly reliant on the orbicularis of the lips and buccinators. In the absence of a cortical relationship, the mesencephalic nucleus, which links the sensory pathway and the motor root, is also reached by the afferent trigeminal fibers [18]. This direct sensory-motor relationship enables the voluntary chewing action to have a reflex component, which modifies the variation of the chewing intensity caused by the ongoing modification of the resistance of the bolus under preparation through proprioceptive perception during the bolus preparation process.

2.2.2 Oral Qualification

The inner bolus can be recognized by the oral cavity in a number of ways. It displays at least four different kinds of perception: chemical, mechanical, unpleasant, and thermal. Different amounts of heat or cold can be perceived by the thermal receptor [19]. They can be added to the enjoyment of the diet when they are appropriate and palatable for the type of meal. They result in rejection when they are severe and harmful. Usually, mechanical, thermal, or chemical hyper-stimuli generated on sensitive afferent pathways cause pain perception, alerting and averting harm. Nonetheless, capsaicin, which is found in many peppers, produces a painful submodality that is frequently interpreted as culinary pleasure. It most likely uses the same pain mechanism. It is possible to observe the bolus's contact with the intraoral structures thanks to mechanical reception. The tongue gathers tactile information by pressing the bolus. This information makes it possible to perceive the bolus's physical properties and determine whether its contents are improper. In order to determine how many motor units must be depolarized in order to generate the appropriate oral pressure to move the contents from the oral cavity to the pharynx, mechanical reception is also in charge of characterizing the volume and viscosity of the oral bolus. Different methods are used by the chemical receptor to identify flavors. The pairing of a primary messenger (taste protein) with a secondary messenger (cyclic adenosine monophosphate, or cAMP), whose concentration rises and causes membrane depolarization, seems to be how sweetness is detected. It is thought that the intracellular metabolic pathways that produce natural sweeteners are different from those that are triggered by artificial sweeteners. The latter would use inositol triphosphate (IP3) as a secondary messenger to act on the calcium channels and cause depolarization and calcium input into the cells. By linking the same primary messenger (taste protein), the IP3 secondary messenger causes an increase in calcium and releases a neurotransmitter without depolarizing the membrane, identifying the bitter taste. The direct transport of sodium through the depolarizing membrane channels creates the salty sensation. By obstructing the potassium channels, the hydrogen from sour or acid tastes enters the cell and promotes membrane depolarization. Other tastes, such as metallic, astringent, and more recently, umami (monosodium glutamate), have been proposed as main, even if sweet, salty, sour, and bitter are thought to be basic. The first four, however, were the ones that eventually resisted as basic. It's unclear if and how the basic tastes—sweet, salty, sour, and bitter—can be combined to create the palate, or the entire gustatory sense. Each of us has a unique palate, which is a combination of our social and educational backgrounds, basic tastes, tactile and temperature sensations, and undoubtedly the impressions made possible by our senses of sight and smell. Priority has been given to the tongue's ability to perceive tastes in the oral cavity. According to the classic description, the front tip of the tongue has the ability to select for sweet flavors, the sides sequentially taste salty and sour, and the posterior central portion tastes bitter. These sequential zones are located on either side of the anterior two-thirds of the tongue. This idea, which is already up for debate, demonstrates that the tongue can detect all of the fundamental flavors in every part of the body, with the bitter flavor being the most expressive. The physical components of the tongue that are involved in the chemical senses (taste) are the filiform, fungiform, foliate, and circumvallate papillae. The gustatory buttons on these papillae are incrusted. Gustatory buttons are either nonexistent or very uncommon in filiform papillae. There aren't many in fungiform ones, but there are a lot in foliate papillae and particularly in circumvallate ones. Along with the tongue papillae, the palate and vallecula also include buttons that are regarded as gustatory. On the pharyngeal areas, where taste is initially not sensed, buttons that resemble those classified as gustatory in morphology have been discovered. Even when the mouth cavity is anesthetized, vagus nerve conduction can detect the bitter taste that has been transmitted to the throat in the vallecula. To the best of our knowledge, only the morphological kind of receptors recognized as gustatory have been characterized or observed in the oral cavity. The mouth cavity, however, contains a number of additional sensations. It is said that certain receptors must be triggered. However, there is no proof that a particular receptor is just in charge of identifying one kind of input. Other oral cues may also be able to reach receptors that are considered gustative. The presence of receptors in the pharynx (apart from the vallecula) and larynx that resemble the gustatory receptor in morphology, where tastes are not felt as palate, supports this theory. Additionally, there are accounts of gustatory perceptions that involve thermal stimulation of the tongue, such as the evocation of acidic or salty perceptions with intensification of chilling and sweet perceptions by heating the front edge of the tongue from a cool condition.

2.2.3 Cranial Nerves

Trigeminal (V), facial (VII), glossopharyngeal (IX), vagus (X), accessory (XI), which is typically over-looked, and hypoglossal (XII) are the cranial nerves linked to the swallowing process [20]. It should be noted that because of the dual-side innervation, the swallowing process involves pairs of struc-tures, both physically and/or functionally. The tongue, palate, pharynx, and larynx are anatomi-cally distinct functional pairs with autonomous innervation on each side. The trigeminal (V), facial (VII), and glossopharyngeal (IX) nerves send information to the brainstem from receptors on either side of the oral cavity. These mixed neurons control both motor command (efferent pathway) and sensibility (afferent pathway). The lingual nerve connects the trigeminal (general sensitivity) and facial (taste) nerves, supplying the afferent pathways of the anterior two-thirds of the tongue. The glossopharyngeal nerve conducts both taste and general sensibility at the back portion of the tongue. The trigeminal, facial, and glossopharyngeal nerves on both sides will form ganglionar synapses that resemble the posterior roots of the spinal cord in their afferent paths toward the brainstem. The trigeminal ganglion (Gasser), the geniculate ganglion, the glossopharyngeal gan-glion, and the rostral ganglion (upper one) are all synapses of the trigeminal nerve's afferent route. Three branches make up the trigeminal nerve (V): the lower (mandibular), middle (maxillary), and upper (ophthalmic). The inferior is mixed, whereas the upper and middle are only sensitive. The face is innervated in transverse bands of representation by the sensitive fibers of the three branches. The top lip, cheeks, hard palate (mouth mucosa), upper arcade teeth, and rhinopharyngeal mucosa are all sensitively under the middle branch (maxillary) of the oral cavity. The sensitivity of the lower arcade teeth and lower mucosa of the mouth, as well as the overall sensitivity of the anterior two-thirds of the tongue, are caused by the sensitive part of the lower branch (mandibular). The posterior part of the brainstem, which includes the medulla oblongata (spinal tract nucleus of the cranial nerve V), the pons (main sensory nucleus of the cranial nerve V), and the midbrain (midbrain nucleus of the cranial nerve V), is where all sensory pathways from the trigeminal ganglion to the brainstem terminate. The sensitive fibers split centrally into long, descending branches that help to sense pain, temperature, and tact as well as providing collateral paths to the spinal nucleus of the cranial nerve V. The short, ascending branches terminate in the main sensorial nucleus, which attends to tactile sensibility. Proprioceptive fibers from the trigeminal nerve's midbrain nucleus are thought to be able to integrate crucial chewing reflex arcs when they form a synaptic connection with its motor nucleus in the upper part of the pons. Even during the purposeful bolus chewing preparation, these arcs permit reflex regulation of chewing strength depending on differences in bolus consistency, unless specifically required. The trigeminal nerve's motor root leaves the ventral part of the pons and passes through the mandibular root to innervate the mylohyoid, anterior digas-tric belly, tensor muscle of the palate, and chewing muscles. Taking into account both its motor root and the sensitive root provided by the intermediate (Wrisberg) nerve, the facial nerve (VII) is a mixed nerve. It is in charge of the taste of the front two-thirds of the tongue on each side. In order to form synapses on the geniculate ganglion, this afferent, preganglionic pathway leaves the tongue and travels via the lingual nerve (association of nerves V and VII) and then the tympanic cord nerve (facial branch). The mucosa of the nasal cavities and soft palate receives sensitive innervation from the postganglionic fibers (afferent visceral special-gustative route) that synapse in the medulla oblongata's solitary tract nucleus through the intermediate nerve. These fibers are linked to the general afferent visceral fibers. Starting from the upper salivary nucleus on either side of the top part of the medulla oblongata, the parasympathetic efferent fibers of the facial nerve go through the intermediate nerve and then the tympanic cord nerve to form synapses in the submandibular gan-glion. They then encourage the submandibular and sublingual glands to secrete saliva through postganglionic fibers. The nucleus of the facial nerve's motor portion is located on the ventral part of the pons. Along with the vagus (X) and accessory (XI) nerves, the glossopharyngeal (IX) nerve emerges from the skull. The glossopharyngeal nerve's visceral general afferent and visceral special afferent fibers are connected. The posterior third of the tongue and the oropharynx mucosa's gen-eral sensitivity are caused by the visceral general afferent fibers, whereas the posterior third of the tongue's taste is caused by the unique visceral afferent fibers. The higher ganglion forms connec-tions with these preganglionic fibers. The solitary tract nucleus is where the postganglionic fibers will terminate. The medulla oblongata contains two separate nuclei that supply the glossopharyngeal nerve's efferent pathways: the ambiguous motor (special visceral efferent) nucleus and the salivary inferior (parasympathetic) nucleus. Following synapses with the optic ganglion, from which postganglionic fibers arise to innervate the parotid gland, the parasympathetic fibers stimulate salivary secretion. The stylopharyngeus muscle is the sole motor function of the glossopharyngeal nerve. Yet, it has already been identified as the motor for the superior pharyngeal constrictor muscle, whose function was formerly ascribed to the vagus nerve, which supplies all pharyngeal constriction muscles with motor innervation. From the cervical region to the abdomen (transverse colon), the vagus (X) nerve has connections. The medulla oblongata's solitary tract nucleus is connected to its sensory afference, or sensory route. The parasympathetic fibers (visceral general efference) originate from the dorsal motor nucleus of the vagus nerve, whereas the ambiguous nucleus in the ventral part of the medulla oblongata provides the visceral special efference (motor route). Similar to the intermediate part of the facial nerve and the glossopharyngeal one, the postganglionic fibers of the vagus nerve's visceral special afferent (taste) and visceral general afferent (sensibility) pathways terminate at the solitary tract nucleus following synapses in a peripheral ganglion (lower or caudal). The visceral special afferent pathway leads taste inputs from receptors on the vallecula and from a tiny posterior portion of the tongue adjacent to the vallecula, whereas the visceral general afferent fibers conduct impulses associated with the sensitivity of the pharynx, larynx, trachea, and esophagus. From the vagus dorsal motor nucleus, the visceral general efferent (parasympathetic) fibers of the vagus nerve emerge in a single-trunk, descending tract that emits branches in the cervical, thoracic, and abdominal regions before terminating. These preganglionic fibers will form synapses near or even inside the visceral walls in the peripheral ganglia of the parasympathetic vegetative or autonomous nervous system. The striated muscles of the pharynx, larynx, and esophagus are innervated by the visceral special efferent (motor) fibers of the vagus, which have their origin in the ambiguous nucleus. Special visceral efferent fibers from the ambiguous nucleus (motor to striated muscles of branchial origin) are presented by the accessory (XI) nerve, which is not always thought of as one of the nerves involved in swallowing control. These fibers would join the vagus nerve's unique visceral efferent fibers. The striated parts of the throat, larynx, and esophagus would therefore be innervated by the accessory (XI) nerve in addition to the vagus (X) nerve. The presence of parasympathetic fibers (general visceral efferent) in the accessory nerve, which originate in the dorsal nucleus of the vagus and accompany the vagus nerve fibers, would indicate a potential second relationship between the vagus and auxiliary nerves. Each side of the medulla oblongata contains a unique nucleus on the ventral-medial section of the motor hypoglossal (XII) nerve. It is in charge of the intrinsic and extrinsic muscles of the tongue. Furthermore, the geniohyoid muscle, which is one of the muscles that causes the hyoid-laryngeal displacement, is innervated by a branch of the cervical plexus, often C1, which is formed by fibers from the cervical plexus in conjunction with the hypoglossal nerve. The pharyngeal reflex phase, in which afferent information from the pharynx reaches the brainstem and generates efferent stimuli to the pharyngeal structures involved in this phase of the swallowing process, is thought to be caused by the pharyngeal plexus (glossopharyngeal, vagus, and accessory through vagus). The brainstem, particularly the sensitive (solitary tract) nucleus, would receive afferent impulses from the pressure transfer from the oral cavity to the pharynx through distention. The ventral motor (ambiguous) nucleus of the brainstem produces efferent motor stimuli to the pharyngeal structures from the sensitive nucleus via interneurons of the reticular formation. Without taking into account the palate tension caused by the trigeminal nerve, a number of structural movements that begin during the voluntary oral phase continue until the end of the pharyngeal phase. These movements include hyoid-laryngeal elevation, swallowing apnea, and tongue posterior projection to the pharynx. Thus, we can consider the pharyngeal phase to be dependent on the cranial nerves V, VII, IX, X, XI, and XII of both sides because the pharyngeal reflex phase incorporates a number of oral phase features.

2.2.4 Base Nuclei, Cortex, Cerebellum, and Brain

The medulla oblongata, pons, and midbrain combine to form the brainstem. It includes the swallowing-related nuclei of the cranial nerves [21]. The motor and sensory nuclei are situated anteriorly and posteriorly, respectively, on both sides. The brainstem's sensory and motor nuclei are connected via neurons and reticular formation pathways. Through base nuclei, these are also linked to peripheral effectors such as muscles and salivary glands, as well as to peripheral receptors, the cerebellum, and the sensory and motor regions of the cerebral cortex. Information about stimuli is received by the brainstem, which then sends out routes for distribution and integration. The brainstem's sensitive nuclei will obtain information about peripheral sensitivity from peripheral receptors through general afferent pathways (V, VII, IX) and taste through special afferent pathways (VII, IX, X). The cortex identifies and evaluates every bolus characteristic during the oral phase, informing the brainstem of the pattern that the oral effectors should use. Both intrinsic and extrinsic tongue muscles will be stimulated by the brainstem via the motor hypoglossal (XII) nerve. Motor fibers of visceral special efferent nerves (V, VII, IX, X, and XI) will stimulate the other swallowing muscles as well as those involved in the pharyngeal phase. Additionally, visceral general efferent parasympathetic routes to the salivary glands (nerves VII and IX) are depolarized by the brainstem. Through fibers from the vagus dorsal nucleus, the vagus (X) and maybe the accessory (XI) transmit preganglionic parasympathetic fibers to the autonomic digestive system. The routes of swallowing cranial nerves connect to the cerebellum in the brainstem. Through the inferior, middle, and superior cerebellar peduncles, the swallowing cranial nerves enter and exit the cerebellum. Only afferent impulses are received by the medium, primarily efferent signals by the superior, and primarily afferent signals by the inferior. Base nuclei and the cerebral cortex are connected to brainstem and cerebellar nuclei via particular longitudinal routes. The cranial nerves' routes during the swallowing process can be affected in this way by interference from the cerebellum and cerebral cortex. Apart from regulating muscle tone and balance, the cerebellum also controls the temporal order of the synergistic contraction of the many skeletal striated muscles, which can cause a fraction of a second delay in motor impulses. Additionally, it can regulate the relationship between agonist and antagonist muscles and works by coordinating the motor activity from one movement to the next. The cerebellum can also modify the motor actions generated by other brain regions as needed. The cerebellum and cortex are connected by descending and ascending cerebellar circuits. The so-called cortex-pons-cerebellar pathway begins in the premotor and motor cortex and extends to the pons's nuclei before reaching the cerebellum's contralateral hemisphere. In order to transmit messages to other areas of the brain, the indications that enter the cerebellum attach to its nuclei. The cerebellar pathway begins in the cerebellar cortex, connects with the dentate, one of its primary nuclei, travels to the thalamus, and then returns to the cerebral cortex to help coordinate the motor activity patterns that the cerebral cortex has initiated. The cerebral cortex has bilateral representations for the motor control of swallowing. Due to its bidirectional representation, peripheral stimuli are received by both brain hemispheres, yet one is acknowledged to be more dominant. This dominance presupposes that the dominant hemisphere suppresses the contralateral hemisphere's function under physiological circumstances. It has been noted that the contralateral hemisphere can improve its representation in cases of dysphagia caused by involvement of the dominant hemisphere, with apparent functional recovery. We can choose whether or not to ingest the oral content because the oral phase is voluntary. The lower part of the precentral gyrus (frontal cortex) and postcentral gyrus (parietal cortex), where the central sulcus divides sensitivity (somatosensory cortex) from motor control (somatomotor cortex), is the cortical region with the oral control capacity. The intraoral qualification will have visceral afferent general and particular impulses conducted through base nuclei up to the cerebral cortex. It is connected to sensory pathways of the cranial pairings V, VII, and IX, with nuclei in the brainstem. Under cerebellar mediation, efferent direct or indirect orders (using the base nuclei) travel from the cortex to the brainstem's motor nuclei, where the motor pathways of these nerve pairs regulate the peripheral effectors' dynamics. The cerebral cortex receives afferent routes from nerves V, VII, and IX. Secondary dorsal tracts provide tactile sensitivity channels from the trigeminal (V) sensory nucleus to the thalamus and cortex. The secondary ventral tract carries touch, pain, and temperature channels from the spinal nucleus of cranial pair V to the thalamus and cortex. Sensitive fibers from the solitary tract nucleus travel through the medial lemniscus and thalamus to connect the facial (VII) and glossopharyngeal (IX) nerves to the cerebral cortex. With bilateral (mostly cross) connections of the cortex-nuclear tract (voluntary), the cerebellum regulates the efferent routes from the cortex to the brainstem motor nuclei of these three pairs of cranial nerves. Both the motor neurones of pair IX in the ambiguous nucleus and the motor nucleus of nerves V and VII will be connected to the brainstem by these voluntary routes.

2.2.5 Voluntary Oral Phase

Once the bolus has been prepared and qualified, it will often be placed on the tongue (organized) and transferred (ejected) to the pharynx during the nutritive swallowing that occurs after chewing [22]. The afferent pathways of nerves V, VII, and IX (mixed pairs) carry information to the cortex during the voluntary oral phase of swallowing. This information enables the cortex to activate the motor sections of these mixed nerves in conjunction with the hypoglossal (XII–motor pair). Afferent routes lead from peripheral receptors to the brainstem. The thalamus and cortex receive touch (as well as volume and viscosity), temperature, and potentially nociceptive sensations from the sensory nuclei of the cranial pair V via the secondary ventral and dorsal routes. The solitary tract nucleus in the dorsal part of the medulla oblongata is reached by afferent general (sensitivity) and special (taste) routes that are guided by the cranial nerves VII and IX. This is followed by afferent pathways connecting to the base nuclei, such as the thalamus, and then to the cerebral cortex on the postcentral gyrus of both hemispheres. From there, efferent pathways lead to the brainstem motor nuclei (V, VII, IX, XII). Both afferent general (sensitive) and special (taste) and efferent special (motor) and general (parasympathetic) routes connecting both sides of the cortex and brainstem come and depart as direct and cross paths, according to the hemisphere dominance. By combining the cranial nerves that function in the oral phase, this arrangement provides each cerebral hemisphere with access to the entirety of the information gathered in the oral cavity. This allows effective directives from each hemisphere to reach both sides of the brainstem. The peripheral information travels to the motor cortex, where it is regulated and retransmitted to the base nuclei and brainstem after the base nuclei have activated the sensory cortex on both sides. The latter would result in an oral dynamic that would expel its contents into the pharynx through the efferent pathways of the trigeminal, facial, and hypoglossal nerves. Despite the dominance of one hemisphere, both are fully aware and capable of performing their entire range of duties. There is proof that the non-dominant (non-damaged) hemisphere can be more represented when the dominant hemisphere is wounded, which is linked to apparent function recovery. The corpus callosum has channels that connect the hemispheres by going from side to side. Therefore, in healthy people, a connection that travels through the corpus callosum allows the dominant cortex to inhibit the contralateral one. Excitatory routes from the dominant motor cortex to the base nuclei of the contralateral hemisphere can also be taken into account. Despite the inhibition of the non-dominant hemisphere's motor and sensory cortex, this architecture would account for both the integrated bilateral stimulus that is observed and the function recovery that has already been demonstrated in cases of dominant hemisphere lesions. The existence of these excitatory routes in both directions might also be assumed. There are also connecting channels that lead to and depart from the cerebellum between the brainstem and the cortex. These pathways are thought to be able to control the sequencing and intensity of muscle contractions. In this manner, the motor nuclei of the cranial nerves V, VII, IX, and XII will form synapses with the cerebellar pathways that link to efferent voluntary (cortex-nuclear) routes. The oral effectors receive efferent impulses from these nuclei, which provide them with signaling of appropriate contraction intensity and sequence. The cerebellum and brain coordinate these signals. In order to produce the required oral ejection, the bolus volume and viscosity will interfere with the muscle contraction intensity, which is determined by the cortex based on the oral qualification. However, all sequences involving the oral phase will share the effectors' contraction activation sequence, indicating that the neural organization has a preset sequence. Temperature and taste had no effect on the cortical definition of the intensity of mouth muscle activity. This finding indicates that, within acceptable bounds, chemical, thermal, and most definitely pain perception do not impede oral activity, which is controlled by mechanical reception, specifically volume, and viscosity, which will influence the number of motor units that must be depolarized for an efficient oral phase. Information transmission and maintenance during the reflex phase of swallowing will depend on the production of the required and sufficient muscle contraction intensity. The brain regulation of the reflex pharyngeal phase will respond to the stimulus of the pressure intensity transmitted by the oral phase. The oral phase should have some influence on the esophageal phase, which is also reflex. The following is a description of the fundamental mechanics of the oral phase of swallowing: by contracting their chewing muscles, the dental arcades make contact with one another (pair V). In order to stop pressure from escaping from the oral cavity during the bolus transference to the pharynx, the arrangement of the dental arcades enables skin-inserted muscles in the orbicularis oris (pair VII) and specific buccinators to create intraoral pressure resistance. The tongue (pair XII) will be able to evacuate the bolus due to the pressured and resistive oral cavity, which will then convey the bolus and pressure to the throat. At the start of the pharyngeal phase, the levator veli palatini muscle will project the soft palate superiorly and posteriorly against the pterygo-pharyngeus fascicle, the first fascicle of the pharynx superior constrictor muscle, while the tensor veli palatini muscle (pair V) will provide resistance to the soft palate as part of the oral phase actions. Because the suprahyoid muscles reverse the tweezers action between the larynx and vertebral body, they raise the hyoid and larynx, opening the pharyngoesophageal transition. The cranial nerves V and VII, as well as C1 through the ansa cervicalis, are primarily responsible for the elevation of the hyoid and larynx, which serves to reverse the tweezers action caused by the larynx's apposition against the spine. Beginning at the end of the oral phase, the hyoid elevation continues to be active until the end of the pharyngeal phase. The pharyngeal distal resistance will decrease when the longitudinal stylopharyngeus muscle (IX) contracts. Swallowing apnea, also known as preventative apnea, occurs near the end of the oral phase and may be caused by the respiratory center located on the floor of the fourth ventricle in the brainstem. At the start of the pharyngeal phase, vocal fold adduction will take place sequentially, but with an independent mechanism of apnea. By assimilating the reflex pharyngeal phase coordination, all oral events continue to occur throughout the pharyngeal phase.

2.2.6 Primary Voluntary Oral Cortical Phase

Without any qualifying intraoral substance, this kind of oral phase replicates all dynamic events seen in the nutritive oral phase of swallowing [23]. The efferent cortical motor area mimics an oral ejection with the same properties and via the same efferent pathways as if the imagined bolus could be exposed to oral receptors. This occurs as if the cerebral cortex imagined a bolus with such well-known traits. Therefore, the afferent communication from the oral receptors to the sensitive cortex is not an essential component of this sort of neural regulation. The order from the motor brain to the mouth effectors will be precisely the same in this manner.

2.2.7 Semiautomatic Oral Phase

The brain control that takes place during the act of swallowing nutrients is momentarily replaced by this kind [24]. When the nutritional oral phase's characteristics are repeatedly certified and accepted as normal and within reasonable bounds, it takes the place of the voluntary control of that phase. In these situations, a semiautomatic control that is processed at the subcortical level (base nuclei) may take the place of swallowing control if attention has been diverted to another topic that requires cortical action. Given the suggested structure for the integration of base nuclei and cortex, we can conclude that the base nuclei dominate the oral phase, retaining their integrative function while suppressing input from the periphery at the level of the base nuclei. However, the base nuclei are still capable of reactivating cortical control at any moment, especially if alterations are noticed. Similar to inhibitory control, the dominant hemisphere regulates this semiautomatic process from its base nuclei via the corpus callosum.

2.2.8 Later Oral Gulps Phase

Oral phase swallowing in consecutive gulps indicates the intake of liquids, which in healthy people requires the depolarization of fewer motor units because the required ejection force doesn't require much work [25]. This oral phase swallowing type is controlled similarly to nutritional swallowing, at least for the initial gulp. Even though the substance to be consumed is liquid, it must be properly qualified because it may have unexpected or different properties from its appearance. During the initial swallow, taste, warmth, and viscosity are evaluated. If approved, they quickly go on to semiautomatic coordination, which is comparable to what occurs in a nutritious diet. Without requiring any additional cerebral attention, the semiautomatic dynamics can begin here, and the fundamental perception of the gulps' properties is retained. Similar to nutritional swallowing, voluntary cortical control can be immediately restored if desired or if an irregularity is noticed.

2.2.9 Oral Spontaneous Phase

The swallowing that takes place to clear the oral cavity of the saliva produced and released in distinct yet constant amounts is known as the spontaneous oral phase [26]. Without conscious control, this kind of oral phase recurs continuously throughout the 24-hour day, whether the person is awake or asleep. These swallowing attempts provide a mechanical sequence that is comparable to other oral cavity-originating swallowing types. Its trigger mechanisms are different in a few ways, though. It is reasonable to suppose that this kind of swallowing results from the airways' defense mechanism against aspirations and respiratory system compromise. Saliva adsorbed to the mucous membrane has been shown to be able to lubricate the vocal folds and laryngeal vestibule without causing discomfort. Additionally, upon swallowing with the adducted vocal folds, the volume of stored saliva would be crushed between the vestibular folds and the epiglottic tubercle, returning any remaining saliva to the pharynx. One could assume that this physiological permeation of the airways is what causes spontaneous swallowing. Although it has a different trigger mechanism, most likely related to airway protection, the semiautomatic swallowing seen in the nutritious swallowing sequence appears to be the same as the repeated spontaneous swallowing that takes place while the person is awake or asleep and without conscious control. Saliva serves a variety of purposes, including lubricating mucosal membranes for appropriate transport and preparing chewing boluses. The salivary glands continuously create saliva in terms of volume and physical-chemical properties, and the cranial nerves VII (facial) and IX (glossopharyngeal) mediate this process through parasympathetic fibers. Saliva is distributed over the oral, pharyngeal, and even vestibular mucosa during spontaneous swallowing, which humidifies these membranes and most likely aids in keeping the mucus fluid over the laryngeal ventricles. Continuous airflow from inhalation and expiration dries the mucosa, but spontaneous swallowing maintains the mucous membranes' moisture content. Controlling the small volume of liquids adsorbed to the laryngeal vestibule walls and eliminating any overflow over this mucosa are two other benefits of spontaneous swallowing. The epiglottic tubercle presses on the adducted vestibule folds during swallowing, creating a virtual vestibule lumen and expelling any surplus to the pharynx.

2.2.10 Pharyngeal Phase and Neural Control

There is no direct cerebral command or voluntary control during the reflex pharyngeal phase [27]. The oral phase transfers the pharyngeal pressure stimulation, which initiates this phase. Following bolus qualifying in nutritional swallowing, the oral ejection will convey the qualified information (bolus and pressure) to the pharynx, particularly with regard to volume and viscosity (mechanoreceptors). From there, the brainstem (solitary tract nucleus) receives the perceived input. Based on the values certified and conveyed by the oral phase, a motor reflex reaction in the brainstem, particularly in the ambiguous nucleus, would produce consecutive muscle contractions in the delay line. The sequential dynamics of the pharynx contractile activity are produced by the delay line, which is the contractile sequential muscular response of the pharyngeal muscles to a single pressure stimulus. The delay line leaves the pharynx and travels to the posterior sensory portion of the brainstem before returning to it via a ventral motor pathway. The pharyngeal phase is not directly influenced by the motor cortex, although it is possible to sense the transmitted material, such as its temperature. This type of perception indicates afferent sensitivity, which may be used to give tolerance limits for oral transmission. The pressure that distends the pharynx, with or without contents, is the stimulus that initiates the pharyngeal phase, not the contact created by food passing through it. Food and pressure are transferred during nutritional swallowing, but pressure is only during cortical swallowing. The pharyngeal response is comparable to that of nutritional swallowing, suggesting that the pressure exerted on the pharyngeal walls is what triggers the pharyngeal motor activity. Sensitive afferent fibers of the pharyngeal plexus (cranial nerves IX, X, XI) detect and transmit the pharyngeal distention pressure to the brainstem. Based on the pressure value conveyed from the oral cavity to the pharynx, the glossopharyngeal (IX) and vagus and auxiliary (X and XI) nerves in the oropharynx and the laryngopharynx, respectively, carry the stimulus to the brainstem dorsal area (solitary tract nucleus-sensitive). The reticular system of the brainstem contains interneurons that integrate the dorsal (sensitive) and ventral (motor) regions. A single tract nucleus receives a distinct stimulus, and the motor reflex response is made up of multiple muscles acting sequentially at various periods, resulting in a delay line of sequential contraction. The successive contraction of muscles in the pharyngeal phase (delay line) can be explained by a control of the cerebellum over the brainstem-determined pharyngeal reflex responses. One of the cerebellum's primary roles is to coordinate the temporal sequence of the synergic contraction of the various skeletal striated muscles. It can also produce a delay in the muscle contraction sequence by causing motor impulses to be delayed by fractions of a second. We assume that the sensory-motor connection in the brainstem would be carried out by different amounts of synapses between interneurons connecting sensitive and motor nuclei, generating different transfer times between the solitary tract nucleus to the ambiguous one. The delay line seen in the swallowing pharyngeal phase would be configured as a result of a signal that was interpreted by the pharyngeal receptors and sent to the solitary tract nucleus as unique. This stimulus would then be retransmitted to the ambiguous nucleus, passing by an increasing number of distinct interneurons. The pharyngeal phase integrates or assimilates the oral phase developments already underway as its functional component, in addition to the order and force of muscle contraction dictated by the brainstem from pressure reception. Both the pharyngeal phase and the oral phase will conclude together. Thus, during the pharyngeal phase, the brainstem combines the oral and pharyngeal phase sequences. The pharyngeal plexus, which is made up of the glossopharyngeal (IX), vagus (X), and accessory (XI) nerves, initiates the pharyngeal phase. The trigeminal (V), facial (VII), glossopharyngeal (IX), and hypoglossal (XII) nerves, as well as certain cervical plexus components (C1, C2), are secondary to this. The geniohyoid muscle, one of the muscles involved in the elevation of the hyoid-laryngeal complex, is accessed via the ansa cervicalis, which is formed by the cervical plexus and the hypoglossal nerve on either side. Not typically included in the list of nerves related to swallowing, the accessory (XI) nerve is acknowledged to have unique visceral efferent (motor) fibers that originate from the ambiguous nucleus that would subsequently be connected to the vagus nerve, which would also exhibit this type of fiber. Therefore, in conjunction with the vagus nerve, the accessory (XI) nerve is also in charge of motor innervation of the musculature of the palate, pharynx, larynx, and esophagus. The palatoglossal muscle, innervated by the motor component of the pharyngeal plexus (X, XI), adjusts over the tongue on both sides during the pharyngeal phase to stop pressure from returning to the oral cavity. The potential pressure escape from the oropharynx to the rhinopharynx is prevented by the tension (V) and elevation of the palate (X, XI) against the first fascicle (pterygopharyngeal) of the upper constrictor muscle of the pharynx, which is innervated by the cranial nerves X and XI. Each of the pharynx's superior, middle, and inferior constrictor muscles is made up of separate components with unique insertions. Each of these components is placed in the posterior median line of the pharynx (pharyngeal raphé) on one side and in anterolateral fixed places on the other. They are able to contract in sequential mode as a result of their motor units being individually tailored. There are two portions (chondropharyngeal and ceratopharyngeal) in the middle, two parts (thyreopharyngeal and cricopharyngeal) in the inferior, and four parts (pterygopharyngeal, buccopharyngeal, mylopharyngeal, and glossopharyngeal) in the superior. Two fascicles, the upper oblique and the lower transverse, are present in the cricopharyngeal, and their fibers appear to cross in the midline. Muscular absence results in an architecturally less-resistant region between the two cricopharyngeal muscle fascicles. The entire oropharyngeal extension is occupied by the superior constrictor's four components. In order to isolate and stop pressure escapes from the oropharynx to the rhinopharynx, just the first segment of its upper (pterygopharyngeal) section must perform apposition against the palate. The pharynx can simultaneously receive oral pressure without encountering any resistance. Since the pharynx wall lacks a circular muscle, pharyngeal peristalsis is not produced by the successive contraction of the superior, middle, and inferior constrictors. A constrictor muscle contraction causes a pressure sequence to be generated in the cranial-caudal direction when the pharyngeal contiguous cavities close, with the exception of the pharyngoesophageal transition, which opens due to the elevation of the hyoid and larynx. By opening the pharyngoesophageal transition, this pressure series moves the temporary bolus from the pharynx to the permissive, less resistive esophagus. Peristalsis is by definition a sequential expression generated by the circular layer of muscles. Thus, it is not appropriate to classify this cranial-caudal pressure sequence with distal reduced resistance and no muscle circular layer as peristalsis or peristalsis-like, as is commonly defined. The cranial nerves V and VII as well as the (C1) cervical plexus, which is related to the hypoglossal nerve via the ansa cervicalis, innervate the suprahyoid muscles. The mylohyoid and anterior belly of the digastric muscles are innervated by the mylohyoid branch of the mandibular nerve (mixed root of trigeminal–V); the facial nerve (VII) innervates the posterior belly of the digastric and the stylohyoid muscles. Through the hypoglossal (XII) nerve, the ansa cervicalis (typically C1) innervates the geniohyoid and thyrohyoid muscles. The additional infrahyoid muscles are innervated by the cervical plexus (often C2) via the ansa cervicalis. The infrahyoid group modulates the suprahyoid muscle group, which is in charge of the hyoid and larynx's upward and forward motion. By doing this, the pharyngoesophageal transition is opened and the larynx is moved away from the vertebral body. Furthermore, depending on the bolus volume and viscosity, the suprahyoid group can maintain this open position while moving the larynx away. The contraction of the longitudinal pharyngeal muscles, the palatopharyngeal muscle, innervated by motor fibers from cranial nerves X and XI, and the stylopharyngeal muscles, innervated by the glossopharyngeal (IX) nerve, also aids in the opening of the pharyngoesophageal transition. A preventative apnea, also known as swallowing apnea, develops as a final act while still in the oral phase. It is absorbed by the pharyngeal phase and lasts until its conclusion. Independent vocal fold adduction (X, XI) and vestibular fold closure with the bolus passage through the already open pharyngoesophageal transition are linked to the airways resistance caused by apnea. By elevating the hyoid and larynx, the pre-epiglottic fatty cushion is compressed, causing the vestibular folds to adduct. This compression occurs within the pre-epiglottic fibrous area. The lateral portions of the tapering end of the epiglottis, which correspond to the protrusion of the vestibular folds on both sides, are the space's point of least resistance. As a result, the vestibular folds medially move and end up in apposition against the epiglottis tubercle due to the compression created by this fatty cushion on the epiglottis's sides. When it is its turn, the tongue-everted epiglottis travels posteriorly, adjusting its tubercle against the vestibular folds that have now been adduced. The bolus is forced from the pharynx into the esophagus at the same time by the sequential, cranio-caudal contraction of the constrictor muscles, including the cricopharingeal one (nerves X and XI). Both the reflex pharyngeal and esophageal phases exhibit anatomical and functional relationships. Skeletal striated muscles, such as those of the mouth and throat, form the first 10 cm of the esophagus. In fresh anatomical specimens, a muscular distinction is visible macroscopically in the distal extremity of this striated segment by 2 or 3 cm. This muscular distinction is defined microscopically as a mixture of skeletal striated muscle (long and multinucleated fibers) and short and mononucleated smooth muscle fibers, where the first ganglion of the myenteric plexus appears. The distal pharynx, where a tweezer action seals the pharynx between the larynx (cricoid cartilage) and the cervical lordosis at the level of the fifth to sixth cervical vertebrae, is the high-pressure zone known as the upper esophageal sphincter. The cricopharyngeal muscle, which is a component of the inferior pharyngeal constrictor, is typically thought to be the cause of this elevated pressure. This idea is a serious misinterpretation of the region's anatomical and functional features. The thyropharyngeal and cricopharyngeal fascicles make up the skeletal striated muscle that serves as the inferior constrictor of the pharynx. The organization of the cricopharyngeal fascicle consists of two fiber parts: an upper, oblique and a lower, transverse. The top one attaches on the posterior pharyngeal raphé on both sides of the cricoid cartilage, where its fibers extend from the bottom upward and from lateral to medial. The lower or transverse portion intercrosses at the midline, where the raphé is invisible, and inserts on either side of the cricoid cartilage in a transverse manner. At the level of the transverse cricopharyngeal portion, the pharyngeal lumen is about 17 mm wide. This area lacks a muscular ring, which is more accurately described as a muscular half-curvature. An anatomically less-resistant point, known as the Killian zone, is created by the divergence of the oblique and transverse parts of the cricopharyngeal muscle. It is in this zone that the posterior pharyngeal diverticulum, also referred to as Zenker's diverticulum, can occur. Because of the tweezer action created by the vertebral body and the larynx, this anatomically less-resistant location also happens to be the point of higher pressure levels. The pharynx and esophagus are intercommunicated by the open pharyngeal-esophageal transition, which enables the flow of contrast material to fill both cavities nearly simultaneously during the videofluoroscopic examination. It is evident that during the pharyngeal phase, there is a relationship between the esophageal and pharyngeal cavities and the contrast medium. As a result, the esophageal and pharyngeal phases almost begin at the same time, indicating a definite functional link between them that is as consistent, if not more so, than that between the oral and pharyngeal phases. This fact indicates that the conduction of the contents transferred by the oral phase is the responsibility of the pharyngeal and esophageal phases.

2.2.11 Esophageal Phase and Neural Control

The bolus conveyed by pharyngeal pressure is the result of the successive contraction of the pharyngeal muscles [28]. The striated muscle of the upper part of the esophagus is also caused by the unique visceral efferent innervation carried out by the vagus nerve, which originates in the ambiguous nucleus. Primary peristalsis is the process by which the bolus is carried out into the esophagus by successive contractions in a distal direction. In contrast to striated muscle, this type of muscle can be stimulated by the mechanical relationship between the bolus and smooth muscle in the esophageal wall. The smooth muscle of the esophageal wall will depolarize syncytially, meaning that contraction is processed throughout the muscular layer's extension as the depolarization of the muscle cells is freely transferred from one to the other. The transfer of contents from the pharynx to the esophagus while in its striated segment can therefore be thought of as a hypothetical mechanism that is carried out similarly to that which occurs in the pharynx, via depolarization of motor units. However, the bolus can stimulate the myenteric plexus from this point on, causing syncytial contraction, once it crosses the striated/smooth transition. This syncytial depolarization can result in the longitudinal layer contracting, which lowers the esophageal resistance overall, increases its compliance, and leads to—or at least contributes to—the gastroesophageal transition opening that coincides with the start of primary peristalsis. Another possibility is that, in conjunction with primary peristalsis, the circular musculature depolarizes and contracts during the bolus passage through the striated/smooth transition. The bolus passes down the esophagus as a result of this contraction, which presses the esophageal lumen downward. The unique visceral efferent (motor) pathway of the vagus nerve innervates the striated muscles that create the pharynx and the first segment of the esophagus. The general visceral efferent (parasympathetic) pathway, which is preganglionic to the myenteric plexus, is also present in this cranial nerve. Another theory is that myenteric postganglionic stimulation, in conjunction with the general visceral efferent pathway (parasympathetic motor to smooth muscle) of the vagus nerve, along with the unique visceral efferent pathway (motor to striated muscle), achieves the motor coordination of the esophageal smooth muscles. The stomach is not always reached by the contents that are transmitted from the pharynx to the esophagus, especially those that contain solid particles. They can selectively activate the submucosal plexus, which then sends an activation instruction to the myenteric plexus, causing muscle contraction from the retention point on. Occasionally, they halt at the level of the smooth muscle of the esophagus. Secondary peristalsis is the term for this downward contractile wave that ultimately transports the remaining contents of the esophagus to the stomach. The general visceral efferent pathway (parasympathetic fibers) has been thought to originate in the posterior motor nucleus of the vagus as preganglionic fibers that will connect to the esophageal wall's intraparietal ganglia. From there, postganglionic fibers will connect to visceral effectors that release neurohormones that can affect the smooth portion of the esophagus's tonus and motility. The distal circular muscula-ture is thought to be involved in the resting tonic contraction of the esophageal distal extremity. In conjunction with intrinsic and extrinsic nerves, hormones would control this resting tonic contrac-tion, producing pressure readings of about 20 mmHg. According to this widely accepted theory, the gastroesophageal transition opens to the necessary muscle relaxation that would accompany primary peristalsis. This relaxation would be brought on by vagus fibers, which would prevent the circular musculature from contracting tonically. It may be mediated by vasoactive intestinal polypeptide (VIP) neurotransmitters and nitric oxide (NO). Despite popular belief, a muscular ring with the traditional features of smooth muscle sphincters has not been found in the distal part of the esophagus. Without muscle thickening, the gastroesophageal transition exhibits positive resting pressure, which disappears during the main peristaltic wave that transports the bolus to the stom-ach. This transition, known as the cardia, has been classified as a physiological sphincter because of the lack of understanding of the morphology that causes its high pressure. A total of around 27 potential pathways, either alone or in combination, have been proposed as a result of this circum-stance, including those affecting the regional muscle organization. The esophagus, as we already know, has two layers: an external layer that is longitudinal and an internal layer that is circular. When it contracts, the external layer lowers the esophageal tube's resistance, while the internal layer forces the bolus to contract sequentially. It is plausible that the arrangement of the esophageal muscle layers is such that the internal layer exhibits short-pitch spiral fibers and the external layer long-pitch spiral fibers. This morphology, which is linked to the idea of energy preservation, enables us to acknowledge that the external layer's contraction could extend the esophagus, lowering flow resistance and most likely opening the gastroesophageal transition as well. The meal would then be propelled downward by the internal layer's successive contractions. Therefore, there would be no energy expenditure during the resting esophagus stage. The myenteric plexus would be activated during the bolus's passage into the esophagus by the esophageal peristalsis, which would cause the gastroesophageal transition to open. The fact that the esophagus reacts differently to pure pressure distension than it does when the solid bolus is present supports this theory.

2.3 FLUOROSCOPIC EVALUATION OF NORMAL SWALLOWING FUNCTION
2.3.1 Oral Phase

During the bolus preparation, an oral liquid bolus is often placed on the dorsum of the tongue, with the tip of the tongue pushed against the back of the upper incisors on the upper gum ridge [29]. This first bolus placement results in the occurrence of the typical tipper-type swallow. The major-ity of the bolus is situated in the central groove of the tongue and in a concave area like a spoon in the middle of the tongue. The back section of the tongue raises up and presses against the soft palate, which in turn moves downward to prevent the food from leaving the mouth too soon and entering the throat too early. The closure of the posterior tongue against the soft palate serves as a glossopalatal sphincter. Some individuals display a dipper-type swallowing pattern where the food bolus is initially positioned below the front part of the tongue, namely within the front sub-lingual groove. With the bolus in this position, the tongue at the commencement of swallowing must descend beneath the bolus to scoop it to a supralingual position. With this movement, the tip of the tongue makes contact with the back part of the upper incisors, and the swallowing actions, characterized as dipper-type and tipper-type, continue in a similar fashion. The front two-thirds of the tongue rises as a rounded mass and establishes consecutive peristaltic contact with the hard palate, creating a V-shaped arrangement in the tail of the food bolus. The tongue moves backward in a piston-like manner to push the bolus into the oropharynx. Simultaneously, the base of the tongue descends and slides toward the front to widen the hypopharynx and provide a pathway via which the bolus can pass into the pharynx. At the same time, the roof of the mouth lifts upward to open the area of the glossopalatal sphincter, making it easier for fluid to pass between the mouth and throat. Simultaneously, the palate makes contact with the posterior pharyngeal wall in order to create a seal that separates the nasopharynx from the oropharynx, thus preventing the backflow of nasal contents. The sealing motion of the palate involves more than just a simple upward action resembling a swinging trap door. Instead, the lateral walls of the nasopharynx, which consist of the superior pharyngeal constrictors, also come together to create a strong circular seal. Aside from the elevation of the soft palate, many other processes take place to provide space for the ingested bolus to enter the oropharynx. In the sagittal plane, the pharynx expands as the posterior tongue, hyoid, and larynx travel upward and forward. Essentially, the bolus descends down the ramp, formed by the flattening and forward motion of the posterior tongue, and enters the chute. In addition, the contraction of the pharyngeal levators, such as the stylopharyngeus muscle, helps to widen the width of the pharynx.

2.3.2 Pharyngeal Swallowing Phase

Upon entering the oropharynx, the bolus is propelled through the oropharynx into the hypopharynx by the rapid backward movement of the posterior tongue resembling a piston. The posterior chamber accommodating the posterior lingual piston is created by the posterior pharyngeal wall, which becomes rigid due to the successive contraction of its three constrictors (superior, middle, and inferior) [30]. Therefore, the movement of the food bolus through the pharynx is a result of the posterior tongue pushing and the consecutive contraction of the pharyngeal constrictors in a downward direction. The bolus tail in the pharynx has a V-shaped pattern, much like it does in the oral cavity. Due to the faster movement of the bolus head compared to the bolus tail, the bolus stretches in the pharynx, exerting a force that aids in the opening of the upper esophageal sphincter (UES), and quickly reaches the proximal esophagus. The UES opening often occurs in a wide and unimpeded manner. The size of the sphincter opening is directly proportional to the volume of the barium bolus that is swallowed. Typically, the oral phase and pharyngeal phases of swallowing are so closely connected that the first oral phase seamlessly transitions into the subsequent pharyngeal phase. It is believed by some that the act of swallowing begins with the oral phase, which is triggered when the back of the tongue presses on the tonsillar pillars or when a mass of food is delivered into the back part of the throat (oropharynx). A potential alternative is that the connection between the oral and pharyngeal stages of swallowing is primarily controlled by the brainstem swallowing center. The typical pharyngeal phase of swallowing includes (1) the closure of the palate, (2) the movement of the bolus down the pharynx, (3) the closure of the glottis to prevent inhalation, and (4) the opening of the UES and the passage of fluid across the transsphincteric region. We suggest that the normal opening of the UES involves four components: (1) a temporary relaxation, lasting approximately 0.5 seconds, of a UES that is normally contracted; (2) the UES becoming more stretchable and less resistant to expansion when it is relaxed; (3) the anterior movement of the hyoid bone, which pulls the larynx forward and exerts pressure on the relaxed and stretchable UES; and (4) the radial pressure exerted by the bolus of food or liquid that is approaching, causing the fully relaxed UES to expand once it has been initially opened by the traction of the hyoid bone. Manometric investigations reveal that the UES during nesting shows a high-pressure zone that is greater in the posterior and anterior regions compared to the lateral regions due to the cricopharyngeal arrangement. Pressure sensor measurements taken across the UES suggest that the cricopharyngeus muscle is the primary component of the UES. During the process of swallowing, the UES experiences a decrease in pressure, accompanied by a relaxation of its underlying electromyographic activity. The flaccid compliant cricopharyngeus muscle may be easily elongated by applying modest pulling force in newly dissected anatomical specimens. During the initiation of swallowing, the hyoid bone moves upward and forward due to the contraction of the suprahyoid muscles. The larynx is able to move in conjunction with the hyoid bone due to the interconnections formed by the thyrohyoid membrane and the paired thyrohyoid muscles. Consequently, the larynx shifts forward in conjunction with the anterior displacement of the hyoid bone. Therefore, the hyoid bone applies force to the larynx, causing it to move forward and apply force on the cricoid cartilage. This, in turn, applies forward force to the UES. The anterior traction force results in an initial relaxation of the UES, causing it to open by approximately 6 mm. After the UES has opened, the barium bolus that was swallowed starts to pass into the sphincter section. When the barium bolus enters the sphincter segment, the pressure from the bolus causes the UES segment to expand even further. During the process of swallowing, there are cases when a little and temporary swelling of the cricopharyngeus muscle can be observed. The temporary and fast disappearance of the depression in the cricopharyngeus is a typical occurrence. Typically, nevertheless, the UES section opens completely without any sign of a cricopharyngeal depression. The duration of the UES opening and the width of the UES are directly influenced by the volume and viscosity of the bolus. The superior movement of the hyoid bone lasts approximately 1.2 seconds. It occurs throughout both the oral and pharyngeal phases of swallowing and continues from the beginning to the completion of the swallow. The opening and shutting of the UES occur when the hyoid and larynx are in close proximity or at the highest point of their movement in the oral cavity. In the pharyngeal phase of swallowing, the laryngeal vestibule shuts for approximately 0.6–0.7 seconds, starting shortly before the opening of the UES. The closure of the vestibule primarily relies on the movement of the epiglottis, which is mostly controlled by the contraction of the thyrohyoid muscles. The movement of the epiglottis during swallowing happens in two distinct steps. First, the epiglottis changes from an upright to a horizontal posture, induced mostly by elevation of the hyoid and larynx as well as by contraction of the paired thynohyoid muscles. The rotation of the free edge of the epiglottis is primarily achieved by the aryepiglottic and thyroepiglottic muscles. This occurs when the epiglottis is in a horizontal position, with the arytenoids acting as a pivot point. The contraction of these muscles also functions as a sphincter at the opening of the larynx. The flexible epiglottis swiftly rotates in a downward motion. Occasionally, an elongated epiglottis might be physically obstructed from moving downward due to the posterior pharyngeal cervical wall, cervical spine, or a nasogastric tube that is in place. The initiation of vestibular closure is marked by the horizontal displacement of the epiglottis, which functions in a bellow-like manner to expel gas swiftly from the vestibule. Therefore, the first closure of the vestibule results in the expulsion of a burst of gas into the pharynx, which serves to hinder the entry of ingested substances into the respiratory passage. Solely relying on vestibular closure does not ensure the absence of barium penetration. Occasionally, in healthy individuals, a small amount of barium can be observed entering the vestibule during one or two barium swallows, especially during the first swallow. These penetrations are often quickly cleared during the act of swallowing.

2.4 NORMAL VARIANTS OF PHYSIOLOGIC SWALLOWING

Normal asymptomatic individuals may have morphologic variations such as a postcricoid impression, pharyngeal outpouches, tiny cervical web, and a small posterior impression of the cricopharyngeus when swallowing. In the past, the postcricoid sensation was sometimes misdiagnosed as a tumor. However, it was later discovered that this impression is a regular occurrence during the pharyngeal phase of swallowing [31]. At first, the feeling was ascribed to a postcricoid plexus of veins. From our perspective, the postcricoid impression appears to be a mere folding of the mucosal tissue, as there are no large veins positioned after the cricoid lamina. Mucosal webs, which are thin and measure around 1–2 mm in height, are typically seen on the front wall of the cervical esophagus. These webs are often discovered incidentally and do not have any clinical importance. More prominent and widespread webs that round the circumference of the esophagus may lead to significant constriction of the inner passage, resulting in difficulty swallowing solid foods, known as dysphagia. The majority of pharyngeal outpouches are temporary and are discovered by chance in individuals without any symptoms. Pharyngeal pouches often manifest and vanish early in the pharyngeal stage of swallowing. A common morphological anomaly observed in asymptomatic individuals is a small indentation caused by the cricopharyngeus muscle. This indentation can occur at various times, such as early, late, or during the opening of the UES and the flow of barium. These subtle imprints can be erased by a significant amount of barium, such as 15 out of 20 mL. There is a belief that any action performed by the cricopharyngeus is considered aberrant. We believe that a slight cricopharyngeal impression is within the usual range and does not result in any clinical complaints. Further study is required to address this problem.

2.5 SWALLOWING IN GERIATRIC PATIENTS

Age-related changes occur in the structure and function of the mouth, throat, and esophagus. It is important to consider these variations in the condition of older individuals (primary aging) while conducting clinical and radiological assessments [32]. These modifications often do not hinder the process of swallowing and hence do not cause any symptoms. Nevertheless, the addition of disease processes, known as secondary aging, can lead to substantial deterioration. To comprehensively understand swallowing in older individuals, it is necessary to distinguish between anticipated age-related alterations and those induced by pathological conditions. Regrettably, the presence of subclinical illness, particularly cerebral vascular disease, complicates the process of making this differentiation. Based on information from other organ systems, there is an approximate annual decrease of 1% in function starting at the age of 30. Aging is a gradual decline in overall bodily function, leading to a reduced ability to respond to stress and an increased susceptibility to age-related diseases. The senescent alterations in oropharyngeal function can be described as somewhat less effective. Nevertheless, the correlation between symptoms and morphodynamic anomalies, particularly in the setting of compensation and decompensation, is highly intricate.

The oral cavity experiences significant alterations as one ages. These modifications consist of a rise in the quantity of connective tissue in the tongue, absence of teeth, and decreased chewing power. Studies have demonstrated that in the pharynx, the elderly exhibit less anterior elevation of the larynx and experience a notable delay in the pharyngeal swallowing phase. Above the age of 60, research has demonstrated a deceleration in the pharyngeal peristaltic action. However, a different study demonstrated that this assumption is incorrect and instead revealed a broader range of individual differences within older individuals. Nevertheless, there is no notable alteration in the pharyngeal peak pressure, duration, or the pace of contraction propagation. Consequently, older individuals in good health do not experience any lingering buildup in the throat following the act of swallowing.

2.5.1 Oral Phase

Research has demonstrated that the pressure exerted by the tongue during swallowing remains consistent in older adults compared to younger individuals. However, when individuals are requested to exert their maximum strength, the pressure recording significantly increases in young people, but in the elderly, this additional potential does not appear to be present. Prior studies have demonstrated a decline in lingual peristaltic pressure as individuals age.

2.5.2 Pharyngeal Phase

The most notable occurrence detected during videofluoroscopy is the inadvertent entry of a bolus into the airways. The time and magnitude of bolus misdirection are crucial factors to consider; however, they might vary significantly. In older individuals, it is frequently seen that they consume a disproportionately large amount of food or drink, or consume it excessively quickly, during unregulated administrations. This leads to the interruption of the sequential process including the intake, delivery, movement, and closure of the larynx. Certain patients have aspiration just during the initial dose of liquid barium, whereas others initially appear to be in reasonably normal condition until a small quantity of barium penetrates, causing a significant decline in their condition and subsequent aspiration before, during, and after some of the following swallows. The misdirection of a bolus, especially in older individuals, mostly occurs due to malfunction in the oral stage, even if it happens during the pharyngeal stage. Another frequent observation in older individuals is the inability to control the movement of food during the act of eating and holding the food in the mouth. These individuals have an insufficient glossopalatal seal. Lingual motions can be dyskinetic or disorganized, causing disruption to the glossopalatal seal. Alternatively, there may be a lack of oromotor activity in trying to control the bolus after it is swallowed. Transitional dissociation is the third oral stage cause of misdirection. This indicates that the bolus is situated at an incorrect location at an inappropriate moment. During swallowing, the hyoid bone in young individuals begins to travel forward (from its initial location at the back) before the apex of the bolus reaches the level of the faucial isthmus. This movement may be observed in a true lateral projection. The initiation of anterior migration of the hyoid bone is postponed as one gets older. It is frequently observed in individuals over the age of 75 to have a delay of more than 0.5 seconds in the forward migration of the hyoid bone after the bolus has passed the faucial isthmus. The study revealed that 50% of cases of aspiration were caused by dysfunction at the oral stage, 30% were due to pharyngeal dysfunction, and 20% were a result of combined dysfunction. The predominant oral stage anomaly observed was the inability to maintain control or confinement. Many patients exhibited transitional dissociation. Equally prevalent was the act of consuming a significant amount of food at once or consuming it quickly. The predominant anomaly observed in the pharyngeal stage was incomplete transfer, namely retention. The occurrence of a partial failure to close the larynx was seen with lower frequency. There is no discernible correlation between a patient's particular ailment and the irregularities observed during a barium swallow procedure. Consequently, the identified dysfunctions lack specificity in terms of their underlying causes. It is necessary to regularly examine for oral stage abnormalities during videofluoroscopy due to the frequent occurrence of mouth dysfunction. Dysphagic individuals may have aspiration due to the presence of anterior osteophytes that are greater than 10 mm and cause obstruction in the throat. The presence of concurrent clinical illnesses and diseases, such as stroke and partial laryngeal resection, heightens the likelihood of aspiration in individuals with smaller osteophytes of the cervical spine. Pneumonia frequently occurs in the aged population, often as a result of impaired airway closure during the act of swallowing, known as penetration or aspiration. Nevertheless, the causal link and its effects are intricate, and only a limited number of studies have adequately examined this matter. The most likely explanation is that the infection occurs when contaminated saliva enters the lower airways through the larynx.

There is a disagreement among experts on the impact of aging on deglutitive pharyngeal pressure. Although one study indicated the absence of a pressure disparity, others have demonstrated variations. Nevertheless, there are several methodological disparities that hinder the process of comparison. One study showed that the peristaltic pressure wave, including its amplitude and length, was notably higher in the older population compared to younger individuals. The changes that occur with age, which might be perceived as improvements, may be seen as compensatory reactions to the decreasing size of the aperture in the throat and esophagus during swallowing in older individuals. Shaker has offered a study that provides support for this notion. According to this study, the intrabolus pressure in the pharynx was notably greater in older individuals compared to young patients. This difference was observed while swallowing in both upright and supine postures, as well as with both liquid and mashed potatoes. This may suggest that the pharyngoesophageal segment (PES) in the elderly is not adequately distended.

2.6 THE PHARYNGOESOPHAGEAL SEGMENT

A comparison was made between older and younger subjects regarding the pressure of the pharyngoesophageal sphincter. Cook et al. observed no significant alterations in resting PES pressure, as measured by a sleeve device, in individuals below the age of 55. Wilson et al. reported a similar observation in individuals who were under the age of 62 and in good health. In contrast, Fulp et al. demonstrated that individuals over the age of 62 who are considered to be in good health have a lower resting pressure in their PES compared to younger individuals who served as controls. Shaker et al. examined how the process of getting older (specifically, in individuals aged 70 years and older) affects the pressure of the PES when at rest, as well as its reaction to the introduction of air into the esophagus and the expansion of a balloon within it. The findings of this study suggest that the process of aging has a substantial impact on reducing the resting PES pressure [33]. Many studies demonstrated that the elderly had typical pressure responses in the PES during swallowing and when the esophagus was distended with air or a balloon. Thus, the elderly maintain the protective function of the PES in preventing the backflow of stomach acid into the pharynx. Further investigations have demonstrated the presence of pharyngeal weakness in older patients suffering from dysphagia. In their investigation, they also determined that 75% of cases of aspiration were caused by inadequate pharyngeal constrictions, which indicated pharyngeal weakness.

2.7 THE AGING ESOPHAGUS

The term "presbyesophagus" is commonly used to characterize anomalies in esophageal motility that occur in elderly people. However, further investigations demonstrated that dysmotility is not a result of aging itself. Esophageal illnesses are prevalent among individuals of all age groups, including the elderly. Certain illnesses, including adenocarcinoma, become more common as individuals age. It is important to consider that an older patient with suspected achalasia is significantly more prone to having a distal esophageal cancer compared to a younger patient. Additionally, older patients with long-standing achalasia may develop a secondary cancer. The manifestation of symptoms in the elderly tends to be more intricate for commonly recognized disorders. Hence, differentiating between chest discomfort caused by esophageal dysmotility or gastroesophageal reflux illness and coronary artery disease might pose significant challenges. Furthermore, older individuals with long-standing chronic diseases are at a higher risk of experiencing problems. This assertion has validity in the case of Barrett's esophagus and cancer of the esophagus. Esophageal dysmotility is a significant issue in older individuals. The symptoms are often associated with improper movement of ingested particles down the esophagus. The cardinal symptoms consist of chest discomfort and/or vomiting. The primary challenge in differential diagnosis is identifying any potential mechanical blockage, such as reflux, strictures, or cancers. Typically, strictures cause symptoms while consuming solid foods but not when consuming liquids. The symptoms of dysmotility are often the same for both liquids and solids. Endoscopy should always be taken into account while dealing with individuals in this particular age bracket. If it is not recommended or unavailable, the radiologic investigation must include an assessment of the structure or form. The elderly frequently have a high number of nonpropulsive, often recurrent contractions. Additionally, the occurrence of tertiary contractions, delayed esophageal emptying, and esophageal dilation is frequently observed. Research has demonstrated that the strength of contractions in the lower part of the esophagus is considerably greater in older individuals compared to younger ones. Curiously, the amplitude of contractions in the proximal esophagus did not show any increase as individuals became older. Previous studies have demonstrated that there is no significant difference in the resting pressure of the lower esophageal sphincter between young and older individuals.

2.8 SWALLOWING IN PEDIATRIC AND INFANT PATIENTS

While a comprehensive analysis of swallowing in children and babies is not within the scope of this book, it is necessary to briefly address infantile-type swallowing. In babies, the tongue is disproportionately large and completely occupies the oral cavity, while the hyoid bone is positioned at a higher height in relation to the jaw. During nursing, the mouth is engaged in an oral suckle which involves the compression of the nipple and the application of oral suction. The fluid from each suckling is spat back into the pharynx. When the pharynx is filled, it initiates a pharyngeal swallow. Typically, there are two or three suckles that occur before each pharyngeal swallow. During the pharyngeal swallow, the hyoid bone exhibits anterior movement due to its preexisting elevated position. Infants are able to breastfeed and swallow while breathing via their nose due to the elevated resting posture of their hyoid, epiglottis, and larynx. As the individual matures, the hyoid bone moves downward and the pharynx expands in size. Additionally, the tongue becomes comparatively smaller due to the uneven growth of the mandible and tongue. These advancements are accompanied by the capacity to masticate and handle food within the oral cavity. These developmental modifications facilitate the administration of larger amounts of substance into the pharynx and the production of speech resonance in the pharynx. Curiously, the way adults swallow is similar to how infants do it, since the hyoid and larynx briefly move to a higher position during the swallowing process.

REFERENCES

1. Erhart EA. *Neuroanatomia simplificada*. 6th ed. São Paulo: Roca; 1986.
2. Ertekin C, Aydogdu I. Neurophysiology of swallowing. *Clin Neurophysiol*. 2003;114:2226–44.
3. Miller AJ. Deglutition. *Psysiol Rev*. 1982;62:129–84.
4. Rosso ALZ. Controle neural da deglutição. In: Costa MMB, Carrara-de-Angelis E, Barros APB (Orgs.), *Temas em deglutição & disfagia: abordagem multidisciplinar*. Rio de Janeiro; 1998. p. 13–16.
5. Roman C. Neural control of deglutition and esophageal motility in mammals. *J Physiol*. 1989;81:118–31.
6. Bieger D. Rhomboncephalic pathways and neurotransmitters controlling deglutition. *Am J Med*. 2001;111:85S-89S.
7. Machado A. *Neuroanatomia funcional*. 2nd ed. Atheneu, Editor. São Paulo; 1993.
8. Guyton AC, Hall JE. *Textbook of medical physiology*. 10th ed. Philadelphia, PA: Saunders Elsevier, 2011.
9. Jean A. Brain stem control of swallowing: neural network and cellular mechanisms. *Physiol Rev*. 2001;81:929–69.
10. Ertekin C. Electrophysiological evaluation of oropharyngeal dysphagia in Parkinson's disease. *Mov Disord*. 2014;7:31–56.
11. Jean A, Car A, Roman C. Comparison of activity in pontine versus medullary neurons during swallowing. *Exp Brain Res*. 1975;22:211–20.
12. Jean A. Brainstem organization of the swallowing network. *Brain Behav Evol*. 1984;25:109–16.
13. Kessler JP, Jean A. Identification of the medullary swallowing regions in the rat. *Exp Brain Res*. 1985;57:256–63.
14. Umezaki T, Matsuse T, Shin T. Medullary swallowing-related neurons in the anesthetized cat. *Neuroreport*. 1998;9:1793–8.
15. Ertekin C. Neurogenic dysphagia in brainstem disorders and EMG evaluation. *J Basic Clin Heal*. 2017;1:1–10.
16. Jean A. Control of the central swallowing program by inputs from the principal receptors. A review. *J Auton Nerv Syst*. 1984;10:225–33.
17. Aydogdu I, Ertekin C, Tarlaci S, Turman B, Kiylioglu N, Secil Y. Dysphagia in lateral medullary infarction (Wallenberg's syndrome): an acute disconnection syndrome in premotor neurons related to swallowing activity. *Stroke*. 2001;32:2081–7.
18. Jean A, Dallaporta M. Electrophysiologic characterization of the swallowing pattern generator in the brainstem. *GI Motil*. 2006;9:1–37.
19. Ertekin C, Pehlivan M, Aydogdu I. An electrophysiological investigation of deglutition in man. *Muscle Nerve*. 1995;18:1177–86.
20. Ertekin C. Voluntary versus spontaneous swallowing in man. *Dysphagia*. 2011;26:183–92.
21. Ertekin C, Aydogdu I, Yüceyar N. Effects of bolus volumes on the oropharyngeal swallowing: an electrophysiological study in man. *Am J Gastroenterol*. 1997;92:2049–53.
22. Miller AJ. *The neuroscientific principles of swallowing and dysphagia*. San Diego, CA/London: Singular Publication Group; 1999.

23. Jean A, Car A. Inputs to swallowing medullary neurons from the peripheral afferent fibers and swallowing cortical area. *Brain Res.* 1979;178:567–72.
24. Perlman AL, Schlze-Delrieu KS. *Deglutition and its disorders: anatomy, physiology, clinical diagnosis and management.* San Diego: Singular Publication Group; 1997.
25. Ertekin C, Aydogdu I, Yüceyar N, Tarlaci S, Kiylioglu N, Pehlivan M. Electrodiagnostic methods for neurogenic dysphagia. *Electroenceph Clin Neurophysiol.* 1998;109:331–40.
26. Jean A, Amri M, Calas A. Connections between the medullary swallowing area and the trigeminal motor nucleus of the sheep studied by tracing methods. *J Auton Nerv Syst.* 1983;7:87–96.
27. Costa MMB. *Disfagia oral e ou faríngea e os distúrbios referentes.* Rio de Janeiro: Medbook; 2013. p. 180–95.
28. Machado A. Nervos cranianos. In: *Neuroanatomia funcional.* 2nd ed. São Paulo: Atheneu; 2006. p. 119–28.
29. Chusid JG. *Neuroanatomia correlativa e neurologia funcional.* 18th ed. Rio de Janeiro: Guanabara Koogan; 1985.
30. Pansky B, Allen DJ. Cranial nerves. In: *Review of neuroscience.* New York: MacMillan Publishing; 1980. p. 223–54.
31. Guyton AC. Os sentidos químicos. In: Guanabara Koogan (ed.), *Tratado de fisiologia médica.* Rio de Janeiro: Guanabara Koogan; 1992. p. 512–14.
32. Rhodes RA, Pflanzer RG. Sensory systems. In: *Human physiology.* 3rd ed. Philadelphia: Saunders; 1996. p. 252–97.
33. Lent R. Os sentidos químicos. Estrutura e função do sistema gustatório. In: Lent R (ed.), *Cem bilhões de neurônios: conceitos fundamentais.* São Paulo: Atheneu; 2001. p. 324–30.

3 Clinical Evaluation of Pharyngoesophageal Disorders

3.1 OVERVIEW

This chapter's goal is to present a multidisciplinary diagnostic work-up, with a focus on a systematic and useful radiological approach. More than 5% of people worldwide have swallowing issues, and up to 50% of patients in hospitals suffer from them. Numerous anatomical structures make up the swallowing tract. Food, both liquid and solid, must be appropriately moved from the mouth into the throat and then down the esophagus and into the stomach. Deglutition may therefore be impacted by a wide range of illnesses, leading to a multidisciplinary work-up of dysphagic patients. The preferred technique for examining the entire swallowing system in a "one-stop shopping" way is videofluoroscopy (VF) of deglutition. VF can show abnormal morphological features and serve as a foundation for choosing a more specific work-up [1].

3.2 HISTORY-TAKING FROM THE RADIOLOGIST'S PERSPECTIVE

While radiologists often interact with patients less directly than primary clinicians, understanding the clinical history is essential for optimizing imaging strategy, tailoring protocols, and improving diagnostic accuracy. A focused and relevant clinical history, either obtained through referral notes or direct communication, provides crucial context for interpreting imaging findings in pharyngo-esophageal disorders.

Key elements of history-taking relevant to radiologic assessment include:

- *Asking for the main symptom*: Characterizing the primary symptom (e.g., dysphagia, odynophagia, regurgitation, weight loss, aspiration, globus) helps guide the appropriate, tailored barium swallow protocol for the specific patients, adding maneuvers that may not be performed during routine examinations.

- *Swallowing phase involvement*: Asking whether symptoms arise during the oral, pharyngeal, or esophageal phase assists in focusing the attention more on the specific section of interest, even though we advise carrying out thorough examinations in each patient.

- *Onset and duration*: Acute symptoms may suggest infection, trauma, or foreign body, while progressive symptoms raise suspicion for malignancy or stricture.

- *Associated symptoms*: Hoarseness, chronic cough, recurrent pneumonia, and gastroesophageal reflux offer clues to underlying pathologies and guide further examinations and referrals.

- *Surgical or radiation history*: Prior head and neck surgery, cervical spine instrumentation, or radiotherapy can alter anatomy, affect swallowing, or predispose to strictures and may influence image interpretation.

- *Neurological history*: Stroke, neurodegenerative disorders, and cranial nerve palsies are relevant to motility assessments and should be considered when planning dynamic imaging protocols.

Radiologists benefit from integrating this clinical history with imaging requisitions, especially in cases where subtle findings or functional impairments must be correlated with patient-specific risk factors. When history is lacking, we encourage radiologists to communicate with referring clinicians or review the electronic health record to ensure a comprehensive and context-sensitive evaluation.

3.3 SIGNS OF DISORDERS OF SWALLOWING

In order to customize the examination and match the particular radiological findings to the patient's symptoms, the first step in investigating individuals with swallowing issues is always to establish their medical history. The duration and onset of swallowing disorders, the pattern of swallowing events, the location of symptoms, the consistency of foods that cause difficulty swallowing, aspiration, regurgitation, coughing, pneumonia, prior upper gastrointestinal tract surgery, neurological diseases, and other information should all be included in a questionnaire that aids in organizing the patient's medical history [2]. The patient's history must be divided into useful categories in order to facilitate an appropriate flow of diagnostic procedures and therapeutic ideas. We may delve more into the "art and science of history-taking in the patient with dysphagia" as we gain more experience with this patient group. The imaging specialist must critically incorporate the patient's history into the interpretation of the study and use it to inform the design of the VF assessment. Do the patient's symptoms make sense in light of the VF findings or other test results? Inquiries should

DOI: 10.1201/9781003508113-3

focus on whether the symptoms or syndromes covered in greater depth in the following sections are present when the patient has referred their issue.

3.3.1 Dysphagia

Eating and drinking are performed for nourishment, hydration, social, and personal enjoyment without compromising one's respiratory tract. Dysphagia is the term used to describe any subjective sensation of disruption of this process. Rarely occurring, isolated oral dysphagia is caused by neurogenic diseases or decreased salivary flow. Salivary flow is also impacted by medication (anticholinergics, antihistamines, antidepressants, antihypertensives, and diuretics), and neuroleptic medications may also impede or interfere with the oral phase of swallowing. The most common cause of pharyngeal dysphagia, which is characterized by the patient's perception of difficulty passing the bolus through the suprasternal notch, is neuromuscular abnormalities that result in weakening and/or incoordination of the striated swallowing muscles. Structural narrowings such as a mucosal web, Zenker's diverticulum, surgical abnormalities, or a tumor are less common. Patients with esophageal dysphagia may pinpoint the site anywhere from the suprasternal notch to the epigastrium, where the material appears to adhere to the swallowing tract. Patients typically lack the ability to distinguish between an esophageal lesion's proximal and distal sites. For instance, symptoms above the suprasternal notch are frequently caused by achalasia or a Schatzki ring at the level of the esophagogastric junction. Lower esophageal rings or strictures with fewer than 2 cm of residual lumen are common causes of intermittent esophageal dysphagia for solid meals. In esophageal cancer, solid food dysphagia frequently progresses quickly within three months. Esophageal dysphagia for fluids only signifies esophageal motor abnormalities in the absence of any indication or evidence of aspiration. The latter can also cause solid food dysphagia, depending on how severe the motility problem is. During a meal, regurgitation of previously consumed food can occur for any reason or in any location. Late regurgitation of undigested food is common in achalasia or Zenker's diverticulum. The hallmark of gastroesophageal reflux disease (GERD) is heartburn accompanied by complaints of sour and/or bitter substance. Moreover, the most common cause of "non-cardiac chest pain" is GERD. Once a cardiovascular problem has been ruled out, the esophagus needs to be examined. Proton pump inhibitor medication for three weeks may be a useful diagnostic and treatment strategy. Odynophagia is the term for painful swallowing; a dull or squeezing sensation is linked to esophageal spasm, while a "sharp" pain is typically indicative of ulcerative mucosal lesions of the pharynx or esophagus.

3.3.2 The Globus Sensation

Globus is a prevalent issue that affects roughly 5% of people with general otolaryngologic disorders. These patients often complain of a "lump in the throat," a sore throat, frequent clearing of the throat, fullness, and the feeling of a foreign body. Symptoms usually appear sporadically. When eating, the symptom usually improves, but dysphagia is often present as well. Evidence of esophageal motor dysfunction was found in 47% of 150 individuals with globus as the only symptom, in which VF might show abnormal functional and/or morphological findings. Manometry revealed that 87% of patients had a high incidence of esophageal motility problems in this context. The globus feeling appears to be a laryngopharyngeal irritation symptom that is not unique to GERD but is influenced by it. The pathophysiology of globus is still up for debate. Pharyngeal and/or esophageal diseases should be ruled out based on the particular history, and the term "globus hystericus" should be avoided. The diagnosis of "non-cardiac chest pain" is frequently made for people who exhibit no signs of heart disease.

3.3.3 Aspiration

Aspiration is defined as the introduction of food or fluids into the airways below the glottis. Aspiration is suspected in cases of recurrent pneumonia, coughing, or choking right after swallowing. If there is no or little cough reflex, silent aspiration may occur. People who aspirate are more likely to experience severe respiratory consequences, such as aspiration pneumonia and airway blockage. The effects of aspiration are influenced by the amount, the depth of aspiration (trachea or distal airways), and the physical characteristics of the aspirate. Aspiration of stomach or esophageal contents can occur retrogradely or anterogradely during or immediately after eating. Patients who are at risk of aspiration must be identified by the radiologist. A customized VF study prevents extreme aspiration during the assessment.

3.3.4 Odynophagia

Pain during swallowing typically indicates mucosal inflammation, infection, ulceration, or malignancy. It may also result from esophageal candidiasis in immunocompromised patients or postradiation mucositis. CT imaging is to be preferred when infection or abscess is suspected, while endoscopy and contrast-enhanced MRI may be warranted for mucosal evaluation.

3.3.5 Chronic Cough

A frequent symptom in pharyngoesophageal pathology, chronic cough may arise from aspiration, reflux-related laryngeal irritation, or a tracheoesophageal fistula. When these complications are suspected, cross-sectional imaging, particularly CT, is useful for identifying bronchopulmonary complications, fistulas, or lymphadenopathy compressing the esophagus or airway.

3.3.6 Regurgitation

Passive return of swallowed contents suggests motility dysfunction, pharyngoesophageal diverticulum (e.g., Zenker's), or obstruction. Dynamic imaging is ideal for characterizing bolus flow and identifying structural abnormalities such as cricopharyngeal bars or strictures.

3.3.7 Weight Loss

Unintended weight loss in the setting of dysphagia or regurgitation raises high concern for malignancy. Cross-sectional imaging with CT or MRI, often combined with endoscopy, is essential for tumor staging, nodal assessment, and surgical planning.

3.4 MULTIDISCIPLINARY ASSESSMENT OF SWALLOWING DISORDERS

When examining patients with swallowing issues, the radiologist should be knowledgeable about the particular methods used in other medical specialties [3]. The use of various clinical tests by different clinical areas differs from one country to another and overlaps significantly. Our goal is to shed more light on therapeutic interactions rather than the distinctions between different clinical disciplines. Mental and social functioning, physical mobility, and the patient's level of nutrition and hydration are all considered aspects of general patient status. A chest examination can identify aspiration-related respiratory function issues or diseases where aspiration may result in serious complications. The musculoskeletal system's dysfunction can hinder normal mobility, the cardiovascular system must be evaluated for potential sources of brain emboli, and several systemic disorders, including scleroderma and muscular diseases, can impact the swallowing process. A thorough head and neck examination is part of the status of speech-language pathologists and otolaryngologists. It is important to check the neck for lumps, particularly adenopathies, an enlarged thyroid, and scars that may indicate surgery on the swallowing structures. Indirect laryngoscopy or fiberoptics should be used to examine the oral cavity, cranial nerve function, palate, pharynx, and larynx in order to check for tumors, mucosal integrity, vocal cord motion, secretion pooling into the piriform sinus or vallecula, as well as sensation and voice. The sounds of swallowing motility and the probing of the elevation of the hyoid and larynx are part of the dynamic clinical inquiry. Stridor is an indication of upper airway blockage and may only be audible with auscultation over the trachea. A well-recognized diagnostic procedure, fiberoptic endoscopic evaluation of swallowing (FEES), allows investigation of morphologic and functional alterations in the larynx, velopharynx, and nose. Through the nose, the lightweight, flexible instruments are inserted. It is possible to incorporate video documentation. Otolaryngologists, speech-language pathologists, and radiologists work together to apply and interpret the results of FEES, which is a complementary technique to VF. FEES can detect aspiration and pharyngeal retentions; however, it does not display the full motion of the bolus and important foodway structures during swallowing. First, VF and FEES outcomes are "diagnostic studies." Second, they enable the physician to create a suitable diet and compensatory techniques to enhance pharyngeal clearance and reduce aspiration. This application of VF and FEES, which include trials to evaluate the efficacy of therapy, are referred to as "therapeutic studies." Neurologists also use FEES. Nonetheless, a key component of the multidisciplinary approach to treating dysphagic patients is the neurologic evaluation. Among the many neurological conditions that may entail deglutition are multiple sclerosis, amyotrophic lateral sclerosis, poliomyelitis, myasthenia gravis, dementia, Parkinson's disease, and cerebrovascular disease. Both general surgeons and otolaryngologists perform invasive treatment of the upper esophageal sphincter (UES), which is commonly utilized as therapy for Zenker's diverticulum. Discussions about various surgical techniques are ongoing. To reestablish a sufficient opening of the pharyngoesophageal segment, myotomy of the UES, myotomy with laser, or myotomy using an endoscopic technique is used, either with or without excision of the diverticulum itself. Esophageal disease diagnosis and treatment are the areas of expertise for gastroenterologists and surgeons. Endoscopy can take biopsies for pathologic diagnosis and can disclose even the smallest mucosal features. However, endoscopy might miss small rings or stenoses that are passable by the endoscope but will obstruct larger solid food boluses. Additionally, endoscopy frequently cannot be sent distal to a narrow stenosis and cannot always show the topographic relationship of stenoses to significant anatomic landmarks. VF can be useful in these situations by assessing the esophagus distal to stenoses, testing for modest stenoses with solid bolus, and offering good topographic overviews. Endoscopy and VF are used to identify benign and malignant macromorphological changes of the esophageal tube. In addition to manometry, the gold standard for diagnosing esophageal motility abnormalities, VF can identify delayed transit for both liquids and solid foods. Videomanometry is the combination of manometry and VF. This technique synchronizes the pressure readings with the videofluoroscopic record of the bolus transit. Scintigraphy is used to assess stomach emptying and esophageal transport. Diabetes is known to cause delayed stomach emptying, which can disrupt esophageal transport and exacerbate symptoms like heartburn, dyspepsia, and epigastric fullness. While VF can characterize the dynamic appearance of the esophagogastric junction during and after bolus passage, pH probe investigations can identify pathologic gastroesophageal reflux [4]. Videofluoroscopic analysis is used to rule out early and late postoperative problems including stenosis, leakage, or perforation in cases of hiatal hernia, cardiac insufficiency, and the esophagogastric junction following procedures such as fundoplication, myotomy, dilatation, gastric banding, and others. The preferred diagnostic test for obtaining a comprehensive picture of the entire swallowing tract, identifying macropathologic alterations, and identifying abnormal function is VF. A customized VF examination that is pertinent to the clinical issue might be made to serve as the foundation for additional diagnostic tests or to supplement their findings.

REFERENCES

1. Swallowing Disorders: Symptoms of Dysphagia. New York University School of Medicine. Archived from the original on 14 November 2007. Retrieved 24 February 2008.
2. Sleisenger MH, Feldman M, Friedman LM. *Sleisenger & Fordtran's Gastrointestinal & Liver Disease*, 7th edition. Philadelphia, PA: W.B. Saunders Company; 2002. Chapter 6, p. 63.
3. Dysphagia. University of Texas Medical Branch. Archived from the original on 6 March 2008. Retrieved 23 February 2008.
4. Franko DL, Shapiro J, Gagne A. Phagophobia: a form of psychogenic dysphagia a new entity. *Annals of Otology, Rhinology & Laryngology*. 1997; 106(4): 286–290. doi:10.1177/000348949710600404.

4 Basics of Pharyngoesophageal Endoscopy

4.1 INTRODUCTION

Pharyngeal and esophageal endoscopy are cornerstone procedures in the assessment and management of swallowing disorders [1]. These minimally invasive techniques allow for direct visualization of anatomical and mucosal structures within the upper aerodigestive tract, enabling clinicians to detect abnormalities that may not be apparent on radiologic imaging alone. In patients with dysphagia, persistent throat symptoms, chronic cough, reflux, or suspected malignancy, endoscopy offers a vital diagnostic window into both structure and function (Figures 4.1 and 4.2). The integration of endoscopy into dysphagia evaluation reflects a broader movement toward multidisciplinary, multimodal assessment strategies that combine imaging, physiology, and clinical expertise.

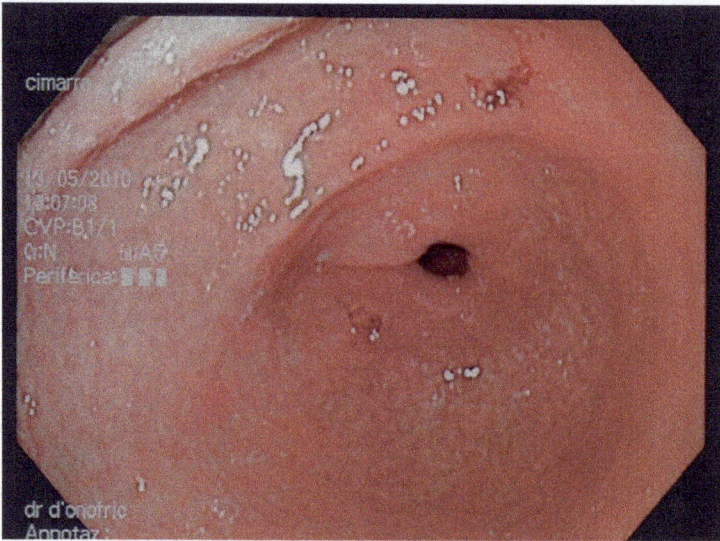

Figure 4.1   Endoscopic view of the gastroesophageal junction in a patient with achalasia.

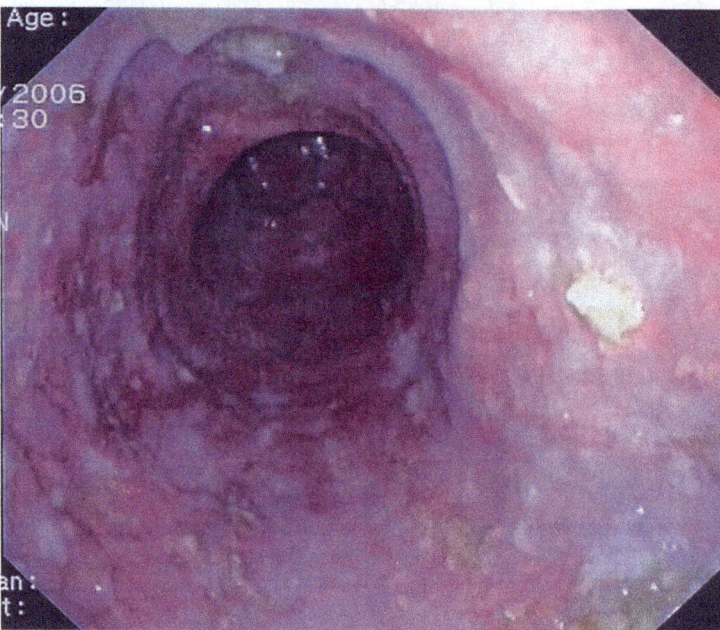

Figure 4.2   Endoscopic view of the esophageal lumen in a patient with esophagitis.

                                                    DOI: 10.1201/9781003508113-4

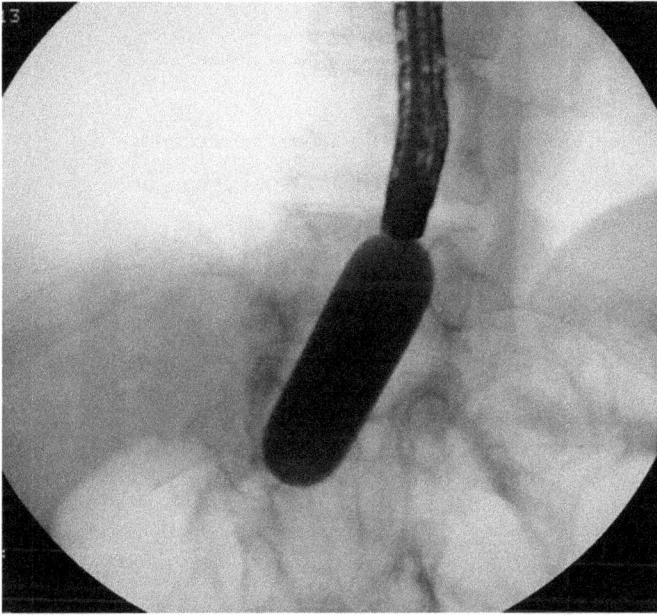

Figure 4.3 Intraoperative fluoroscopy of the gastroesophageal junction balloon dilation.

Whereas radiologic tools like the videofluoroscopic swallow study (VFSS) and modified barium swallow impairment profile (MBSImP) capture the dynamic motion of bolus transit, endoscopy provides static and real-time views of the tissues themselves. The two approaches are complementary, not competing. When used together, they provide a robust understanding of the pathophysiology underlying swallowing difficulties, allowing for more precise diagnosis and individualized treatment.

4.2 OVERVIEW OF PROCEDURES

Pharyngeal and esophageal endoscopy can be performed using flexible or rigid instruments, depending on the clinical indication, provider expertise, and the procedural setting (clinic, operating room, or endoscopy suite) [2]. The primary goals of these procedures are to assess mucosal integrity, identify anatomical or structural abnormalities, and observe the interaction between bolus material and the aerodigestive tract. Endoscopic procedures may also be therapeutic, enabling biopsy, dilation (Figure 4.3), injection, or removal of foreign bodies.

Flexible pharyngeal endoscopy—often referred to as fiberoptic nasolaryngoscopy or video naso-endoscopy—is a well-tolerated, in-office procedure commonly performed by otolaryngologists and some trained speech-language pathologists. It enables visualization of the nasal cavity, nasopharynx, oropharynx, larynx, and hypopharynx. This type of endoscopy forms the basis for the fiberoptic endoscopic evaluation of swallowing (FEES).

Esophageal endoscopy can be performed with a traditional flexible endoscope under sedation (typically by gastroenterologists), or using a smaller-caliber, unsedated transnasal esophagoscope (TNE), a technique increasingly used by otolaryngologists. TNE allows for rapid, office-based inspection of the esophagus and upper stomach without the logistical requirements of sedation, making it especially suitable for patients with upper esophageal symptoms or contraindications to sedatives.

4.3 INDICATIONS FOR USE

Endoscopy is indicated in a broad range of clinical contexts. For pharyngeal endoscopy, common indications include [3]:

- Assessment of structural or mucosal abnormalities such as lesions, masses, or inflammation.

- Evaluation of vocal fold mobility and closure.

- Identification of laryngeal sensory deficits.
- Pre-swallow study screening and post-treatment monitoring.

For esophageal endoscopy, indications include:

- Evaluation of esophageal-phase dysphagia or globus sensation.
- Suspected gastroesophageal reflux disease (GERD) or laryngopharyngeal reflux (LPR).
- Detection and surveillance of strictures, webs, or diverticula.
- Surveillance in patients with Barrett's esophagus or a history of esophageal cancer.
- Investigation of suspected foreign-body impaction or food bolus obstruction.

4.4 PROCEDURAL TECHNIQUE

Procedural success in endoscopy depends on proper patient preparation, adequate topical anesthesia, and skilled technique [4]. In pharyngeal endoscopy, the patient is seated in an upright position, and a topical vasoconstrictor and anesthetic (e.g., oxymetazoline and lidocaine) are administered to the nasal mucosa. The flexible endoscope is gently passed through the most patent nostril and advanced posteriorly to visualize the nasopharynx, soft palate, base of tongue, valleculae, epiglottis, arytenoids, and true vocal folds. The examination may include phonation, breath holding, and dry or actual swallows to assess functional integrity. Real-time video recording is strongly recommended for documentation.

Transnasal esophagoscopy follows a similar initial approach. After topical anesthesia is applied to the nasal cavity and oropharynx, the endoscope is passed into the esophagus with minimal discomfort. The examiner visualizes the upper esophageal sphincter (UES), cervical esophagus, thoracic esophagus, and lower esophageal sphincter (LES). In many cases, entry into the stomach and inspection of the gastric cardia are possible. Advanced procedures may include dilation, brush cytology, or therapeutic injection. Compared to conventional sedated endoscopy, TNE offers improved efficiency and lower procedural risk for suitable patients.

4.5 DIAGNOSTIC UTILITY

Pharyngeal and esophageal endoscopy are powerful diagnostic modalities, capable of detecting abnormalities that may escape other forms of evaluation [5]. Pharyngeal endoscopy enables direct inspection of the oropharyngeal and laryngeal mucosa, vocal fold movement, and secretion management. This is particularly valuable in the setting of hoarseness, chronic throat discomfort, or suspected laryngeal pathology. The use of pharyngeal endoscopy in the context of swallowing disorders allows the examiner to assess for pooling of secretions, structural obstructions such as a post-cricoid web, and signs of laryngopharyngeal reflux, such as erythema or edema of the posterior larynx.

Esophageal endoscopy—especially TNE—offers detailed views of the esophageal lumen and is used to identify motility abnormalities, strictures, rings (e.g., Schatzki ring), webs, diverticula (e.g., Zenker's), hiatal hernias, and mucosal inflammation. In patients with esophageal-phase dysphagia, this technique helps distinguish mechanical obstruction from neuromuscular dysfunction. When combined with biopsy, it also serves as a critical tool for diagnosing eosinophilic esophagitis or malignancy. In selected cases, endoscopy can guide interventions such as esophageal dilation, injection of botulinum toxin into the cricopharyngeus muscle, or foreign-body retrieval.

4.6 COMPARISON WITH RADIOLOGIC STUDIES

While both endoscopy and radiologic studies such as VFSS and MBSImP are used to assess dysphagia, they provide fundamentally different types of information [6]. VFSS captures dynamic bolus transit in real time under fluoroscopy, allowing the clinician to evaluate timing, coordination, residue, and airway protection throughout the oral and pharyngeal phases. MBSImP further refines this analysis into 17 physiological components that can be scored systematically.

Endoscopy, on the other hand, provides static and sometimes real-time mucosal views but lacks the ability to visualize bolus transit unless used as part of FEES. FEES is especially sensitive in detecting laryngeal penetration, aspiration, and residue, often with superior resolution compared to VFSS. However, it does not visualize the oral or esophageal phases and lacks a "white-out" period during the actual swallow.

Transnasal esophagoscopy complements both modalities by visualizing the esophageal mucosa and luminal diameter directly, identifying pathology such as rings, strictures, or malignancy that may not be detected fluoroscopically. Thus, endoscopy and imaging are synergistic, and when combined, they provide a comprehensive assessment of swallowing function.

4.7 RISKS AND CONSIDERATIONS

Although generally well tolerated, pharyngeal and esophageal endoscopy are not without risks [7]. For flexible pharyngeal endoscopy, common side effects include mild discomfort, nasal irritation, and gagging. Rare complications may include epistaxis, vasovagal reaction, or laryngospasm, especially in highly sensitive patients [8]. Adequate topical anesthesia and patient reassurance typically mitigate these effects. Transnasal esophagoscopy shares similar risks, including nasal trauma, sore throat, and discomfort during scope advancement. Although major complications such as esophageal perforation are exceedingly rare in skilled hands, practitioners should be trained in proper technique and emergency management protocols. In sedated endoscopy performed by gastroenterologists, risks include aspiration pneumonia, sedation-related cardiovascular events, and more invasive procedural complications. Contraindications for endoscopy include recent nasal or esophageal surgery, active bleeding disorders, severe coagulopathy, or unstable cardiopulmonary status. Special caution is advised in patients with obstructive sleep apnea, high vagal sensitivity, or anatomical variants that may complicate scope navigation.

4.8 ROLE IN DYSPHAGIA MANAGEMENT

Pharyngeal and esophageal endoscopy serve as indispensable tools in the interdisciplinary management of dysphagia [9]. While not traditionally considered first-line procedures, they are often utilized when radiologic imaging is inconclusive, symptoms persist despite therapy, or anatomical or mucosal pathology is suspected. Their greatest strength lies in their ability to supplement physiological assessments with detailed structural evaluation.

Pharyngeal endoscopy, particularly when conducted as part of FEES, provides immediate bedside assessment of swallowing safety and secretion management. It is especially valuable for patients who cannot be transported to radiology for VFSS, such as those in intensive care or with limited mobility. FEES enables visualization of bolus residue, vocal fold closure, and the presence of penetration or aspiration. Its repeatability and portability make it well suited for monitoring progress across therapy sessions and guiding diet modifications in real time.

Transnasal esophagoscopy has grown in popularity due to its minimal invasiveness and diagnostic power in assessing esophageal-phase dysphagia. It enables direct visualization of lesions, strictures, or mucosal injury due to reflux or eosinophilic esophagitis. In clinical practice, TNE fills a diagnostic gap between oropharyngeal and gastric investigations. When structural issues such as cricopharyngeal hypertrophy, Zenker's diverticulum, or Schatzki rings are identified, endoscopy may lead directly to therapeutic intervention—such as dilation or botulinum toxin injection—without the need for further imaging.

Endoscopy also plays a critical role in cancer surveillance and preoperative planning for head and neck surgery, as well as in the follow-up of patients treated with radiation, where mucosal damage and strictures are common. These insights guide nutritional strategies, the timing of surgical reconstruction, and speech-swallowing rehabilitation protocols.

4.9 CONCLUSION

Pharyngeal and esophageal endoscopy have revolutionized the approach to diagnosing and managing swallowing disorders [10]. These procedures offer unparalleled access to the internal anatomy of the upper aerodigestive tract, enabling clinicians to identify and address structural and mucosal contributors to dysphagia. When used in conjunction with instrumental tools such as VFSS, MBSImP, and FEES, endoscopy allows for a truly comprehensive evaluation that addresses both form and function.

As healthcare moves increasingly toward individualized, multidisciplinary care, the role of endoscopy will continue to expand—enabling earlier diagnosis, more precise treatment, and better long-term outcomes for patients with complex swallowing disorders. Whether performed in an office setting or a specialized endoscopy suite, these procedures embody the integration of diagnostic precision with therapeutic potential. Their adoption within the broader framework of dysphagia assessment represents a significant advancement in the field of aerodigestive medicine.

REFERENCES

1. Langmore SE. *Endoscopic evaluation and treatment of swallowing disorders.* Thieme Medical Publishers; 2001.
2. Aviv JE, Takoudes TG, Ma G, Close LG. Office-based esophagoscopy: a preliminary report. *Otolaryngol Head Neck Surg.* 2001;125(2):170–175.
3. Postma GN, Bach KK, Belafsky PC, Koufman JA. The role of transnasal esophagoscopy in otolaryngology. *Curr Opin Otolaryngol Head Neck Surg.* 2002;10(6):437–442.
4. Belafsky PC, Postma GN, Daniels SK, Koufman JA. Swallowing and the aging adult. *Dysphagia.* 2003;18(4):284–291.
5. Langmore SE, Schatz K, Olson N. Endoscopic and videofluoroscopic evaluations of swallowing and aspiration. *Ann Otol Rhinol Laryngol.* 1991;100(8):678–681.
6. Martin-Harris B, Brodsky MB, Michel Y, et al. MBS measurement tool for swallow impairment—MBSImp: establishing a standard. *Dysphagia.* 2008;23(4):392–405.
7. Rosenbek JC, Robbins JA, Roecker EB, Coyle JL, Wood JL. A penetration-aspiration scale. *Dysphagia.* 1996;11(2):93–98.
8. Bastian RW. Videoendoscopic evaluation of patients with dysphagia: an adjunct to the modified barium swallow. *Otolaryngol Head Neck Surg.* 1991;104(3):339–350.
9. Miles A, Moore S, McFarlane M, et al. The impact of clinical training on the accuracy of endoscopic assessment of swallowing. *Int J Speech Lang Pathol.* 2014;16(6):570–578.
10. ASHA. *Practice portal: Adult dysphagia.* American Speech-Language-Hearing Association. https://www.asha.org/Practice-Portal/Clinical-Topics/Adult-Dysphagia/.

5 Typical Fluoroscopic Results

5.1 PHARYNGEAL AND ESOPHAGEAL TOPOGRAPHIC ANATOMY

Prior to considering the radiologic anatomy, it is necessary to analyze the topographic anatomy of these structures (Figure 5.1) [1]. The patient's habitus affects the length of the upper alimentary tract. The gastroesophageal junction and the incisor teeth are 40 cm apart on average. The esophagus is typically 24 cm long, while the mouth cavity and hypopharynx are about 16 cm long. The esophagus and hypopharynx are flattened anteriorly against the thoracic and cervical spines. The retropharyngeal fat and paravertebral gaps provide posterior cushioning for the hypopharynx, separating it from the cervical spine and the adjacent muscles. While the hypopharynx rests anteriorly on the suspensory ligament and cricoarytenoid muscle of the cricoid lamina, the carotid sheaths are located laterally next to its walls. The thyroid gland partially surrounds the sphincter zone of the cervical esophagus and may extend posteriorly, dividing it from the carotid sheaths. The thyroid gland partially encloses the superior portion of the cervical esophagus laterally, while the remainder is loosely linked anteriorly to the trachea's posterior wall. Laterally, between the trachea and the esophageal wall, lie the recurrent laryngeal nerves. The vagal nerves and esophageal lymph glands are strongly attached to the esophagus below the tracheal bifurcation. Around the level of the fifth thoracic vertebra, the thoracic esophagus extends to the tracheal bifurcation after lying posterior to the trachea. Here, the left major bronchus passes anteriorly above the esophagus. To pass through the esophageal gap at the level of the first lumbar vertebra, the thoracic esophagus enters from the thoracic inlet, which is somewhat to the left of the thoracic spine. It then swings slightly to the right at around the seventh thoracic vertebra. The aortic arch crosses posteriorly and inferiorly alongside

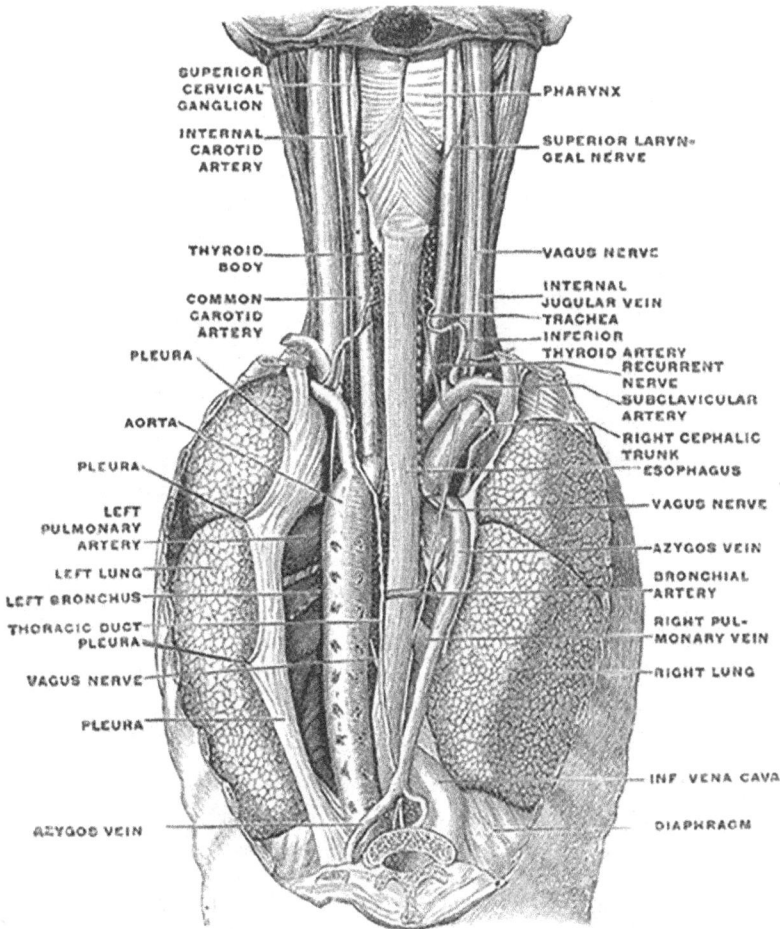

Figure 5.1 Anatomy of the esophagus.

DOI: 10.1201/9781003508113-5

the esophagus at the fourth thoracic vertebra, creating a left-sided depression. Just posterior to the esophagus at the T-S level, the descending aorta swings to the right after following the left side of the esophagus. The esophagus and the pericardial sac that surrounds the left atrium of the heart are in contact below the level of the left main bronchus. The parietal pleura and subclavian veins are next to the esophagus above T4. With the exception of the area where the azygous vein crosses (around T4), the right parietal pleura is located lateral to the esophagus on the right side. Until it passes through the esophageal hiatus of the diaphragm on the left side, the esophagus turns laterally inferior to the seventh dorsal vertebra and comes into contact with the left parietal pleura once more. In the thoracic cavity, the esophagus is flattened anteroposteriorly and has a resting width of around 2 cm. On the underside of the left lobe of the liver, which sits above it anteriorly, the abdominal segment of the esophagus creates a groove.

5.2 PHARYNGEAL AND ESOPHAGEAL RADIOGRAPHIC ANATOMY

Due to the relative ease of direct inspection, radiographic examinations of the oral cavity are rarely performed [2]. Nonetheless, it is the appropriate location to start fluoroscopic observations because it is a component of the upper gastrointestinal tract (Figure 5.2). The tongue is in direct contact with the hard palate while the mouth is closed and at rest. The front part of the tongue drops to provide space for the thick barium bolus as the mouth is opened to absorb it (Figure 5.3). The bolus is then collected in a V-shaped groove at the center of the tongue. When the jaw and mouth are closed and the tongue pushes the bolus against the hard palate, the mandibular teeth are braced against the maxillary teeth to start the swallowing action. The bolus is propelled into the hypopharynx by this stripping action. After being properly prepared by salivation and placing the bolus in the tongue's central groove, a portion of a big, thick barium bolus is retained in the lateral buccal region and ingested by repetitive tongue activity. Drinking barium through a straw or glass causes the fluid to pool at the front of the mouth while the tongue is lowered a significant distance. Periodically, propulsion persists without any jaw or tooth bracing. The next consideration is the radiologic evaluation of the cervical esophagus, orohypopharynx, and oral cavity as shown on lateral and anteroposterior films of this area prior to, during, and following a barium swallow. In this regard, the

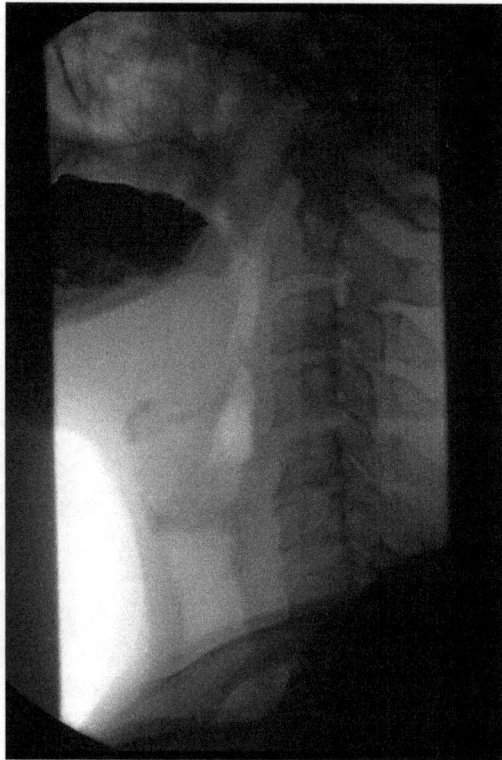

Figure 5.2 Bolus in the mouth.

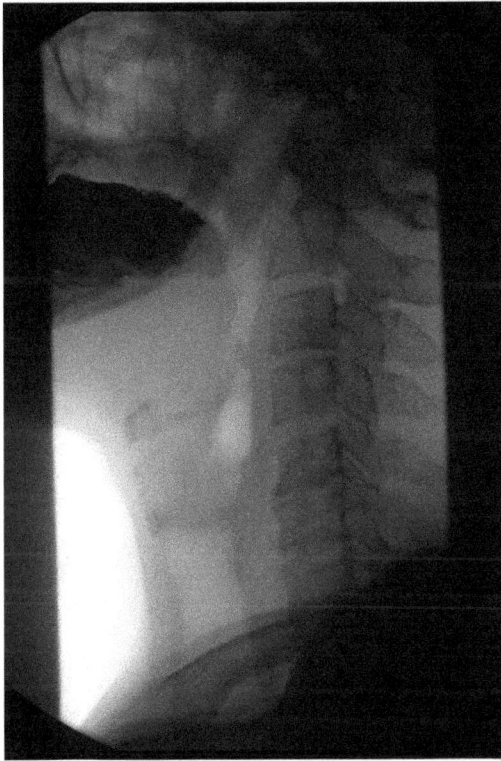

Figure 5.3 Bolus on the tongue.

oral cavity and the lateral routine film of the neck can be separated into many zones for in-depth examination: the oral cavity extends from the uvula or soft palate to the lips. Stretching from the base of the skull to the lowest tip of the uvula, the nasopharynx is located behind the soft palate. The oropharynx reaches the hyoid bone from behind the uvula and soft palate. The hypopharynx reaches the pharyngoesophageal junction from the level of the hyoid bone. One to two centimeters below the pharyngoesophageal junction is the sphincter zone. Stretching from the sphincter zone to the thoracic inlet is the cervical esophagus.

5.2.1 Oral Cavity

The size and position of the tongue, the amount of air in the oral cavity, the size and thickness of the soft palate and uvula, the presence or absence of teeth, dental plates, or fixed dentures, the shape and contour of the oral cavity, including the mandible and maxillae, and the presence or absence of malocclusion are all taken into account on the plain lateral film of the neck. A portion of the roof of the palate is delineated by a barium bolus that is lodged anteriorly after the intake of opaque material but before it is swallowed with the mouth shut. An inferior "ragged" look results from the tongue being flattened and the barium obscuring the floor. The bolus fills the whole oral cavity at the start of the barium swallow and starts to overflow into the valleculae. The palate's whole roof is well defined (Figure 5.4). As it starts its stripping activity, the bolus is now mostly located in the tongue's central groove, which is depressed aside from its anterior region. A coating of barium forms on the dorsal surface of the tongue and the roof of the mouth as soon as the bolus is swallowed with the mouth shut. At the base of the tongue, where it is highly exaggerated all the way down to the vallecula, this barium coating is most noticeable. Because teeth, fixed bridges, dental fillings, and the cervical spine are overlaid, the anteroposterior film of the neck, taken before barium consumption and with the mouth closed, is typically not helpful for this, but we perform it in our clinical routine. The vestibules fill with air during the Valsalva maneuver, and, occasionally, aberrant soft tissue densities can be seen. When the mouth is open, the inner part of the oral cavity and the tongue with its central groove can be clearly seen. Nevertheless, this anteroposterior view is often used to verify the existence of a specific lesion that has already been discovered or, especially in a modified barium swallow impairment profile setting and after barium, to assess the symmetry

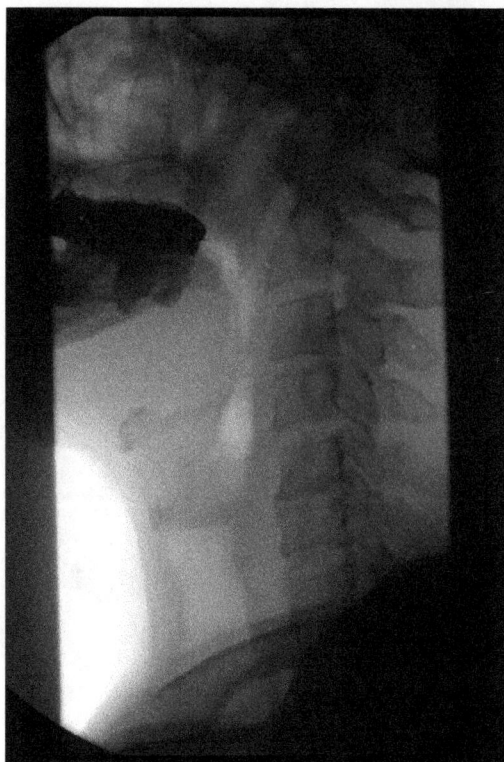

Figure 5.4 Palate roof.

of the swallow. The identification of salivary calculi is another application for this projection. A barium bolus is seen to lie between the tongue's dorsal surface and the palate's roof in the antero-posterior projection (Figure 5.5). Additionally, barium fills the inner oral cavity's lateral recesses (Figure 5.6). Some barium may also be seen in the oropharynx and lateral ventricles upon swallowing. Following swallowing, a residual layer of barium surrounds the posterior molar recesses, the lateral ventricles, and the dorsum of the tongue; the dorsal surface of the tongue and oropharynx is highlighted by a thin layer of leftover barium (Figure 5.7). Sometimes, the bolus is seen as a straight column as it descends into the oropharynx (Figure 5.8). During and after a barium swallow, oblique films of the oropharyngeal region are also highly helpful in identifying anomalies.

5.2.2 Nasal Cavity

With the mouth shut, the nasopharynx is often delineated by air on a simple lateral film of the neck (Figure 5.2). The nasopharynx is a recess that extends into the oropharynx and hypopharynx from the base of the skull, behind the uvula and soft palate. Sometimes a calcified stylohyoid ligament would split it in two. Except for a tiny section just posterior to the uvula at the point of contact between the soft palate and the posterior pharyngeal wall, the nasopharynx is typically not opacified after barium intake, particularly at the height of the swallowing action. This functional point can result in a pseudodiverticulum or a shadow that resembles a beak (Figure 5.9). Barium regurgitation into the nasopharynx is an aberrant finding that suggests inadequate muscular coordination. The nasal cavity and cervical spine's superimposed shadows make it difficult to see the oropharynx and nasopharynx in the anteroposterior view of the mouth.

5.2.3 Oropharynx

A simple lateral film of the neck provides the greatest definition of the oropharynx (Figure 5.2). It is best to take films while at rest and when the dry swallow is at its peak [3]. The air column in this region typically provides a clear outline of the posterior pharyngeal wall, the base of the tongue, the valleculae, and the tip of the epiglottis. The degree of movement can be measured at the height of the swallowing process. It is also possible to identify abnormal soft tissue masses. Delineating

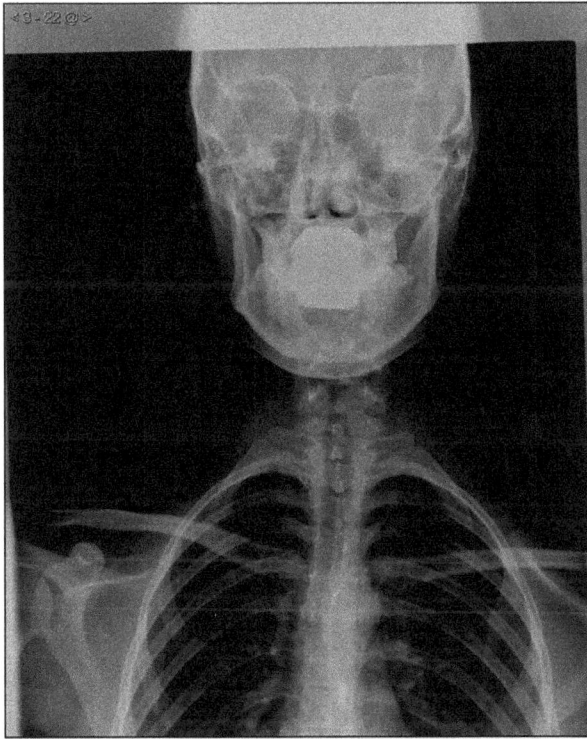

Figure 5.5 Anteroposterior projection.

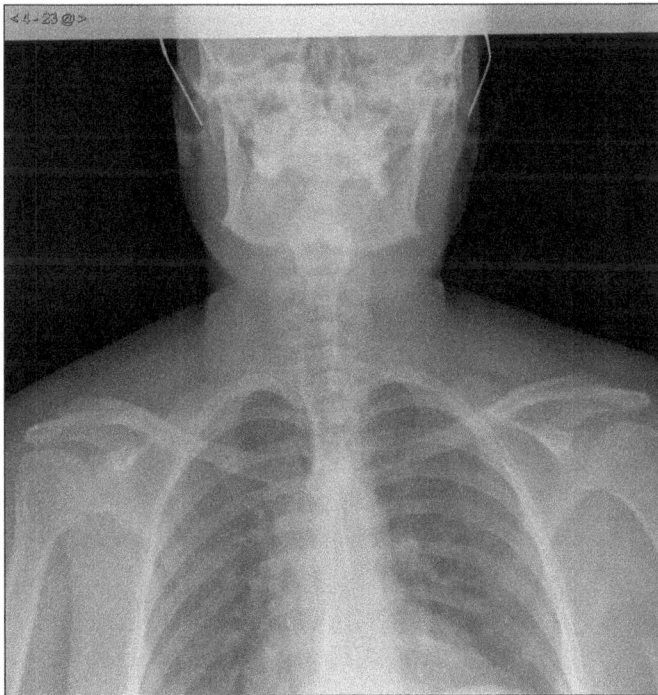

Figure 5.6 Barium fills mouth lateral recesses.

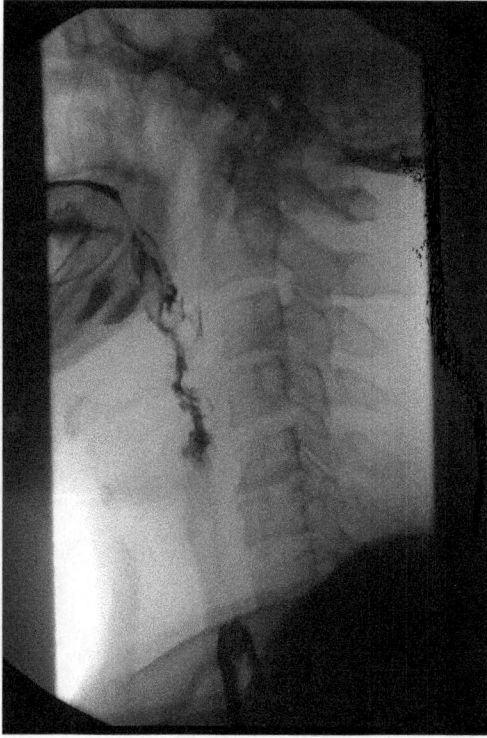

Figure 5.7 Residual barium after swallow.

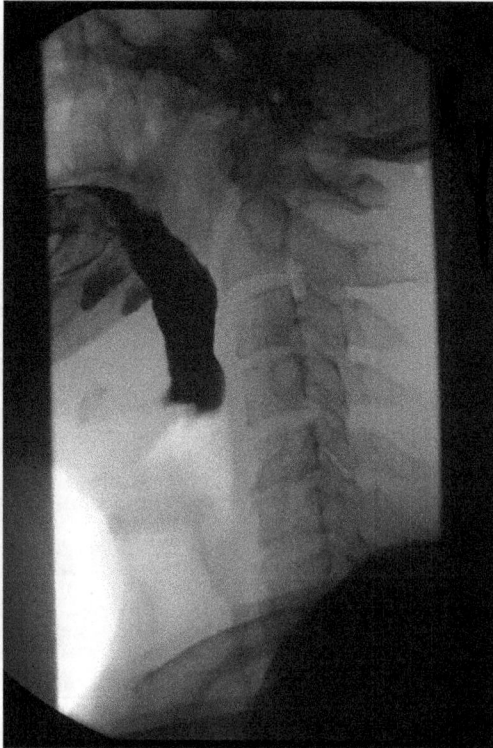

Figure 5.8 Barium column through oropharynx.

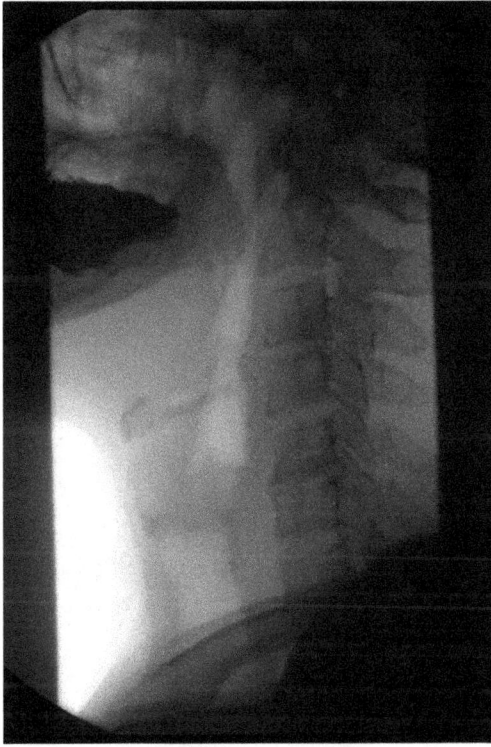

Figure 5.9 Beak-like radio transparency of the nasopharynx.

the surrounding soft tissues can be accomplished with the help of a film made during the Valsalva maneuver, which overdistends the oropharynx with air. Lateral films exposed at the height of a swallow following barium consumption may also show aberrant masses. The inverted epiglottis, which is folded across the glottis introitus, may now be seen outlined inside the barium column due to the opacification of the valleculae (Figure 5.10). The rear surface of the tongue, the valleculae, and the posterior pharyngeal wall will be well defined by any remaining barium after the bolus has been swallowed (Figure 5.11). The mandible's superimposed shadow largely obscures the oropharynx in anteroposterior plain films. A solid, flattened column of barium represents the oropharynx during a barium swallow as it descends to reach the posterior wall of the hypopharynx (Figure 5.12). This region is coated with residual barium following bolus passage; however, the degree of tonicity of the thyrohyoid ligaments, the thickness and length of the patient's neck, the angle of projection, and the amount of residual barium retained in the valleculae all affect how visible the oropharyngeal structures are.

5.2.4 Hypopharynx

There are upper and lower parts of the hypopharynx on the lateral plain neck film (Figure 5.2) [4]. The air-filled top part reaches into the open larynx and trachea and is continuous with the oropharynx. Anteriorly, the valleculae, epiglottis, and laryngeal introitus are typically clearly defined. The pharyngeal and oropharyngeal walls are connected posteriorly. Because the larynx presses against the cervical spine, the inferior part of the hypopharynx is airless. A thickened postcricoid soft tissue density is often how it is seen. Even in the absence of cricoid cartilage calcification, the lower pole of the cartilage extends posteriorly into the subglottic region, creating a soft tissue impression inside the air column. The cervical spine, laryngeal cartilages, and hyoid bone are typically so heavily overlaid in an anteroposterior plain film that the hypopharynx is not clearly defined. The lateral position during bolus ingestion causes the hypopharynx to inflate superiorly and narrow inferiorly where it enters the gaping sphincter, resembling an irregular funnel at the height of swallowing. With the exception of the lowest cricopharyngeal impression (Figure 5.13), which must be distinguished from an advancing peristaltic primary wave often seen at a higher level, the posterior wall

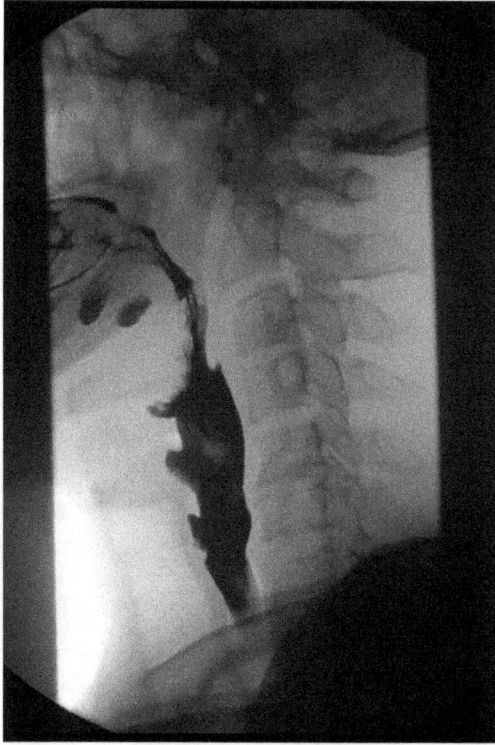

Figure 5.10 Epiglottis.

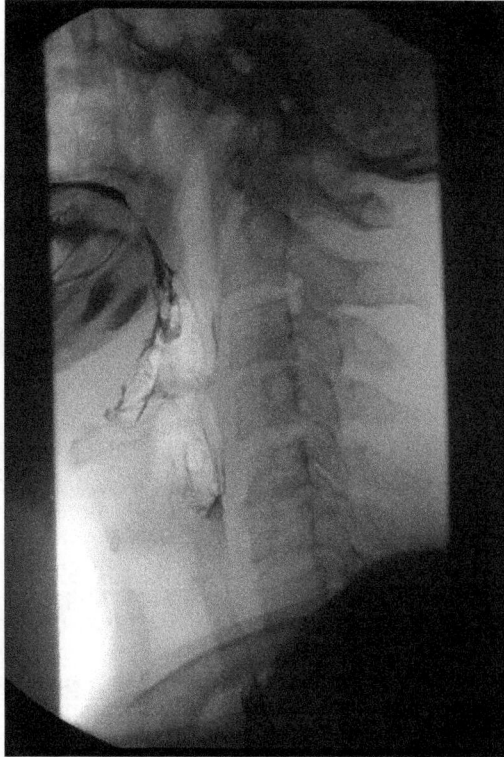

Figure 5.11 Barium residue on the valleculae.

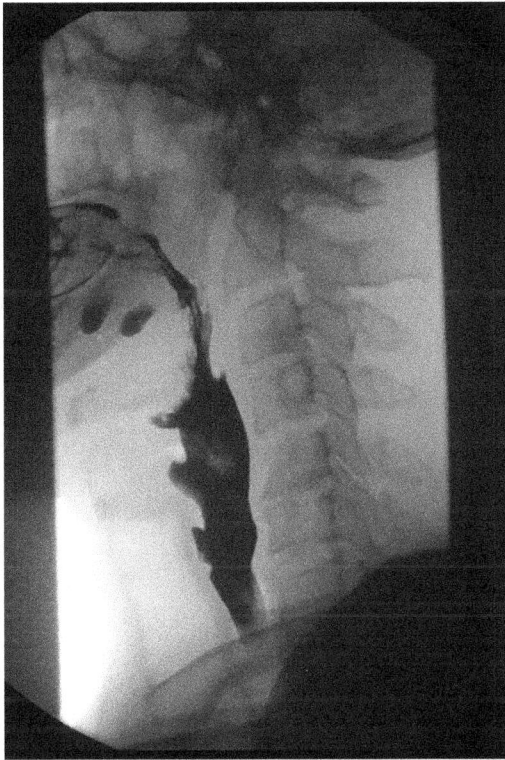

Figure 5.12   Barium through hypopharynx.

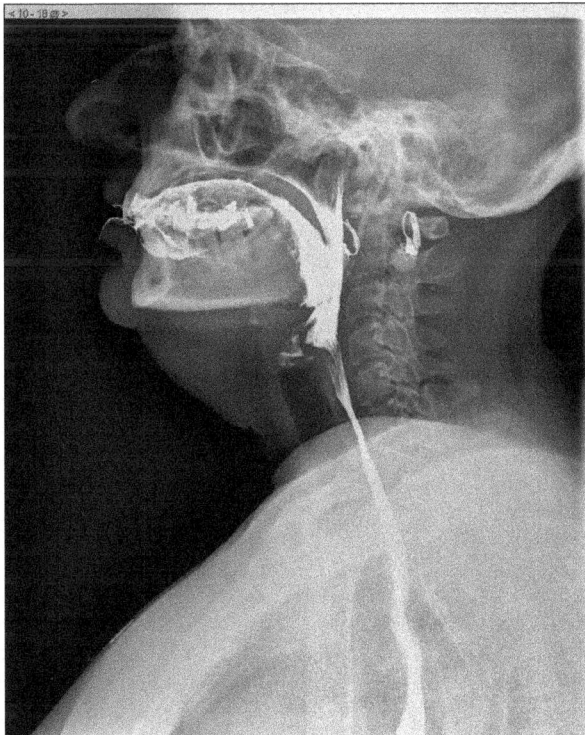

Figure 5.13   Cricopharyngeal impression.

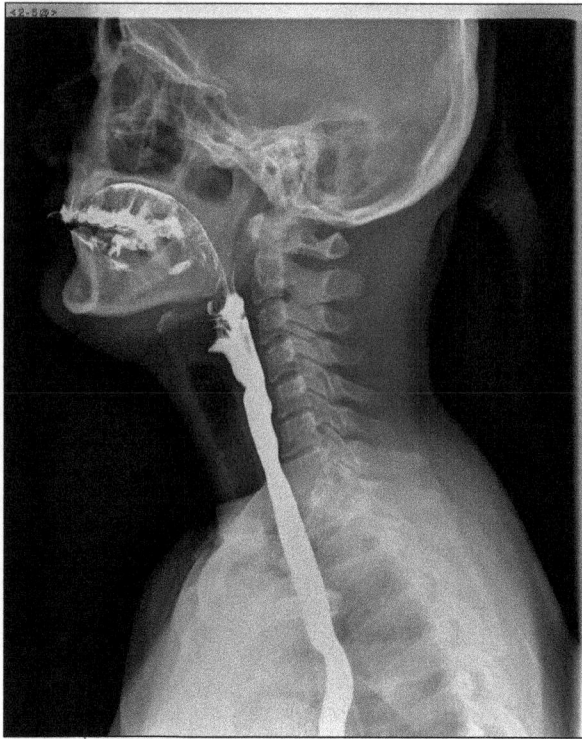

Figure 5.14 Pharyngoesophageal junction.

of the hypopharynx appears smooth and straight. The closed laryngeal introitus causes irregularity in the upper section of the hypopharynx's anterior wall. The impression of the cricoid lamina and the superimposed shadows of the pyriform fossae or lateral channels also generate irregularity in the lower part of the anterior wall. Because of the thickened, redundant mucosa and the engorged venous channels that are frequently present routinely in this location, the impression of the cricoid lamina may seem as an uneven anterior mucosal defect or even mimic a tumor. A tiny irregular incisura or notch at the pharyngoesophageal junction can be seen at the level of the lower pole of the cricoid lamina (Figure 5.14). The posterior cricopharyngeal impression can range from a prominent semilunar indentation to a small anterior bend in the posterior column. The lower or postcricoid part of the hypopharynx is seen as a linear channel coated by the retained barium in the compressed mucosal folds in the lateral view that is taken soon after the barium bolus is consumed with the mouth closed. At the pharyngoesophageal junction, a tiny quantity of retained barium at the lower end of this channel above the typically closed sphincter may resemble a pseudodiverticulum (Figure 5.15). Barium in the hypopharyngeal region opacifies the valleculae, which show up as two opaque pockets on anteroposterior views (Figure 5.16). Because of the "folded over" epiglottis, opacification is not complete below this point. Normal hypopharyngeal bulges, sometimes called "ears," can be seen laterally in the frontal plane views. These "ears" are the result of the thyrohyoid ligaments stretching into the pyriform fossae, which in turn lead into the postcricoid lamina and the last segment of the funnel-shaped segment of the hypopharynx. The region of the pyriform sinuses may occasionally exhibit normal lateral notchings. Due to rotation and the potential asymmetry brought on by uneven barium retention, these notches can be misinterpreted for webs if only one side is visible. Two symmetrical pockets at the base of the tongue are typically the clearest definition of the valleculae (Figure 5.16). The inverted epiglottis may have a star-like appearance when a swallow is at its tallest. If the typical epiglottis is covered with leftover barium when at repose, it may occasionally be delineated (Figure 5.10). The lateral "ears" mentioned previously are emphasized by the lateral air-filled bulges created in the upper lateral channel by films exposed during the Valsalva maneuver (Figure 5.17).

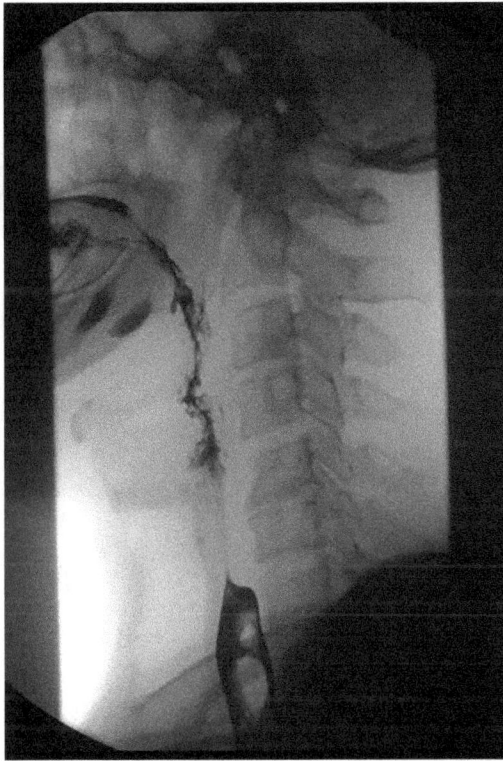

Figure 5.15 Residue at the pharyngoesophageal junction.

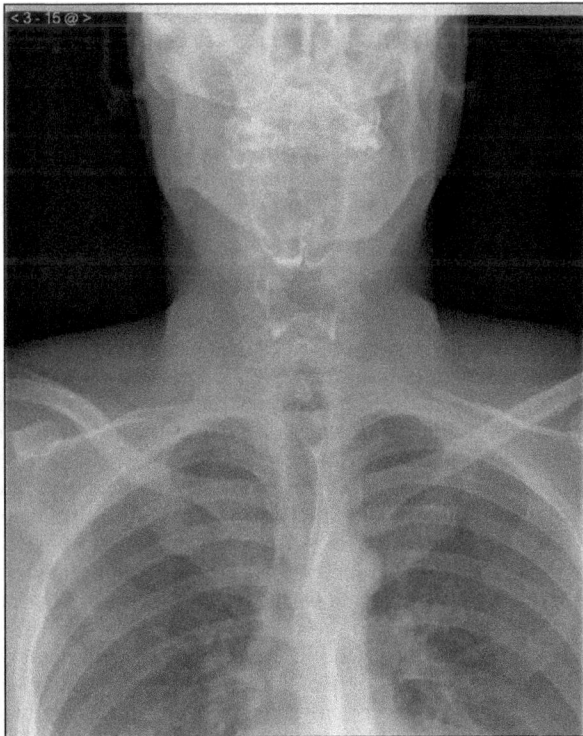

Figure 5.16 Anteroposterior projection.

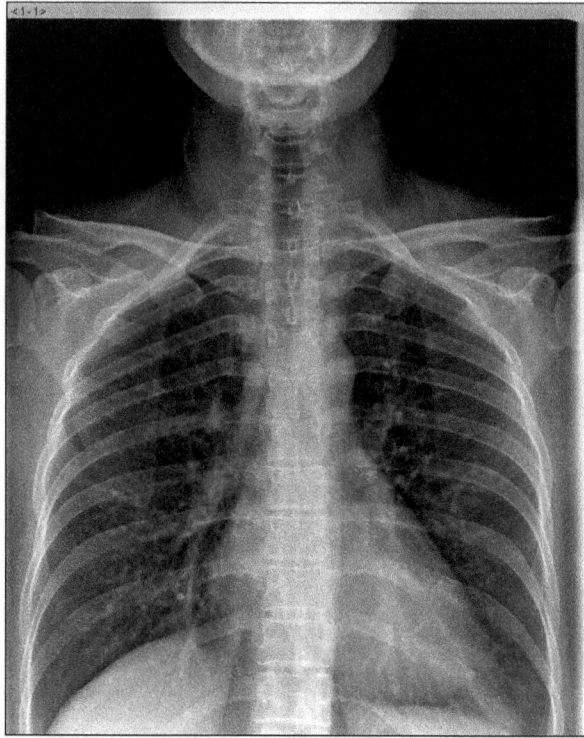

Figure 5.17 Valsalva maneuver, anteroposterior projection.

5.2.5 Pharyngoesophageal Junction

Normally, an opaque substance must be consumed in order to visualize the pharyngoesophageal junction [5]. A posterior depression that represents the cricopharyngeal impression and partially corresponds to the cricopharyngeal muscle may be observed in the lateral images during the height of a barium swallow. The pharyngoesophageal sphincter, which extends 1–2 cm below the cricopharyngeus muscle, is thought to be represented by the cricopharyngeal muscle, according to recent anatomical investigations. It is possible that this posterior indentation is a component of the sphincter's posterior top wall. A tiny quantity of retained barium above the level of the constricted sphincter indicates the pharyngoesophageal junction at rest after the barium bolus has passed (Figure 5.15).

5.2.6 Pharyngoesophageal Sphincter

At around 2 cm in length, the pharyngoesophageal sphincter is the cervical esophageal section that is closest to the throat. The thickened region of soft tissue that is just below the level of the lower pole of the cricoid cartilage and is continuous with the empty lower hypopharynx is known as the sphincter zone in the lateral plain film of the neck when it is at rest. Air trapped in the cervical esophagus can occasionally fill the lower level of the typically contracted pharyngoesophageal sphincter, which is situated several centimeters distal to the lower pole of the cricoid cartilage (Figure 5.18). This contracted section, which corresponds to the sphincter zone, is typically seen in lateral films taken after ingesting a barium bolus (Figure 5.19). The abrupt distension with barium of the cervical esophagus just below the contracted sphincter segment can be used to identify the location of the distal end of the constricted sphincter. Occasionally, a noticeable bulge produced by the barium bolus as it passes through the sphincter at the height of the swallow can be used to identify the dilated sphincter segment. In the partially relaxed sphincter zone, a barium-delineated crinkled mucosal pattern may occasionally be observed (Figure 5.20). As the sphincter closes, this odd abnormality goes away. The visible constricted sphincter sometimes creates a concave depression at and below the level of the cricoid lamina's lower pole during the Valsalva maneuver. Acute flexion of the

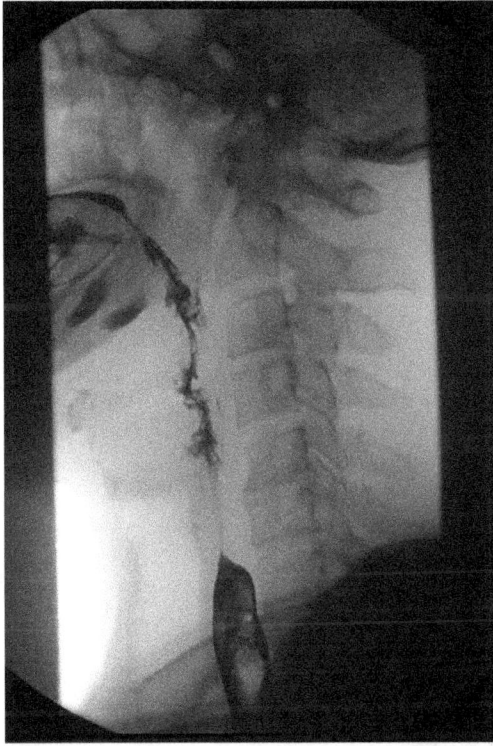

Figure 5.18 Air in the cervical esophagus.

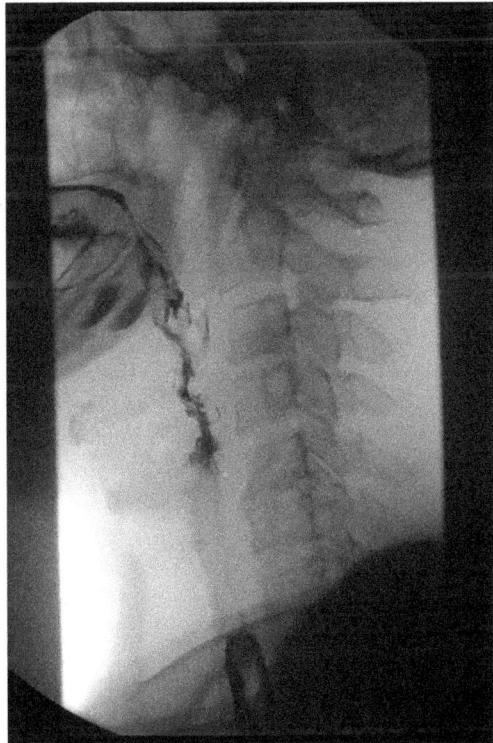

Figure 5.19 Contracted pharyngoesophageal sphincter.

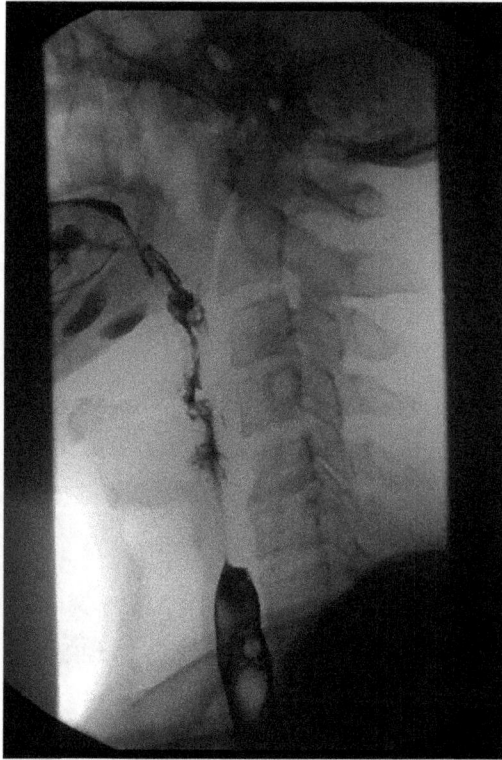

Figure 5.20 Crinkled pattern of the closed pharyngoesophageal sphincter.

contracted sphincter segment as it is displaceable downward by the larynx against the fixed cervical esophagus creates the lower and longer segment of this concavity, while the transverse fibers of the cricopharyngeus muscle create the upper portion. The nonopacified sphincter zone is not visible in anteroposterior images. The sphincter is a constricted, slightly flattened segment located at the level of the sixth and seventh cervical vertebrae after barium consumption. Common observations include distension of the lower cervical esophagus with barium just below the sphincter and stasis of barium at the upper level of the sphincter zone (Figure 5.15). The bolus-stretched dilated sphincter zone at the height of a swallow resembles a funnel's nozzle and infrequently manifests as a localized protrusion. Bilateral distension of the pyriform sinuses and lateral channels is observed during the Valsalva maneuver. When swallowing, the flattened, contracted sphincter zone is visible at a somewhat higher level than when at rest.

5.2.7 Cervical Esophagus (Figure 5.21: 1)

In those with short necks, the clavicle may completely cover the cervical esophageal region beneath the sphincter zone in the plain lateral film of the neck. A column of thickened soft tissue that lies posterior to the trachea and is continuous with the sphincter zone is observed in the typical patient. The connection of the neck's outer long muscles may mask this feature. In order to see if the cervical esophagus contains air, it is retracted superiorly at the height of a dry swallow. Coincidentally, the air-filled lung apices may also extend over the thoracic intake. When barium is consumed, the bolus causes the cervical esophagus distal to the sphincter zone to swell and appear as a solid, opaque column that is continuous with the thoracic esophagus. On rare occasions, the dilated upper sphincter might be seen. Oblique ridges, which may have been created by the underlying muscles, have occasionally been observed above the inlet. Following bolus transit, parallel mucosal folds that are continuous with the thoracic esophageal folds and delineated by barium are observed. The cervical esophagus cannot be seen in anteroposterior views without opaque media. After a barium swallow, the esophagus below the sphincter zone appears as a somewhat left-of-the-midline, dilated, opaque column that is continuous with the thoracic esophagus.

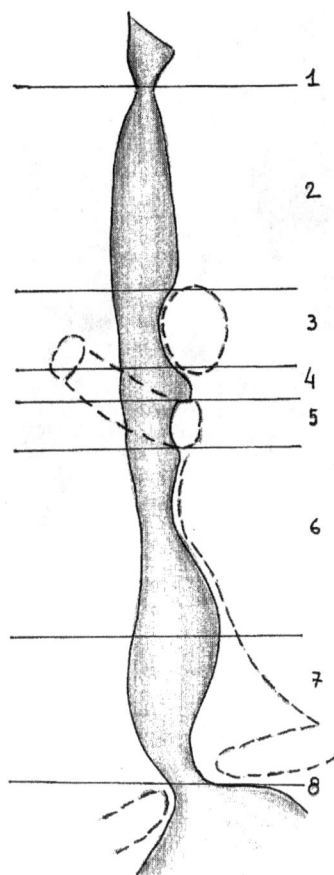

Figure 5.21 Topographic anatomy of the esophagus according to Dr. Marcel Brombart.

5.2.8 Thoracic Esophagus

The following are the segments of the thoracic esophagus [6] as seen in Figure 5.21:

The diaphragmatic tunnel and the abdomen contain a portion of the lower sphincter zone, also known as the abdominal section. The surrounding structures of the thoracic esophagus define its shape and orientation. Normal esophageal indentations and compressions are caused by a number of these structures, which are reviewed to help locate and characterize aberrant findings later on. A tiny quantity of barium should be administered to identify these typical compressions and indentations in order to prevent the esophagus from becoming overfilled and obliterating them.

Paratracheal (2): Spanning from the upper edge of the aortic arch to the thoracic inlet. The thoracic esophagus's supraaortic portion, which runs from the thoracic inlet to the aortic arch, is supported laterally by the pleura and carotid sheaths and their arteries and posteriorly by the prevertebral fascia. This segment runs through the mediastinum somewhat to the left of the trachea and is attached to it anteriorly. On radiologic examination, this segment of the esophagus sometimes exhibits an oblique, linear lucency on its right border due to compression by the trachea (Figure 5.22). In people with narrow thoracic inlets, this observation is more noticeable in the right anterior oblique position.

Aortic (3): Spanning from the tracheal bifurcation's upper border to the aortic arch's top border. The aortic arch impression at the level of the third and fourth thoracic vertebrae is a characteristic of the aortic segment of the thoracic esophagus. A semilunar depression on the left side of the esophagus reflects this aortic impression on radiologic examination (Figure 5.23). The size of the arch and the

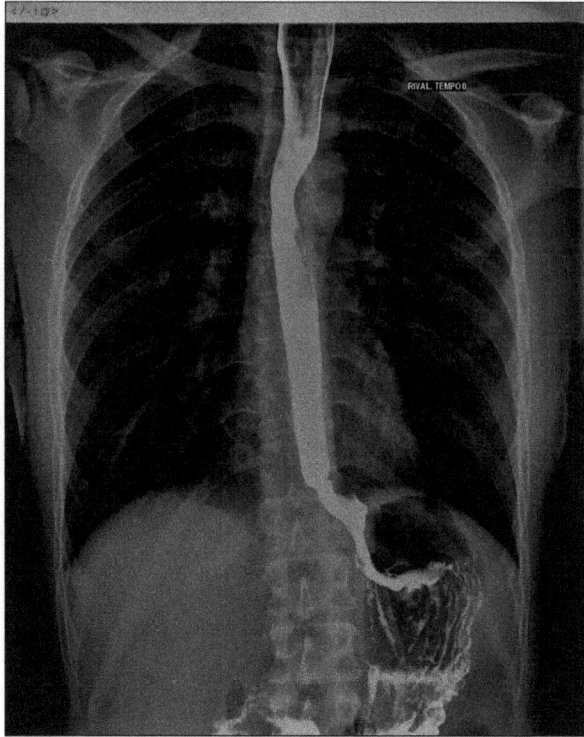

Figure 5.22 Paratracheal portion of the esophagus.

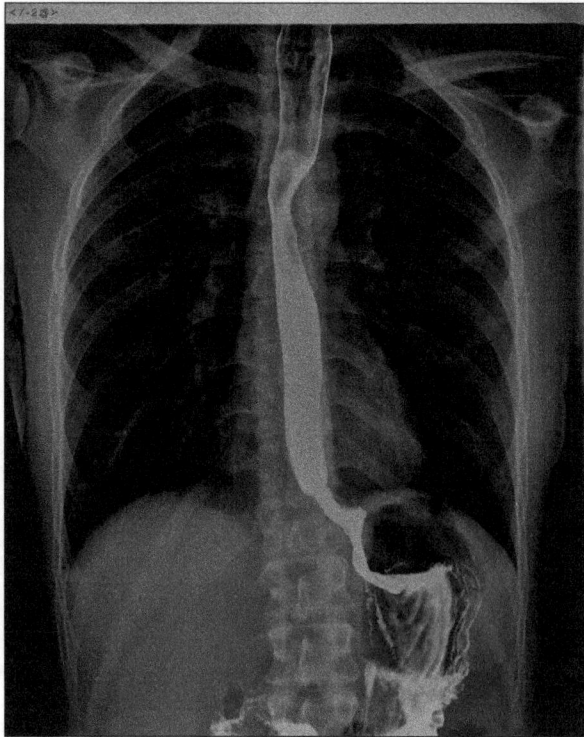

Figure 5.23 Aortic portion.

subject's age affect the degree of indentation. The indentation is slight and unnoticeable in newborns and youngsters whose aorta is underdeveloped. Notching may be observed at the site of compression due to wrinkling of the mucosal pattern in the elderly, especially in the presence of atheromatous alterations. It is recommended to take typical PA frontal, right oblique, left oblique, and lateral views in order to analyze this area and rule out a vascular ring or aberrant arteries.

Aorto-bronchial (4): Between the aortic and bronchial segments.

Bronchial (5): Spanning from the left major bronchus's lower border to the tracheal bifurcation's upper border.

The aortic-bronchial triangle, the bronchial impression, and the interbronchial segment are the three divisions of the thoracic esophageal bronchial segment. The portion of the esophagus that is partially divided by the upper and lower borders of the left main bronchus as it crosses the esophagus from right to left is known as the aortic-bronchial triangle. In older individuals, this segment becomes more noticeable, especially when pulmonary emphysema is present and the bronchial impression is enlarged. A pseudodiverticulum is seen on a barium swallow as a result of the indentations created in this triangle; this is particularly apparent when the swallow is positioned right anteriorly oblique (Figure 5.24). As the left main bronchus descends obliquely to the left and posteriorly from the tracheobronchial bifurcation anterior to the esophagus, it creates the bronchial impression (Figure 5.25). The greatest place to see this depression is between the sixth and eighth thoracic vertebrae. The transparent tubular zone produced by the left main bronchus, which is best seen in frontal and right anterior oblique postures, is accompanied by an area of partial esophageal filling on barium swallow that is proportionate to the extent and degree of the bronchus's impression. The imprint on the esophagus will be larger the more acute the angle at the tracheobronchial bifurcation. The interbronchial segment runs from the upper border of the left main bronchus to the level of the trachea's bifurcation. This area is typically surrounded by chains of lymph nodes.

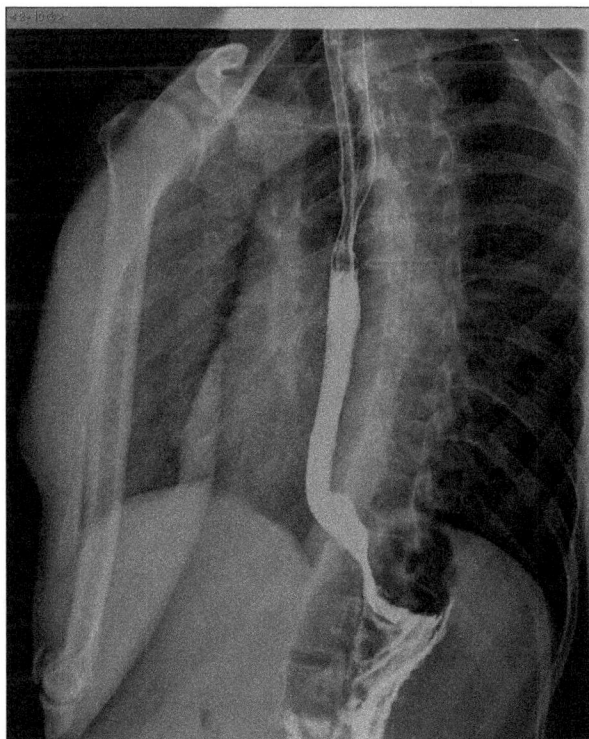

Figure 5.24   Bronchial portion.

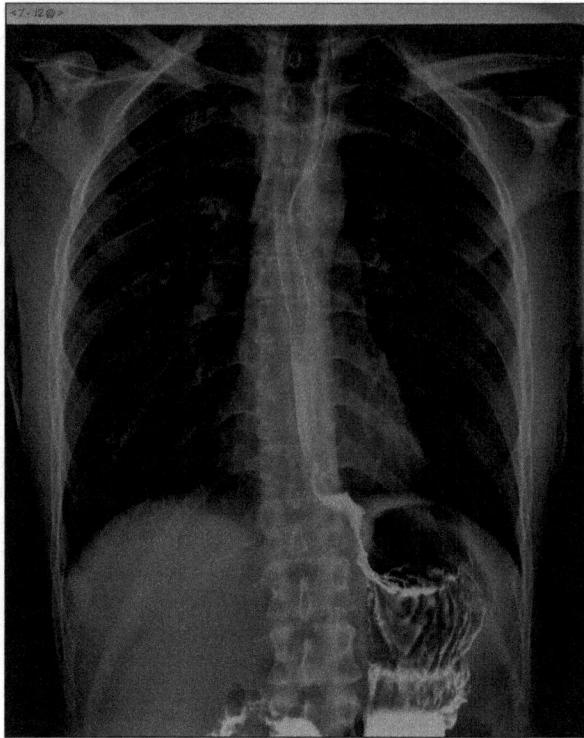

Figure 5.25 Bronchial portion.

Retrocardiac (6): Reaches the level of the left lateral deviation of the lower esophagus from the upper border of the left main bronchus. The part of the pericardial sac that covers the back of the left atrium and left ventricle is near the retrocardiac segment of the thoracic esophagus. In this instance, the esophagus passes from left to right in front of the thoracic aorta. This area often does not induce esophageal compression.

Epiphrenic (7): Spans from the esophageal hiatus's upper diaphragmatic level to the left lateral deviation. As the thoracic esophagus curves once more to the left to enter the esophageal hiatus of the diaphragm, the epiphrenic segment is the most inferior part of the esophagus. The vagal nerves accompany this segment, which also comes into contact with the pleura. A characteristic dilatation, referred to as the "phrenic ampulla," is noted on a barium swallow at the height of sustained full inspiration. The phrenic ampulla represents a physiologic dilatation of the lower end of the thoracic esophagus, observed best in the barium-filled esophagus during sustained inspiration (Figure 5.26). The mucosa of the base of the phrenic ampulla, which is located at the level of the superior attachment of the phrenoesophageal membrane, usually appears puckered. This dilated segment is produced by (a) stasis of barium at this level caused by the occluding action of the inferior pull of the membrane that is fixed to the diaphragm and (b) by the contraction of the lower esophageal sphincter within the esophageal hiatus. The base of the ampulla represents the upper portion of the sphincter zone. The shape and size of the ampulla vary with the degree of distension by the barium within it. The level of the apex of the ampulla depends also on the amount of barium in the distal esophagus. The phrenic ampulla is best visualized in the prone right anterior oblique position and may not even be demonstrated in erect individuals because of the effects of gravity. The ampulla is better demonstrated with thick rather than with thin barium and is more commonly observed in older people. Because the ampulla is produced by normal physiologic and anatomic factors, its demonstrated presence is of no clinical significance.

5.2.9 Lower Esophageal Sphincter Zone

The lower esophageal vestibular complex or the lower sphincter of the esophagus corresponds to Lerche's vestibule, being located partly within the esophageal hiatus and partly within the

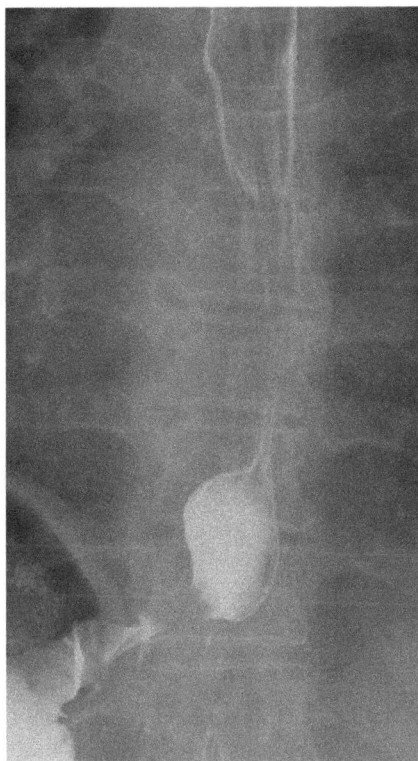

Figure 5.26 Ampulla epiphrenica.

abdomen. This lower esophageal sphincter corresponds to the abdominal segment of the esophagus. The sphincter zone extends from the superior attachment of the phrenoesophageal membrane to the inferior attachment of this membrane, which is at the site of the gastroesophageal junction. The sphincter is normally 2–3 cm long but may be longer, as demonstrated in pneumoperitoneum studies. However, it may appear shorter in the presence of a hiatal hernia. This sphincter is normally contracted, relaxing and opening completely as a bolus approaches it. This opening is caused partly by reflex action and also by the mechanical relaxation of the surrounding phrenoesophageal membrane. The lower sphincter in its dilated phase presents as an ovoid area directly above the gastroesophageal junction (Figure 5.27). The mucosal pattern of the sphincter zone is indistinguishable from the rest of the thoracic esophagus in its relaxed state, consisting of smooth, parallel folds. The radiologic appearance of this segment may vary slightly with position or angulation and is observed best in the prone right anterior oblique position. In anteroposterior views, it can be partially or completely obscured if the gastric fundus is overfilled with barium. In the right anterior oblique position, this sphincter zone can be identified through the air-filled fundus of the stomach. In posterioanterior views the sphincter zone is generally obscured by the barium-filled cardia. The size of this sphincter is also affected by respiratory action because this segment is held in position by the phrenoesophageal membrane within the esophageal hiatus. To some extent, therefore, the position varies with the respiratory phase of the diaphragm. It can also be seen in various stages of contraction or dilation.

5.2.10 Eesophageal Hiatus

As a fixed ring surrounded by the phrenoesophageal membrane, the esophageal hiatus can be seen as an ovoid translucency during radiologic examination, especially with tomography or when pneumoperitoneum is present. The location of the hiatus varies depending on the patient's position and respiratory phase, so it is not always at the point where the esophagus crosses the diaphragm's dome; in fact, it is typically inferior to this site. The thickened lip of the esophageal hiatus may result in a tumor-like indentation of the fundal side of the cardiac incisura.

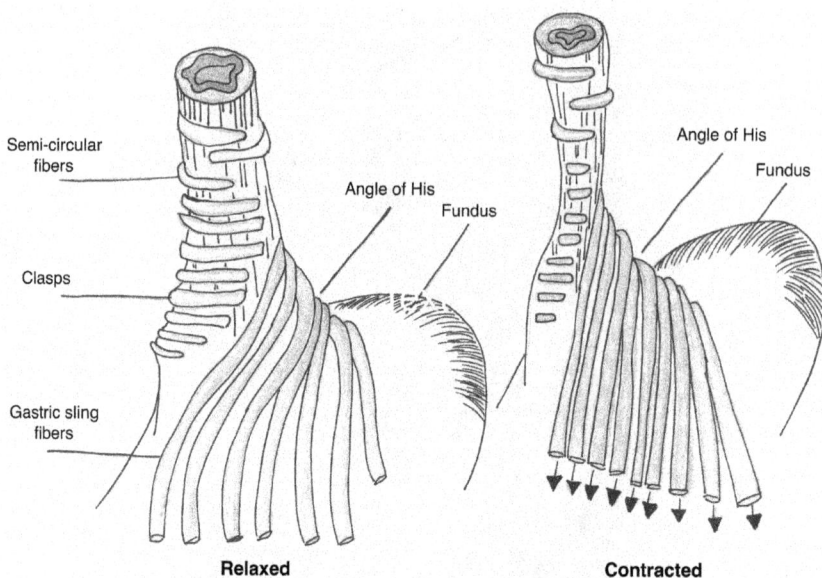

Figure 5.27 Lower esophageal sphincter.

5.2.11 Gastroesophageal Junction

The gastroesophageal junction, also known as the "epithelial line," is the location of the lower attachments of the phrenoesophageal membrane and Lerche's constrictor cardia. It can be seen radiologically as a ring, star, or spherical area through the stomach's air-filled cardia, particularly in the prone right anterior oblique position. Several stages of contraction are frequently observed. The radiologic junction is accompanied by the sign of the burnous, a cloak-like mucosal pattern brought on by contraction of the stomach's underlying oblique fibers (Figure 5.28).

5.2.12 Incisura and Stomach Cardia

The cardia is the portion of the stomach that is directly inferior to the gastroesophageal junction. The fundus represents the lateral and apical region of the stomach and is typically separated by the cardiac incisura. A high cardia can also produce a medial pouch that has been misdiagnosed as a hiatal hernia. The angle formed by the fundus of the stomach and abdominal esophagus varies depending on the patient's habitus from an almost vertical to a horizontal position. In oblique views, the cardiac incisura may appear as a notch or groove separating the barium-filled cardia and fundus (Figure 5.28)

5.2.13 Neck Stripes and Esophagus

The cervical prevertebral fat stripe represents adipose tissue in the retropharyngeal and retro-esophageal spaces. On radiologic examination of a plain lateral film of the cervical region, this stripe is observed as a longitudinal translucent line anterior to the cervical vertebrae. Its importance rests in its altered position secondary to spondylosis deformans, tumors of the cervical vertebrae, hemorrhage, or edema. Inflammatory changes of the prevertebral space may result in the blurring and forward displacement of the stripe. Calcifications posterior to the stripe should not be mistaken for foreign bodies of the orohypopharynx. Certain important mediastinal lines and stripes that can occasionally be identified on a PA view of the chest are related to the esophagus. The posterior mediastinal line is observed in the superior aortic triangle and is formed by the apposition of the pleural surfaces to the esophagus on the right side as projected through the air-filled trachea. The posterior mediastinal line is also referred to as the posterior superior esophageal pleural stripe. The anterior mediastinal line, formed by the combined densities of the visceral and parietal pleura of the right upper lobe, must be differentiated from the posterior mediastinal line. Although this anterior mediastinal line is also projected through the air-filled trachea, it lies more medial and nearer to the midline than the posterior mediastinal line. The posterior inferior stripe is projected

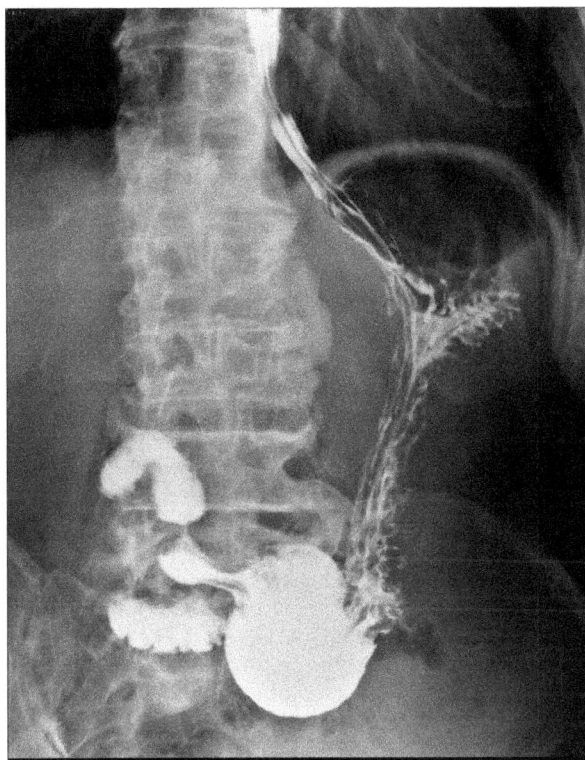

Figure 5.28   Esophageal junction and sign of the burnouse.

in the retrocardiac space and is produced by the intimate contact of the esophagus with the pleura on the right side. These stripes are observed optimally on tomographic examination rather than on plain chest films. Displacement of some of these stripes may occur in the presence of esophageal disorders.

5.3 THE ESOPHAGUS AND OROHYPOPHARYNX AS A FUNCTIONAL UNIT

In connection with these anatomic radiologic observations, the orohypopharynx and esophagus may be described as a physiologic unit as observed during fluoroscopy or during review of motion studies. With the patient in the prone right anterior oblique position, the following observations during fluoroscopy upon ingestion of a barium bolus warrant a detailed description [7].

As the thick barium bolus is held in the oral cavity, it is noted to lie anteriorly in the central groove of the tongue with the mouth and lips closed. As the patient swallows the barium, it is propelled posteriorly by the sweeping action of the tongue, first initiated by a forward and upward motion of this structure against the hard palate. The soft palate or uvula moves posteriorly to abut against a fold of the posterior wall of the pharynx (Passavant's ridge), occluding the nasopharynx. The posterior border of the bolus may appear somewhat irregular in contour as barium fills a small recess posterior to the uvula in the nasopharynx. Opacification of this recess results in a beak-like or pseudodiverticular appearance—a normal finding. As the bolus glides on the posterior wall or root of the tongue, it flattens this structure and pools in the back of the epiglottis filling the valleculae. As the swallowing act progresses, the larynx moves upward and anteriorly under the floor of the tongue, away from the path of the approaching bolus. This permits the epiglottis to be folded over posteriorly by the bolus, forming a partial lid to the laryngeal introitus. The bolus slows momentarily at this site because of the narrowed anteroposterior lumen produced by the folded epiglottis. As the bolus is propelled downward by the contractions of the superior constrictors and passes beyond the level of the epiglottis, this structure returns to its normal position. The bolus then enters the hypopharynx and open sphincter zone. The posterior advancing edge of the bolus passes across a broad indentation of variable length and depth, corresponding to the degree of prominence and contraction of the terminal fibers of the cricopharyngeus muscle (cricopharyngeal impression), just above the sphincter zone. A posterior wall impression in this region may also be produced by spondylosis of the cervical spine. The anterior edge of the bolus is observed posterior to the cricoid lamina. A number of normal irregularities that may produce a variable irregular anterior border can be identified as postcricoid impressions. Occasionally, at the lower pole of the cricoid lamina, a small inconsistent notch or incisura is noted. The bolus is then funneled into the open sphincter zone, with the posterior wall of the hypopharynx acting as a chute. The sphincter occasionally opens with a configuration resembling two open arms. This pattern is more often detected during repetitive swallows, when the mucosal lining has been coated with barium. The filled sphincter zone occasionally appears as a dilated ovoid shadow below the pharyngoesophageal junction. This junction is estimated to be at the level of a small anterior notch, directly below the level of the crico-pharyngeal impression or at the lower pole of the cricoid lamina. As soon as the bolus has passed the sphincter zone, the sphincter contracts, producing a narrowed segment several centimeters long and below the level of the lower pole of the cricoid lamina. Above the level of the contracted sphinc-ter, retained barium may simulate the appearance of a diverticulum at the pharyngoesophageal junction. Below the level of this contracted segment, the esophagus remains distended as the transit of the bolus is slowed at the thoracic inlet. As the bolus enters the supraaortic segment of the thoracic esophagus, an oblique ridge occasionally is noted below the thoracic inlet. This ridge is produced by compression by the trachea as the esophagus veers to the left. This is followed by the aortic impres-sion. The bolus hesitates momentarily at the aortic impression, especially if prominent tortuosity of the aorta exists. As the bolus progresses down the esophagus, the typical concave density of the aortic arch is observed, with its attendant aortic pulsations. Directly below the aortic impres-sion, a pseudodiverticular pocket occasionally may be noted, especially in the elderly, because of retained barium in the esophageal aortic-bronchial triangle. The next impression is that of the left main bronchus as it crosses obliquely against the esophagus, producing a translucent tubular ridge. The bolus then reaches the retrocardiac segment of the esophagus, which is characterized by the presence of cardiac pulsations. Here the barium bolus hesitates again, but momentarily, at the lower end of the thoracic esophagus, above the level of the diaphragm. If the patient then inspires deeply, the bolus usually does not enter the stomach but collects in the lower esophagus above the level of the diaphragm, producing a pear-shaped opacity with its apex at the top—the phrenic ampulla [8]. This ampulla collapses suddenly when normal respiration is resumed. An additional dilated pocket occasionally is noted directly below the phrenic ampulla, corresponding to the dilated vestibule or lower sphincter zone. This secondary pocket is normally within the esophageal hiatus or below the diaphragmatic dome and represents the abdominal esophageal segment. After this segment con-tracts, the bolus has entered the stomach. The contracted lower sphincter is now observed as a nar-rowed segment several centimeters long, similar in appearance to the contracted upper sphincter. The gastroesophageal junction can then be identified as the most distal end of the contracted seg-ment, resembling a small star or a ring density through the air- and barium-coated mucosal pattern of the stomach. This anatomic finding is most apparent after the bolus has descended well beyond the cardia of the stomach. The oblique fibers surrounding the cardia of the stomach occasionally produce characteristic mucosal folds (sign of the burnouse). The cardiac incisura is occasionally noted through the air- and barium-filled stomach as a small vertical notch. Occasionally, a tumor-like indentation is noted on the fundal side of the cardiac incisura, because of a prominent lip of the anterior border of the right crus of the esophageal hiatus of the diaphragm. All these observations are generally not apparent during one primary peristaltic wave, following the synchronous contrac-tions of the constrictors of the pharynx. Additional swallows and changes in position may be neces-sary. As the thick bolus is propelled along, secondary waves appear, permitting complete expulsion of the barium after the bolus has emptied into the stomach. The presence of these secondary waves, producing total expulsion of the barium into the stomach, may be helpful in evaluating the normal functional response of the esophagus and in visualizing the normal mucosal pattern.

5.4 OUTSIDE ELEMENTS IMPACTING THE PHARYNGOESOPHAGEAL MUCOSAL PROFILE

The esophagus is located in the posterior mediastinum, which means that opacification of the esophagus can be used to evaluate a variety of disorders and lesions of this region [8]. This chapter discusses the external and internal factors that mechanically displace, distort, compress, obstruct, or rupture the orohypopharynx and esophagus. The primary external structures and spaces that affect the orohypopharynx are the retropharyngeal space, the thyroid and parathyroid glands, the trachea, and the cervical spine; the structures that surround the esophagus in the posterior mediastinal space include the heart, aortic arch, thoracic aorta, pleura and lungs, mediastinal lymph nodes, and the thoracic spine; the intrinsic abnormalities discussed here include foreign bodies, perforations, erosions, and lacerations.

5.4.1 Retropharyngeal Abscess

In infants up to 6 months of age, the thickness of the retropharyngeal soft tissues varies considerably with crying, phonation, and swallowing. In children, the thickness of the retropharyngeal space is normally about one-third the anteroposterior diameter of the body of the fourth cervical vertebra—a useful index in determining the presence and even the size of any retropharyngeal mass. The most common cause of a retropharyngeal abscess in infants and children is lymphadenitis secondary to acute tonsillitis. Other acute or chronic inflammatory causes, such as an undetected perforation from a foreign body or tuberculous cervical adenitis and retropharyngeal abscess, may be noted anterior to the retrovertebral space when its origin is pharyngeal. The mass is usually painful and in the acute stage can increase considerably in size within a relatively short time. Forward displacement of the larynx, trachea, and epiglottis is common, delineated with a barium swallow when the presence of a fistulous tract is excluded. If the abscess ruptures into the prevertebral space, spread into the mediastinum with resultant mediastinitis may be apparent. In infants, swelling in the prevertebral area must be differentiated from congenital cervical hygroma and in older children from lymphosarcoma. In the adult, an abscess in the prevertebral area is either acute or chronic. It may be secondary to lymphadenitis, although less frequently than in childhood. A chronic process may be caused by tuberculous or by brucellar or pyogenic spondylitis of the cervical spine. The cervical retropharyngeal stripe is blurred or displaced anteriorly by a paraspinal abscess and destructive changes of the cervical spine are noted. A barium swallow outlines a soft tissue mass located posteriorly. Calcified lymph nodes may accompany tuberculous spondylitis. On occasion, a perforated pharyngeal diverticulum may be the cause of a retropharyngeal abscess. On radiologic examination, with barium, part of the diverticulum may be opacified. Fistulous tracts and air in the retropharyngeal space are usually present. A retropharyngeal abscess in adults must be distinguished from a neoplasm. The latter, except for dysphagia, is often clinically silent and radiologically indistinguishable from an infective abscess. A retropharyngeal parathyroid adenoma may also simulate a retropharyngeal abscess.

5.4.2 Enlargement of the Thyroid Gland

The thyroid is located in the region of the pharyngoesophageal sphincter, above the thoracic inlet, and can enlarge uniformly, expanding in all directions, or asymmetrically if only one lobe is affected. The posterior lobes of the gland extend backward on enlargement, partly surrounding both the trachea and esophagus, or may grow posteriorly between the trachea and esophagus; the thyroid may also extend substernally and intrathoracically; calcification may be seen in the thyroid in a number of disorders, such as thyroid adenoma.

5.4.2.1 Thyrotoxicosis

Thyrotoxicosis is usually is associated with a uniform, symmetrical enlargement of the entire gland, resulting in a shallow compression of the trachea followed subsequently by compression of the esophagus. A lateral soft tissue Roentgenogram and anteroposterior view of the cervical region usually demonstrate a soft tissue mass constricting the trachea. Additional films should be obtained upon the ingestion of a barium bolus to exclude compression and/or deviation of the cervical esophagus. Fluoroscopic examination, particularly during a barium swallow, is very helpful in detecting esophageal compression and in confirming the upward and downward movement of the soft tissue mass, synchronous with swallowing. Spasm of the pharyngoesophageal sphincter may be noted if toxic myopathy is present. Following thyroidectomy, regrowth of the gland can take place with recurrent enlargement, particularly in the retroesophageal area. On these occasions, a distinct anterior displacement of the cervical esophagus will be observed.

5.4.3 Benign Nodular Struma

Benign nodular struma is usually asymmetrical. The process grows in one direction either laterally, anteriorly (substernal), or posteriorly (intrathoracic). Lateral enlargement can readily be detected on physical examination. Anterior enlargement usually occurs above the level of the sternal notch but can extend substernally. Posterior enlargement extends around both the trachea and esophagus, resulting in displacement of both structures. Further growth posteriorly may occur between the trachea and esophagus below the level of the sphincter zone, even extending intrathoracically. Radiologic examination with opacification of the esophagus is very helpful in the diagnosis. In the presence of a posterior intrathoracic goiter, a soft tissue mass is usually noted on the right side in the superior mediastinum. On plain films, compression and right-sided displacement of the trachea is noted. Fluoroscopic examination and/or films obtained upon ingestion of a thick barium bolus will show anterior displacement of the upper thoracic esophagus. The thoracic esophagus will be displaced posteriorly and the trachea anteriorly. The aortic arch may be depressed. A grid film of the superior mediastinum may delineate the reflection of the mediastinal pleura, below the level of the goiter. On fluoroscopy, the goiter is observed to move with swallowing, although this feature also may be simulated by an enterogenous cyst. Obstruction of the superior vena cava with resultant venous engorgement may also be present. A goiter must be differentiated from aneurysm of the innominate artery or aortic arch, neurogenic tumor, teratoid lesion, thymic mass, enlarged metastatic nodes from a bronchogenic carcinoma, or even a primary bronchogenic carcinoma itself. An intrathoracic goiter, however, is usually observed at a higher level in the mediastinum than with these lesions just mentioned, and the smooth localized displacement or compression of the opacified esophagus is quite distinctive of a goiter. The presence of a calcified mass in the area of the thyroid is helpful in making the diagnosis of a benign adenoma.

5.4.4 Malignant Neoplasm of the Thyroid

The presence of pin-sized, clumped calcification on films indicates the presence of psammoma bodies, which are associated with papillary carcinoma; on fluoroscopic examination, the soft tissue mass of an enlarged, asymmetrical thyroid gland exhibits rigidity, fixation, and irregularity, which suggest malignancy; and there may be significant compression and even partial obstruction of the cervical esophagus. Malignant changes of the thyroid gland may be difficult to detect.

5.4.5 Tumors of the Parathyroid

When there is clear clinical evidence of hyperparathyroidism, the radiologist plays a crucial role in localizing the parathyroid tumor. The cervical esophagus is slightly deviated in the anteroposterior views with a prominent crescent-like pressure defect of the esophageal wall between C7 and T2 and loss of its normal distensibility. Small thyroid adenomas may show similar findings; these are much more frequently calcified than parathyroid tumors, which are rarely calcified.

5.4.6 Spinal Cord

Spondylosis deformans (degenerative disease of the spine) and/or Forestier disease may demonstrate excessive osteophyte formation which can produce indentations and considerable encroachment on the posterior wall of the pharynx and cervical esophagus (Figure 5.29). Endoscopy in such instances may result in pharyngeal or esophageal tears, particularly if a rigid endoscope is used. In degenerative disease of the spine, the posterior esophageal membranes and fascial sheets may become fused by fibrous adhesions, affecting the musculature of the hypopharynx and cervical esophagus, and resulting in the formation of small localized traction diverticula. Such adhesions may also produce abnormalities of the swallowing mechanism and dysphagia, especially when the sphincter zone is involved. Fluoroscopic examination after a barium swallow is very helpful in determining the degree of fixation of the cervical esophagus affected by the changes of spondylosis deformans. Abnormal fixation with deviation of the pharyngoesophagus to right or left may occur. A cervicothoracic scoliosis also causes displacement and abnormal angulation of the cervical and upper thoracic vertebrae, secondarily affecting the pharyngoesophageal sphincter. Rheumatoid arthritis produces shortening of the neck caused by involvement of the intervertebral small joints and narrowing of the intervertebral disk, resulting in an apparent downward shift of the upper sphincter zone.

5.4.7 Thoracic Spine

Scoliosis, kyphosis, or kyphoscoliosis results in curvatures of the spine and displacement of the esophagus, thoracic aorta, and mediastinal structures. The thoracic aorta is fixed to the thoracic spine because of the intercostal arteries, causing the aorta to follow the spinal curvatures. The esophagus usually accompanies the descending aorta with which it is intimately connected. Depending on the presence or absence of adhesions produced by aortitis, other inflammatory causes, or the aging process, the esophagus, aside from following the aorta and spinal curvature, may remain as a straight tube apparently suspended in the mediastinum. When the esophagus accompanies the

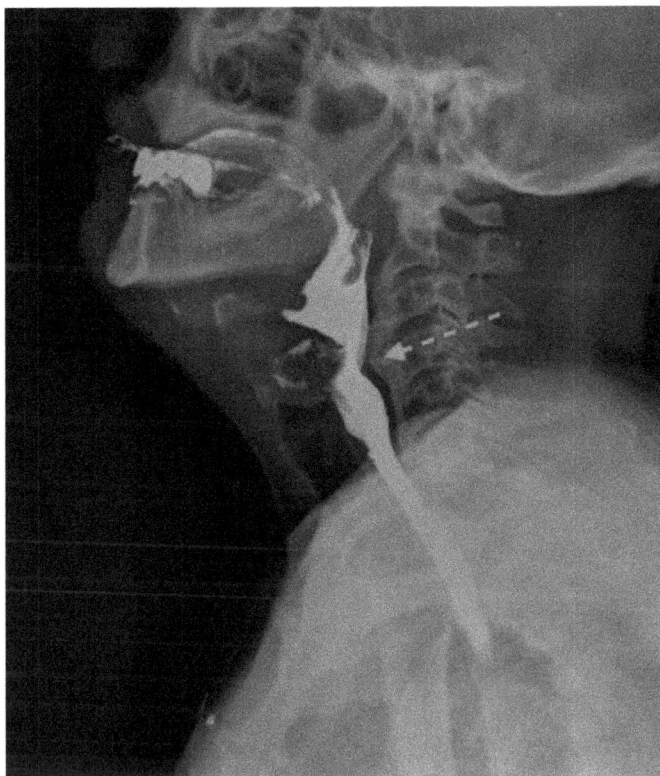

Figure 5.29 Forestier disease.

spine and aorta, it may become redundant and exhibit abnormal kinks and deviations contributed by the effects of the other mediastinal structures. In the presence of kyphoscoliosis and a rigid atheromatous thoracic aorta, the esophagus may be displaced into the posterior portion of the lower left hemithorax, producing a sharp angulation of its distal end. The aorta is then identified in the right anterior oblique position "en face," as a spheroid soft tissue mass or as a calcified density above the diaphragm, displacing the esophagus laterally. In the presence of shortening of the esophagus and laxity of the phrenoesophageal membrane, which is common in elderly individuals, a sliding-type hiatal hernia is usually observed. In infective lesions of the spine, especially tuberculosis associated with a paraspinal abscess, the esophagus becomes fixed in position contiguous with the spinal disorder. Erosions into the esophagus may even result in the formation of an esophageal fistula. Extramedullary hematopoiesis or a fractured vertebral body resulting in a paravertebral hematoma may compress or displace the esophagus. Degenerative changes of the thoracic spine (spondylosis deformans) may also be responsible for esophageal indentations, similar to those seen in Figure 5.29.

5.4.8 Left Atrium

The left atrium is located posteriorly, being in close contact with the middle third of the esophagus. No deviation or compression of the esophagus is created by a normal left atrium. In early enlargement of the left atrium, the anterior wall of the opacified esophagus is observed to be minimally indented. This indentation can escape observation in the standard right anterior oblique position, frequently obtained to detect left atrial enlargement. The presence of left atrial enlargement, however, may be diagnosed more accurately in an upright left lateral chest film, exposed in deep inspiration. With progressive enlargement, an additional posterior displacement of this portion of the esophagus occurs with obliteration of the normal space between the esophagus and spine. With further enlargement, more marked displacement of this segment of the esophagus to the right occurs, with widening of the angle between the right and left main bronchus. These features are best observed in an overpenetrated posteroanterior film of the chest with a barium-opacified esophagus. A fluoroscopic sign has been described which may facilitate the diagnosis of mitral insufficiency.

This is referred to as the posterior wedging sign. Following a barium swallow, the esophagus is noted to be displaced to the right and the descending aorta to the left during ventricular systole in instances of mitral insufficiency. These findings result from the wedging action of a dilated left atrium. Occasionally, the esophagus is displaced to the left because of aortic, esophageal adhesions, or a mobile esophagus. Right atrial enlargement may produce a similar appearance.

5.4.9 Right Atrium

Although it is located posteriorly, the right atrium does not have direct contact with the normal esophagus. A dilated right atrium, which is frequently caused by tricuspid valvular disease, can cause the lower third of the esophagus to be compressed and displaced to the left; this abnormality is best shown in the posteroanterior and left anterior oblique views with an opacified esophagus. Unlike left atrial enlargement, the esophagus is not displaced posteriorly by an enlarged right atrium.

5.4.10 Both Atria

Compression from a tortuous aortic arch may cause left-sided indentation of the mid-esophagus, which usually begins at a higher level than that caused by enlargement of the left atrium, and the cardiac silhouette may be normal. Since these patients are typically older, the aortic arch frequently exhibits calcification in its wall. (See Section 5.4.15 on the aortic arch.) Enlargement of both the right and left atrium will deviate the esophagus posteriorly and to the right, creating a reverse three impression on the opacified esophagus in its middle third.

5.4.11 Left Ventricle

An enlarged left ventricle typically affects the lower third of the esophagus, which is in contact anteriorly with a small portion of the normal left ventricle, lying anterior and to the right of the descending aorta. The esophagus then turns sharply to the left to enter the stomach, leaving a clear space between the esophagus and the spine above the diaphragm. When the left ventricle enlarges, as is frequently seen in hypertensive and arteriosclerotic heart disease, the normally clear lower retrocardiac space disappears and the esophagus is in contact with the heart border down to the diaphragm.

5.4.12 Cardiomegalia

A number of congenital and acquired heart and vascular lesions can cause abnormal esophagograms, but their differential diagnosis is outside the purview of this book. Generalized cardiac enlargement can occur in heart failure, as well as in the presence of specific cardiomyopathies and a variety of systemic disorders (Figure 5.30, with type III achalasia, too). In these cases, the opacified lower third of the esophagus may be indented and displaced, without the typical symptoms of specific chamber enlargement.

5.4.13 Pericardial Effusion

Esophagograms show compression and displacement of the esophagus at a lower level than that produced by an enlarged left atrium, and pericardial effusion causes compression and deviation of the opacified esophagus, as well as the presence of acute cardiophrenic angles, elongation of the cardiac silhouette, and straightening of the left cardiac border in the plain chest film.

5.4.14 Thoracic Aorta and Aortic Arch

Degenerative and involutional changes of the aortic arch affect the normal esophageal indentation. In infants, an aortic impression is generally absent or relatively inconspicuous normally because of incomplete development. However, with increasing age, the aortic indentation becomes increasingly prominent. At the level of the fourth thoracic vertebra, the aortic arch passes inferiorly and posteriorly along the left side of the trachea and esophagus to the vertebral column, where it becomes the descending aorta. A partially obliterated esophageal impression caused by the aorta in the adult may be the result of aneurysm, fusiform dilation of the aorta, an elongated pulmonary artery, an uncoiled aortic arch, mitral disease, a mediastinal mass, spinal deformity, and other pathologic pulmonary or mediastinal diseases. An accentuated aortic arch, which is quite commonly calcified in older individuals and is caused chiefly by atheromatous and degenerative changes, creates the classic "ball-and-socket" appearance, as the aortic knob indents the opacified esophagus (Figure 5.23). The decending thoracic aorta usually becomes uncoiled, elongated, tortuous, and more rigid, depending on the degree and extent of calcific deposits in its wall. Compression

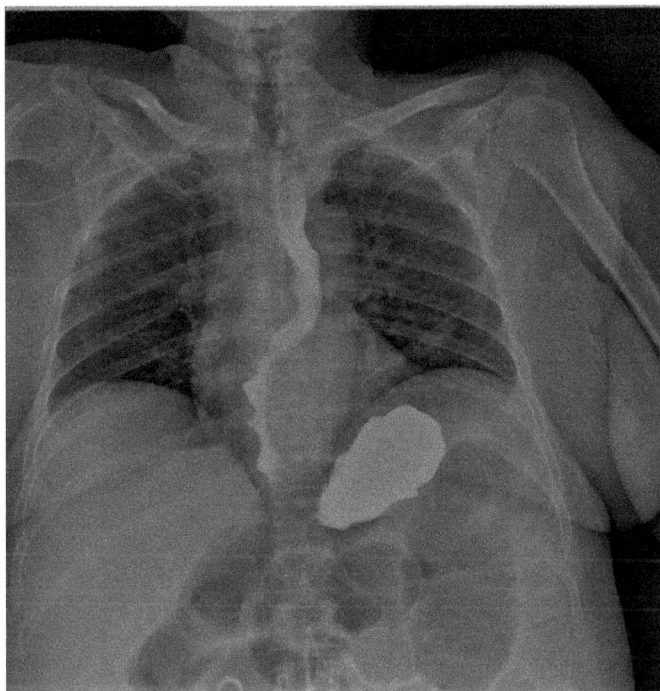

Figure 5.30 Cardiomegalia and achalasia.

of the mid-esophagus in such instances mimics the presence of a vascular ring. The descending aorta in advanced cases may resemble an inverted "S" and can indent the esophagus posteriorly, even narrowing its lower third, causing dilation above. Severe atheromatous changes of the aorta typically produce a rigid tube which may compress the esophagus and produce dysphagia. In the elderly patient, associated motor disturbances also may be present.

5.4.15 Arteria Lusoria

Arteria lusoria, also known as aberrant right subclavian arteries (ARSA), are very common aortic arch anomalies. Generally being the first branch to arise (with the right common carotid as the brachiocephalic artery), in this case it emerges on its own as the fourth branch, distal to the left subclavian artery. It then hooks back to reach the right side with its relationship to the esophagus variable (Figures 5.31 to 5.33).

5.4.16 Aneurysms

Aneurysms are caused by a number of disorders, notably syphilis and arteriosclerosis. Syphilis often involves the ascending aorta because of the underlying aortitis. Saccular or fusiform dilation of the ascending arch may produce compression or deviation of the esophagus. Aneurysms of syphilitic origin also occur in the transverse and descending segments of the thoracic aorta, where they may attain a large size. An aneurysm may produce a solitary compression or multiple ones and even cause obstruction of the esophagus, if large enough. An aneurysm actually may erode into the esophagus, resulting in esophageal perforation. An aneurysm of the transverse arch plainly causes esophageal deviation to the right and posteriorly, in contrast to vascular rings which produce an anterior compression. An elongated aortic arch may also displace the esophagus to the left and posteriorly; this must not be confused with the displacement caused by an enlarged left atrium, that is observed at a lower level. Just superior to the diaphragm, the esophagus lies in front of the aorta and is closely attached to it so that any tortuosity or aneurysmal dilation produces an anterior and left-sided displacement of the distal end of the esophagus. A saccular aneurysm in this area may produce complete obstruction and resemble a mediastinal tumor. An aneurysm may or may not pulsate, depending on the thickness of the wall and the presence or absence of blood clot. Arteriosclerotic aneurysms occur more commonly in the abdominal than in the thoracic aorta. Arteriosclerotic aneurysms generally are smaller than syphilitic aneurysms and aortitis is absent.

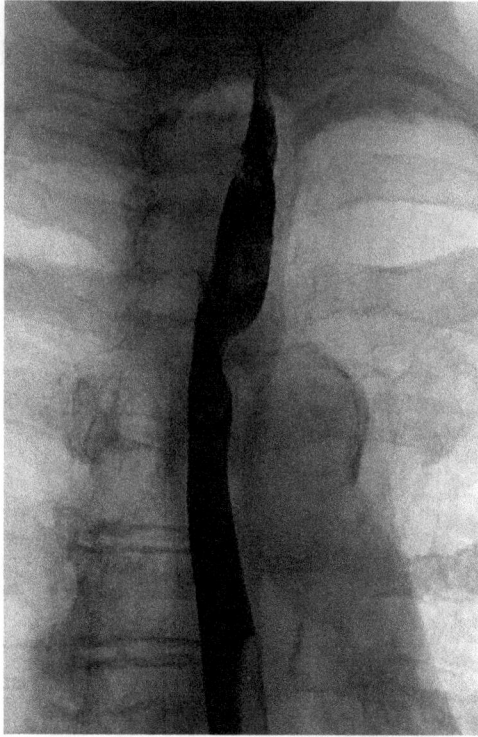

Figure 5.31 Arteria lusoria.

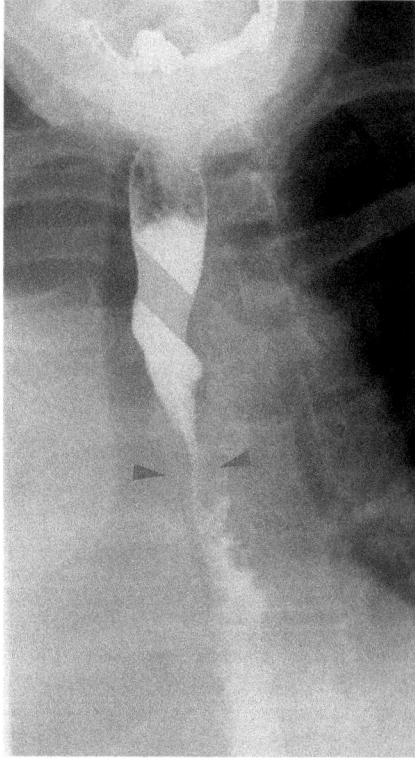

Figure 5.32 Arteria lusoria.

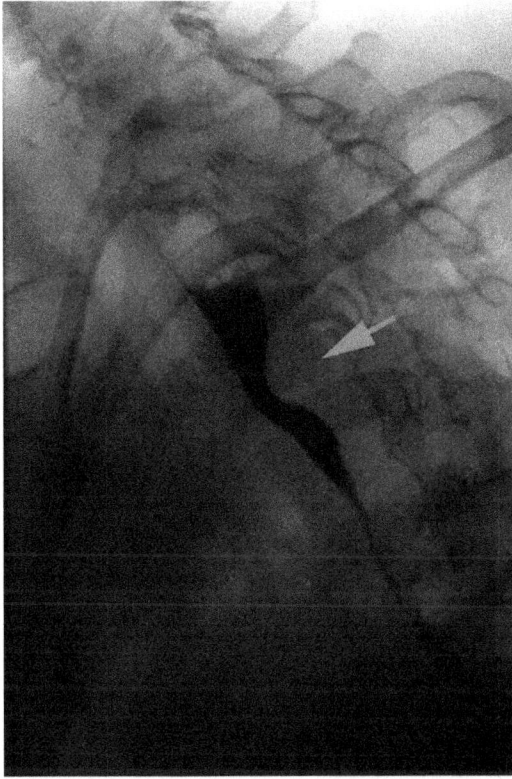

Figure 5.33 Arteria lusoria.

Aneurysms in the transverse arch of the aorta and the descending portion of the thoracic aorta bulging posteriorly may result in extensive erosion of the anterior surfaces of the adjacent vertebral bodies (Oppenheimer's sign). Other less commonly encountered causes of aneurysms of the thoracic aorta exist. Poststenotic aneurysms are usually congenital, being associated with coarctation of the aorta. Mycotic or other infective aneurysms are usually small and are associated with a localized aortitis. Post-traumatic aneurysms often occur in the area of the left subclavian artery. Such aneurysms often calcify in later stages. A hematoma at the site of trauma may simulate an aneurysm on occasion. Dissecting aneurysms may compress or displace the esophagus. The tear in the wall of the aorta in dissections most commonly occurs in the ascending aorta, often extending down into the abdominal aorta. The tear in a dissecting aneurysm may communicate with the pericardial sac, the pleural cavity, or the mediastinum.

5.4.17 Aortitis

The aorta is typically dilated, adhesions form between the esophagus and aorta, fixing the adjacent area of the esophagus to the aorta, and irregular indentations along the esophagus below the level of the aortic arch. Aortitis is caused by a number of diseases, such as syphilis, rheumatic fever, septicemia, scarlet fever, and meningitis.

5.4.18 Pleural Effusion

Depending on the location and volume of fluid, the opacified esophagus in pleural effusion may be moved to the left or right.

5.4.19 Pleural Adhesions

The upper thoracic esophageal segment (and trachea) is typically pulled to the right by fibrotic bands in pleuropulmonary adhesions, particularly from chronic pulmonary tuberculosis. This frequently results in a sharp angulation and, on occasion, even serrated irregularities of the lateral border of the adjacent esophageal segment. If the lower esophageal segment is on the left side, pleural adhesions and organized pleural effusions may affect it, preventing normal distensibility and slowing the rate of emptying; occasionally, a segment of the esophagus may be fixed, and pseudo-diverticular formation of the esophagus may even result; and if a hiatal hernia is present, pleural fibrotic changes may result in incarceration of the hernia, which also produces abnormal contours of the herniated segment of stomach.

5.4.20 Atelectasis

In cases of complete collapse, the mediastinal structures are displaced to the ipsilateral side, and atelectasis can cause aberrant displacement of the esophageal segment on the side of the collapsed lung or pulmonary segment.

5.4.21 Pneumothorax

The esophagus frequently shifts to the contralateral side during a pneumothorax, although the degree of the deviation is determined by the air pressure inside the pleural cavity.

5.4.22 Emphysema

The usual bronchial esophageal impression is more prominent in pulmonary emphysema, especially in older patients, because the over-aerated lungs tend to limit the esophageal distensibility during swallowing, which hinders the normal pace of barium transit.

5.4.23 Acquired Bronchoesophageal and Acquired Tracheal Fistulae

Acquired tracheal and bronchoesophageal fistulae are complications caused by a number of disorders. The etiologic factors include neoplasms, infection, and trauma. Neoplasms may be of esophageal or mediastinal origin. Erosion may occur into a bronchus (or esophagus). Infection (and inflammation) of mediastinal nodes, usually caused by tuberculosis, histoplasmosis, and sarcoid, may produce involvement of the esophagus, trachea, or main bronchi causing indentations and even erosions and development of fistulae. An esophageal diverticulum may rupture or erode into the wall of the trachea or bronchi. Foreign bodies, instrumentation, surgical procedures, caustic burns, crushing, and penetrating injuries may also produce fistulous tracts between the esophagus and the bronchial tree. An examination following ingestion of a thin barium mixture during fluoroscopic examination usually demonstrates the fistulous tract. In young adults with frequent, recurring pulmonary infections, a small, congenital bronchoesophageal fistula, previously undetected, may be present. In older patients who develop pulmonary complications, e.g., pneumonia, following chest surgery, a fistulous tract should be suspected (Figure 5.34).

5.4.24 Mediastinal Adenopathy

Mediastinal adenopathy is the most common cause of mediastinal masses. The main mediastinal glands are grouped into the paratracheal, parabronchial, hilar, and bifurcation nodes. However, not all these glands, if enlarged, may show esophageal involvement on radiologic examination. Enlarged carinal or bifurcation nodes are not identified on plain chest films but can be observed to compress or displace the opacified esophagus anteriorly and to the right below the level of the tracheal bifurcation, particularly in lateral and anterior oblique views. Widening of the carinal angle also may be noted but must be differentiated from an enlarged left atrium, where the esophageal displacement is mostly to the right and posterior. Enlarged carinal nodes, in addition to causing semilunar indentations of the wall of the esophagus, produce irregularity and rigidity below the level of the bronchus. Enlarged lymph nodes can be caused by lymphoma, metastatic disease, infective agents, and chronic granuloma. Lymphoma, particularly Hodgkin's disease, constitutes a common cause of enlarged lymph nodes. Multiple lymph nodes, usually in the anterior mediastinum and less commonly in the mid-mediastinum, are involved in lymphoma. On occasion, a large solitary mass of nodes produces displacement and compression of the esophagus. On radiologic examination, enlarged nodes characteristically produce semilunar indentations of the esophagus that may simulate benign intramural lesions. However, such nodal indentations do not move with the esophagus as do intramural esophageal lesions. Enlarged metastatic nodes are a frequent cause of mediastinal nodal enlargement and may occur at various levels. Metastatic nodes are chiefly observed in the interbronchial segments, whereas inflammatory nodes are located primarily at the level of the tracheal bifurcation. Metastatic hilar nodes commonly have their focus of origin in carcinoma of the bronchus, gastrointestinal tract, prostate, and kidney. Metastatic nodes caused by bronchogenic carcinoma affecting the esophagus are usually located in the middle mediastinal compartment and may compress the esophagus by direct extension. The primary lesion may be so small as to be

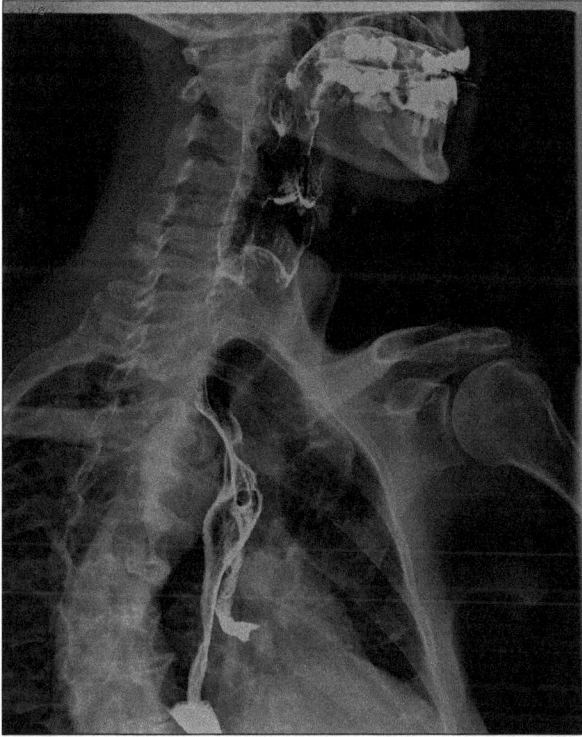

Figure 5.34 Esophageal fistula.

unnoticed except for the appearance of enlarged hilar nodes (particularly in oat-cell carcinoma). Any of the main mediastinal nodes can be involved, with resultant displacement of the aortic knob or distortion of the left bronchial impression on the opacified esophagus. Other mediastinal tumors affecting the paraesophageal nodes are located mainly in the mid or posterior mediastinum. Such enlarged lymph nodes can be caused by granulomas, such as tuberculosis, histoplasmosis, or sarcoid. These nodes often not only compress the esophagus but actually invade the esophageal wall, producing erosions and esophagobronchial fistulae. The distinction from a primary lesion of the esophagus may be difficult. On occasion, granulomatous, even calcified mediastinal nodes may be observed in the anterior mediastinum without effect on the esophagus. A localized tubercular granulomatous nodal mass without pulmonary involvement is uncommon. It usually presents as a loculated mediastinal mass displacing and compressing the esophagus. The accompanying fibrosing mediastinitis results in fixation of the segment of the affected esophagus involved.

5.4.25 Neurogenic Neoplasms
The posterior mediastinum is the most common location for neurogenic neoplasms. There are three primary types of neurogenic neoplasms: neurofibromas, which are also linked to von Recklinghausen's disease; ganglioneuromas, which are derived from sympathetic nerves; and pheochromocytomas, which are derived from paraganglion cells. The latter two types are more common in children who may have malignant potential. On radiologic examination, all three types show a well-defined, spheroid homogeneous density in the paravertebral region, along with evidence of erosion of the posterior ribs and occasionally the thoracic vertebrae, as well as compression and displacement of the esophagus. Ganglioneuromas are typically longer than neurofibromas.

5.4.26 Mediastinitis
Acute mediastinitis is typically secondary to an extension of an inflammatory process from the hypopharynx, lungs, pleura, pericardium, or from an esophageal perforation; the radiologic findings vary depending on the location and nature of the underlying causes, which are discussed in the section on esophageal perforations, but generally speaking, obstruction and compression of the

esophagus occur and widening of the mediastinum is noted; special diagnostic procedures may be required for a proper diagnosis. Chronic mediastinitis is frequently secondary to granulomatous lesions, such as tuberculosis, histoplasmosis, or sarcoidosis, which ultimately cause fibrosing changes, with fixation and narrowing of the esophagus, and may have traction diverticula, particularly in the mid-esophagus.

5.4.27 Fibrotic Diseases

Fibrosclerosis can be the result of a chronic granulomatous infection; it can also be the end result of a chronic granulomatous infection, which can be multifocal and possibly associated with orbital pseudotumors and Riedel's thyroiditis; it can also be the result of extensive hypertrophic changes of the cervical vertebra, which can produce direct compression of the hypopharynx and/or cervical esophagus with anterior displacement of the larynx and hypopharyngeal pseudodiverticula and irregularities of the posterior pharyngeal wall. Fibrosclerosis can be indistinguishable from a chronic mediastinitis, and it can also be secondary to an acute spondylitis.

5.4.28 Trauma

A spontaneous, localized mediastinal hematoma secondary to hemophilia or other blood coagulating disorders produces similar radiologic features, characterized by a localized area of restricted mobility and distensibility of the esophagus without direct involvement or distortion of the esophageal wall and mucosal pattern. Similarly, blunt trauma (e.g., auto accident) or penetrating injuries (e.g., stab wounds) can cause mediastinal hemorrhage from a major vessel, resulting in a uniform, symmetrical widening of the mediastinum or a localized mass (hematoma) that compresses and restricts the esophagus's normal distensibility.

5.5 RUPTURES, EROSIONS, AND PERFORATIONS OF THE ESOPHAGUS

In a normal esophagus, esophageal perforations are caused by direct trauma (e.g., during instrumentation) or by the ingestion of a sharp foreign body; in a normal esophagus, esophageal erosions through the esophageal wall also result in perforations, but these are typically secondary to a preexisting disease process; in a normal esophagus, esophageal ruptures are typically an abrupt process secondary to a sudden increase in intraluminal pressure; in a normal esophagus, such as a severe abdominal blow; in a preexisting condition, such as a peptic ulcer, esophageal diverticulum, or hiatal hernia; in a diseased esophagus, a spontaneous esophageal rupture can be the result of severe vomiting, retching, or straining.

5.5.1 Incisions

Esophageal perforations in the hypopharyngeal area are primarily caused by ingestion of sharp foreign bodies and are most prevalent in children. Rigidity of the cervical spine with extensive cervical degenerative vertebral changes can facilitate esophageal perforation in the adult during esophageal endoscopy. A bubble of gas is first noted in the soft tissues outside of the hypopharyngeal wall, at the site of the perforation, on a plain lateral film of the cervical region. A thickening of the retropharyngeal soft tissues is noted next, with forward displacement of the larynx and/or trachea. If the perforation is contained within the retropharyngeal space, a localized abscess forms. If the perforation extends into the prevertebral space, the infection can spread inferiorly into the mediastinum and produce an acute mediastinitis. Some degree of subcutaneous and mediastinal emphysema is usually present. A contrast swallow may reveal the presence of the perforation site. Where frank perforation is suspected, an aqueous contrast medium is preferable, because it is readily resorbed outside the lumen. Before endoscopy is attempted, therefore, the hypopharyngeal area should always be examined Roentgenologically and fluoroscopically with a barium swallow to exclude any diverticula. The Roentgenologic findings of perforations will be the same as just described. Instrumentation can produce not only actual perforations but also mucosal and/or submucosal tears. These can be detected during opacification studies of the esophagus. Such tears are visualized on a barium swallow as extraluminal parallel channels of barium or irregularities in the mucosal pattern of the wall of the hypopharynx with intramural extension of the medium. These tears are most common in the hypopharyngeal area, above the esophageal sphincter. The sphincter itself may be in spastic contraction during the examination, producing a temporary obstruction. Repeated attempts at passing an endoscope can produce such tears, especially when there is fixation of the hypopharyngeal wall by fiberosclerosis or chronic spondylitis. Incomplete rupture of the esophagus following instrumental trauma may also produce intramural seepage of barium following a barium swallow, with the appearance of a double lumen separated by a translucent stripe, referred to as the "mucosal stripe sign." The lumen itself becomes cleared of barium, with the extraluminal, intramural barium retained excessively long within the esophageal wall. Spontaneous recovery usually takes place.

5.5.2 Erosions

Esophageal erosions with perforation can be caused by a variety of factors, including esophageal erosions resulting from damage to the esophageal wall caused by the ingestion of alkali or acid solutions; esophageal erosions with sudden rupture into the esophageal wall, particularly in children; esophageal erosions caused by undetected foreign bodies; esophageal erosions with a rupture site partially occluded by blood clots; esophageal erosions with a localized, shallow irregularity at the site of the perforation may occasionally be seen on radiologic examination after the ingestion of barium, as a localized, shallow irregularity at the site of the perforation; esophageal erosions occur secondary to Pott's abscess of tuberculous spondylitis, suppurative paraesophageal nodes, or malignant lymphomas; esophageal neoplasms can also be caused by primary esophageal neoplasms; and the presence of a fistulous tract demonstrated radiologically may be diagnostic.

5.5.3 Ruptures

Spontaneous rupture of a normal esophagus may be caused by severe vomiting with a full distended stomach, most commonly following an alcoholic bout. This entity is known as "Boerhaave's syndrome." The perforation is caused by the sudden elevation of intraluminal esophageal pressure associated with a tear usually on the left side of the esophagus and above the level of the contracted lower sphincter. This portion of the lower end of the esophagus has been shown experimentally to have the weakest wall. Spontaneous rupture of the esophagus, however, can also occur at different sites in the presence of a diseased esophagus, stricture, diverticulum, or hiatal hernia. A sudden onset of severe chest pain during or immediately after a vomiting bout is the characteristic clinical manifestation of a spontaneous rupture of the esophagus. On radiologic examination of the chest, mediastinal and subcutaneous cervical emphysema and left-sided pleural effusion are observed frequently. A "V" sign, caused by air outlining the fascial pleural planes and diaphragmatic pleura, has been described. Hydropneumothorax is present if the tear is extensive. An aqueous contrast swallow will show extraluminal contrast in the chest cavity at the site of the rupture and in the mediastinum and/or interpleural space. A neonatal Boerhaave's syndrome has also been reported. It differs from the adult type in that a tension pneumo- or hydropneumothorax is present. It occurs more frequently in females and more commonly on the right side. The right-sided predilection of the tear in infancy results from the position of the lower end of the esophagus; it is situated on the right side, whereas the aorta protects its left lateral wall. The precipitating cause, as in adults, is a sudden increase in esophageal luminal pressure.

5.5.4 Mallory–Weiss Syndrome

An incomplete tear of the esophageal mucosa may occur at the level of the gastroesophageal junction instead of a spontaneous rupture of the esophagus during a severe episode of retching and vomiting, followed almost immediately by hematemesis. This condition is more common in conjunction with a sliding hiatal hernia, in which a sudden distension of the herniated stomach against a contracted sphincter may occur. The tear is typically a long mucosal laceration, and either spontaneous healing occurs or a chronic ulcer may develop at the site of the tear. Radiologic examination at the time of the hemorrhage may show retained barium within the channel, produced by the tear at the gastroesophageal junction. Later in the course of this disorder, if an ulcer develops at the site of the tear, it may be demonstrated on radiologic examination with the ingestion of barium.

REFERENCES

1. Carucci LR, Turner MA. Dysphagia revisited: common and unusual causes. *Radiographics*. 35(1):105–22. doi:10.1148/rg.351130150.
2. Wilkins T, Gillies RA, Thomas AM, et al. The prevalence of dysphagia in primary care patients: a HamesNet Research Network study. *J Am Board Fam Med*. 2007;20(2):144–50. doi:10.3122/jabfm.2007.02.060045.
3. Kuo P, Holloway RH, Nguyen NQ. Current and future techniques in the evaluation of dysphagia. *J Gastroenterol Hepatol*. 2012;27(5):873–81. doi:10.1111/j.1440-1746.2012.07097.x.
4. Domenech E, Kelly J. Swallowing disorders. *Med Clin North Am*. 1999;83(1):97–113, ix.

5. Luedtke P, Levine MS, Rubesin SE, et al. Radiologic diagnosis of benign esophageal strictures: a pattern approach. *Radiographics*. 2003;23(4):897–909. doi:10.1148/rg.234025717.
6. Carucci LR, Turner MA, Yeatman CF. Dysphagia secondary to anterior cervical fusion: radiologic evaluation and findings in 74 patients. *AJR Am J Roentgenol*. 2015;204(4):768–75. doi:10.2214/AJR.14.13148.
7. Ghazanfar H, Shehi E, Makker J, Patel H. The role of imaging modalities in diagnosing dysphagia: a clinical review. *Cureus*. 2021;13(7):e16786. doi:10.7759/cureus.16786.
8. Hillenbrand A, Cammerer G, Dankesreiter L, Lemke J, Henne-Bruns D. Postoperative swallowing disorder after thyroid and parathyroid resection. *Pragmat Obs Res*. 2018;9:63–8. doi:10.2147/POR.S172059.

6 Evolution of Fluoroscopy and Barium Swallow

6.1 INTRODUCTION

The barium swallow examination has evolved since its inception at the beginning of the 20th century, from being considered a rather primitive evaluation of the swallowing function to what is today considered a comprehensive imaging modality that allows the specialist physician to assess both anatomy and function of the oral cavity, pharynx, and esophagus [1]. Our way of describing this is simplified into the words "morphodynamical imaging"; this definition, used rather tentatively at first and especially during our radiology training, should not be thought of as just a pointless way of describing the act of acquiring moving images. A definition is needed to establish, in a clear way, the existence and the importance of an imaging modality that has, albeit in different forms, always been there and can now achieve great results and clinical relevance. The value of a barium swallow is that it is a widely available, rather inexpensive, non-invasive test with which a wide host of pharyngoesophageal morphologic and functional abnormalities can be diagnosed. Technological innovations often tend to shadow the importance and usefulness of what, still to this day, is a basic examination that guides clinical or surgical decisions. Even though our objective with this book is to project the barium swallow into the future, giving it a different dimension and making extensive use, ironically enough, of technological innovations, in the next few pages we will describe the constantly changing and evolving role of imaging in the diagnosis of pharyngoesophageal diseases in the last century, by recalling the evolution of fluoroscopic equipment, radiography, and, last but not least, barium-based contrast media.

6.2 FROM FLUOROSCOPY TO MODERN IMAGING

6.2.1 Evolution of Fluoroscopy and Barium Swallow

While radiography is a technique that essentially acquires static images, by capturing a continuous set of X-ray images, fluoroscopy allows us to assess morphodynamical anatomy in real time, in vivo. Another difference between radiography and fluoroscopy is that the latter has less intrinsic contrast and spatial resolution but, at the same time, a much lower radiation dose per second [2–10]. Considering a 22.83 cm field of view, the radiation dose for fluoroscopy is 0.2–0.3 IGy, while the radiation dose for radiography is much higher at 5–10 IGy. However, a basic principle of fluoroscopy is continuous radiation, while only an instantaneous exposure is needed to produce a spot radiograph; in the end, in a barium swallow examination, the cumulative radiation dose of the fluoroscopy and that of the number of spot radiographs taken are substantially comparable, because it has been estimated that 5–10 spot radiographs hold the same radiation dose as a minute of fluoroscopy at 30 frames per second. In the early 20th century, barium swallows were carried out with primitive fluoroscopes, using a fluorescent screen and an X-ray tube, with the patient placed in between. Usually, the fluoroscopist positioned himself by facing the screen, protected by a leaded glass to decrease his own radiation exposure. The first fluorescent screens were coated with barium platinocyanide and later with cadmium tungstate or zinc cadmium sulfide. The contact between the X-rays passing through the patient and the coating resulted in the emission of very dim visible light, which required the fluoroscopist to wear special glasses, dark- or red-adapted, to be able to adequately view the produced image. Of course, this rather primitive radiographic equipment was able to produce early radiographs, by making the X-rays passing through the patient react with a silver emulsion coating a plate of glass, hence the term "flat plate" that is still colloquially and erroneously used today. A major innovation for both fluoroscopy and radiography was the development and subsequent introduction of image intensifiers during the early 1950s. These devices allowed an electronic magnification of the output of fluorescent screens, dramatically improving the image viewing experience. Conventional image intensifiers have been, even though much more recently, replaced by flat-panel displays. We think it is of utmost importance to know where we have come from, and before going forward, we will now briefly go through these steps of the evolution from the inception of fluoroscopy to modern-day imaging.

6.3 IMAGE INTENSIFIER CHAIN

6.3.1 Generator

A generator is a device needed to produce an electric current, at a specified voltage (kVp) and current (mA), which is then sent to the X-ray tube. While "continuous fluoroscopy" needs a continuous current, "pulsed" fluoroscopy needs just short pulses of current (3–10 ms in length). Blurring artifacts due to motion can be minimized by using short exposure pulses [10–15].

DOI: 10.1201/9781003508113-6

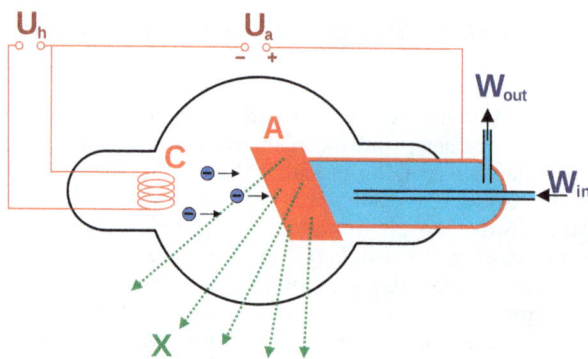

Figure 6.1 X-ray tube.

6.3.2 X-ray Tube
Electric current produced from the generator is made to pass through a heated filament, in order to generate electrons that are subsequently sent toward a positively charged tungsten anode. X-rays are created by making the electrons strike the so-called focal spot, a focal portion on the anode (Figure 6.1). The focal spot used for fluoroscopy, in order to improve geometric sharpness, is much smaller than that used for radiography; which is why radiography requires a much greater number of X-rays, a larger focal spot allowing greater tube currents to generate, minimizing tube heating.

6.3.3 Collimator
In order to reduce the amount of exposed tissue and, of course, decrease the radiation dose to the patient, radiopaque shutters are put in place to alter the shape of the X-ray beam. At the same time, this results in image contrast improvement.

6.3.4 Image Intensifier
An image intensifier is used to capture X-ray images converting them into visible light. Even though image intensifiers are progressively being replaced by new technology, namely flat-panel fluoroscopes, they have been used since the early 1950s and can still be found in many fluoroscopy practices and operating theaters. What happens in an image intensifier is that the X-rays passing through the patient reach a thin titanium plate called the input plate of the intensifier. The emission of light occurs when the X-rays strike the inner surface of the plate and its fluorescent coating, which is generally made of cesium iodide; the light then proceeds to generate electrons by hitting a photocathode layer of antimony. The electrons are subsequently accelerated from the photocathode toward the output phosphor, the electron beam being shaped by focusing electrodes and collimated onto an output phosphor plate. The visible image is the result of the energy conversion generated by the electrons striking the output plate.

6.3.5 Output Phosphor Image Displays
Early fluoroscopes were rather impractical because, in order to view the output image, a lens and mirror system were needed; moreover, light adaptation of the observer for viewing the green-yellow phosphor screen was needed, until, in the 1950s, closed-circuit television was developed and used as a superior method for displaying fluoroscopic images (Figure 6.2). The visible output phosphor image was converted by a television camera into an electronic signal, which was in turn sent directly to a cathode-ray television monitor for viewing. Of course, the result of using this analog television system was that the spatial resolution was reduced to about 1–2 line pairs per mm. The development of a charged couple device camera containing a solid state array of light sensors enabled the images to be stored as digital pixels that could be displayed on a liquid crystal digital monitor with a 1000–2500 matrix size. Returning to early fluoroscopes, another way of recording the images from the output phosphor was to use a roll of film by a photospot camera. The film then had to be processed in a darkroom, and the roll (or selected cut images from the roll) could finally be analyzed by the observer. A dynamic assessment was possible only by analyzing the rapid sequences of static images. In vivo, real-time fluoroscopy finally became possible when video recorder devices were developed, allowing the analysis of anatomic motion at normal speed or in slow motion, a great improvement for the interpretation of movement in comparison to what we have described before.

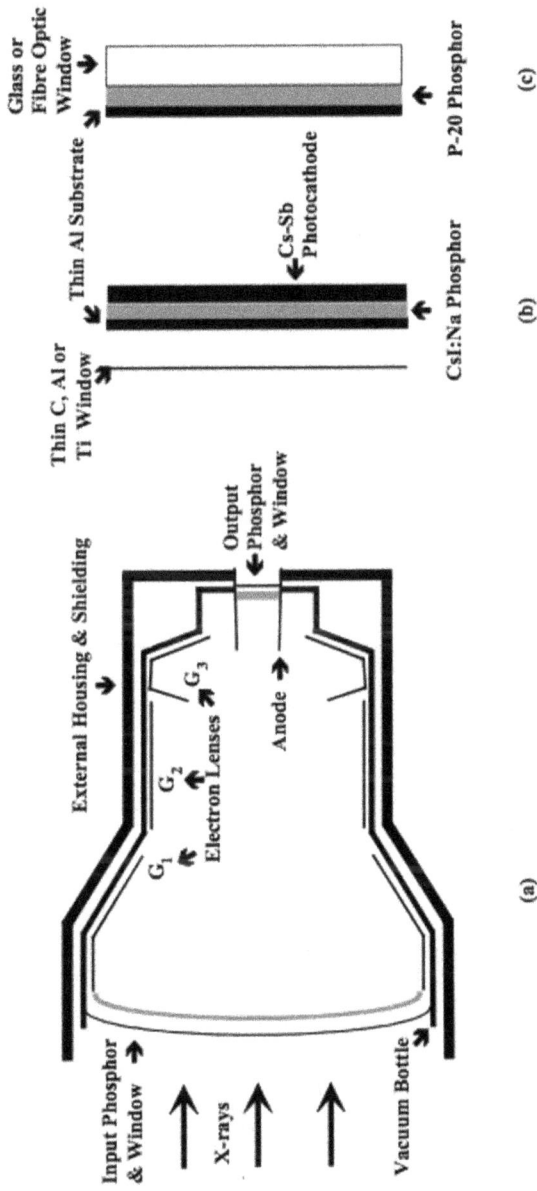

Figure 6.2 X-ray image formation.

6.3.6 Radiographic Image Displays

Radiographic images used to be captured using analog fluoroscopic equipment by manually loading film-screen cassettes [16] (Figure 6.3) into the fluoroscopic unit, exposing the film-screen combination, and then unloading the exposed cassette, only for a new cassette to be loaded and used for another exposure. When in need of rapid sequence images that, however, never can and never will replace a real-time continuous image, one could expose various portions of the cassette to the X-ray beam, obtaining two-on-one or three-on-one spot films. Of course, old-fashioned film-screen cassettes required darkrooms where the exposed films could be processed, back-lit viewers for spot-film analysis, and file rooms for film storage. Cineradiography was the first technique used for real-time acquisition of radiographic images: rapid sequences of radiographs were recorded on 15 or 35 mm film in a movie camera that had previously been installed in the fluoroscopic unit. The film was then obviously processed in a darkroom and made to run through a movie projector, so that image analysis was actually performed on a movie screen. Even though this technique actually had better spatial and contrast resolution in comparison with fluoroscopic images, the whole processing and reviewing was inconvenient and, most importantly, associated with a higher radiation dose to the patient. The final blow that terminated cineradiography was the development of videotape machines, allowing fluoroscopy to be continuously recorded; video systems were, moreover, a lot easier to use [17]. Another huge imaging revolution was the introduction, in the 1990s, of digital radiography that aimed to replace fluoroscopy and analog radiography, enabling much faster acquisition of radiographic and fluoroscopic images. Even though digital images had, of course, less spatial resolution (digital radiographs: 3.5–6 line pairs per mm; analog radiographs: 6–8 line pairs per mm), they had greater contrast resolution. Not needing physical storage like conventional films, digital images are transmitted electronically to a computer-based picture archiving communications system, the so-called PACS, from which they can be selectively retrieved for viewing and interpretation on high-resolution monitors at computerized workstations. The adjustment of image brightness or contrast, with magnification of particular areas of interest, and annotations of image findings for better interpretation and reporting of studies are possible through the post-processing.

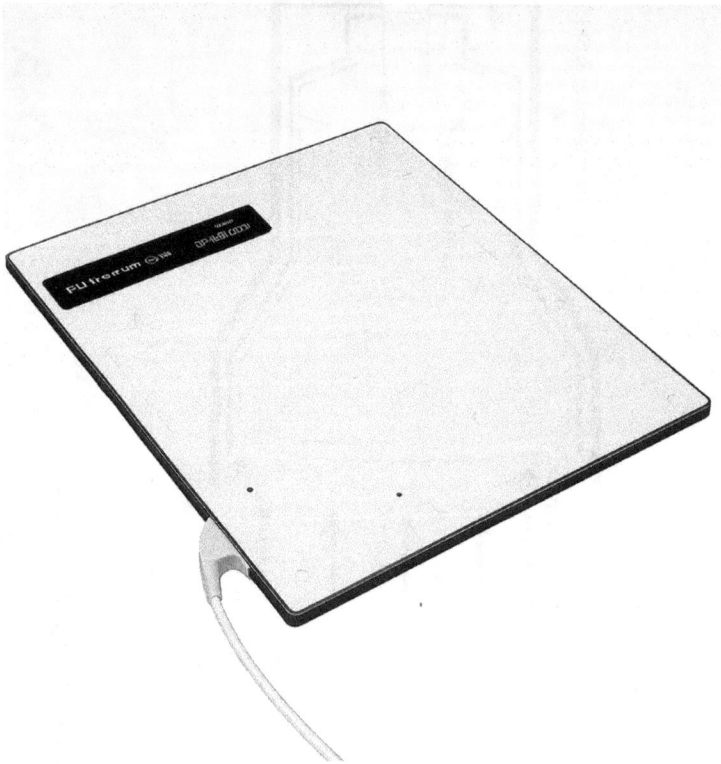

Figure 6.3 Radiographic cassette.

Digital imaging and the use of PACS systems eliminate the need for the production and storage of radiographic films, producing very profitable cost savings. The use of digital fluoroscopic units is particularly convenient due to a wide range of factors: first, shorter exposure times that translate to lower radiation exposure for the patient allowed by the instant display of images on fluoroscopy monitors; second, the shorter exposure also helps decrease motion artifacts and blurring, something of utmost importance when considering pharyngoesophageal imaging [18]. It is also very convenient that digital imaging does not require manual loading and unloading of cassettes, something that is normally done on analog fluoroscopic units, enabling very fast image acquisition, considerably shortening the whole procedure duration. This is important, especially for the morphodynamical study of the pharyngoesophageal tract and, as we will see, for some forms of achalasia, too, especially considering that a swallowed bolus of barium traverses the pharynx and cervical esophagus approximately ten times faster than the thoracic esophagus. Image acquisition speed, however, is still not fast enough to display motion accurately, because modern digital imaging systems are only enabled to capture a maximum of 8 images per second.

6.3.7 Flat-panel Fluoroscopes

When compared to an image intensifier, a flat-panel fluoroscope is something quite different. X-rays passing through the patient are captured by a large array of photodiode cells; subsequently, the flat-panel processes digitizes the X-ray image. Current flat panels measure about 25–40 cm and generally contain from 1.5 to 5 million detectors. After the X-rays pass through the patient, they are made to hit the cesium iodide scintillator layer of each detector; this generates light, in proportion to the amount of X-ray flux, that then hits the photodiode/transistor layer of the detector. The change in charge of each photodiode is then read by the electronic portion of the detector. While the electronic detector proceeds to read each photodiode, row by row, the fluoroscope generates a digitized image, so that it can be displayed on a high-resolution monitor (Figure 6.4) [19]. Even though very much depending on the field of view and the number of raster lines on the monitor, many television systems have a spatial resolution ranging between 0.5 and 1.5 line pairs per mm, a value much lower than the 5 line pairs per mm, the spatial resolution of the output phosphor of a standard fluoroscope. Spatial resolution in flat-panel displays is actually determined by the detector size, with

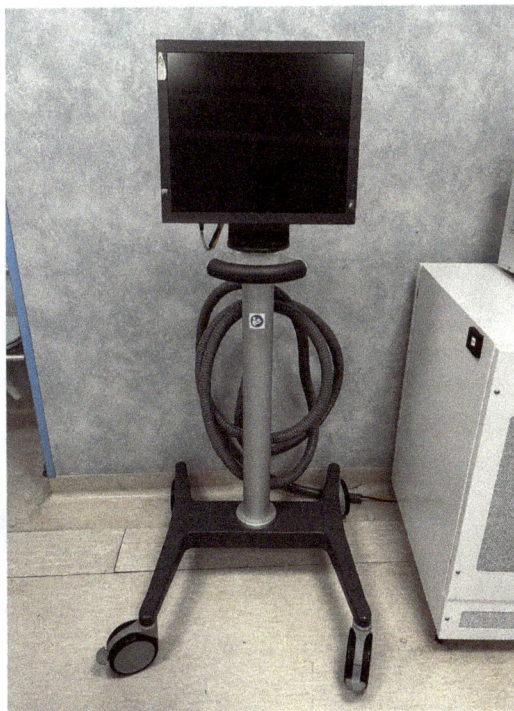

Figure 6.4 Flat-panel fluoroscope.

a current limit of about 2.5–3 line pairs per mm; in comparison, spatial resolution for analog radiography is 6–8 line pairs per mm. Flat-panel detectors enable the depiction of extremely dense and radiolucent structures, much better than image intensifiers; at the same time, the dynamic range of flat-panel detectors is higher than that of image intensifiers. As mentioned, the spatial resolution of flat panels depends very much on detector size and is, at least theoretically, independent of the field of view. So, using smaller fields of view, through collimation we are able to select information from the central portion of the flat panel and subsequently view it on the entire monitor. Using larger fields of view, data generation is so much higher that this forces the grouping of signals from four detectors. This reduces both data volume, spatial resolution, and at the same time, image mottle. Modern fluoroscopy can provide 30, 15, or 7.5 fluoroscopic frames per second and 2–4 radiographic images per second. Continuous motion is perceived by the eye at 30 frames per second; at lower settings, of course, the image is not perceived as continuous. Nowadays, fluoroscopy can be acquired, sent to the PACS, and stored, to be reviewed on the currently available high-resolution monitors. At the same time, alternatively, fluoroscopy can be stored and reviewed on dedicated digital recorders.

6.3.8 Fluoroscopy Versus Radiography

A controversial argument among radiologists dedicated to gastrointestinal tract imaging is the various advantages and disadvantages of fluoroscopy and radiography [20]. Radiography yields higher resolution and greater anatomic detail than fluoroscopic images. Cineradiography allows a better study of motion but yields lower resolution than static images and is, however, associated with larger radiation doses to the patient. Fluoroscopy studies, either analogically or digitally acquired, have the great advantage that they can be viewed in forward or reverse, also in slow motion; the stop-frame images obtained through fluoroscopy have much lower resolution than digital radiographs. This argument about fluoroscopy versus radiography is still very much ongoing today, especially for the study of the pharynx; while some think that the analysis of function should have more emphasis, others give more importance to the assessment of structural abnormalities, at the expense of the dynamic, functional analysis [21,22]. The good news is that modern flat-panel fluoroscopes produce better, improved fluoroscopic images that allow for a dynamic study of motion, even though static digital images yield a little lower resolution than conventional films. The possibility we have right now to acquire and store fluoroscopy images, cine-sequences that can be played over and over again for careful interpretation, is the actual founding principle of this book and the beginning of a new era for morphodynamical imaging (Figure 6.5).

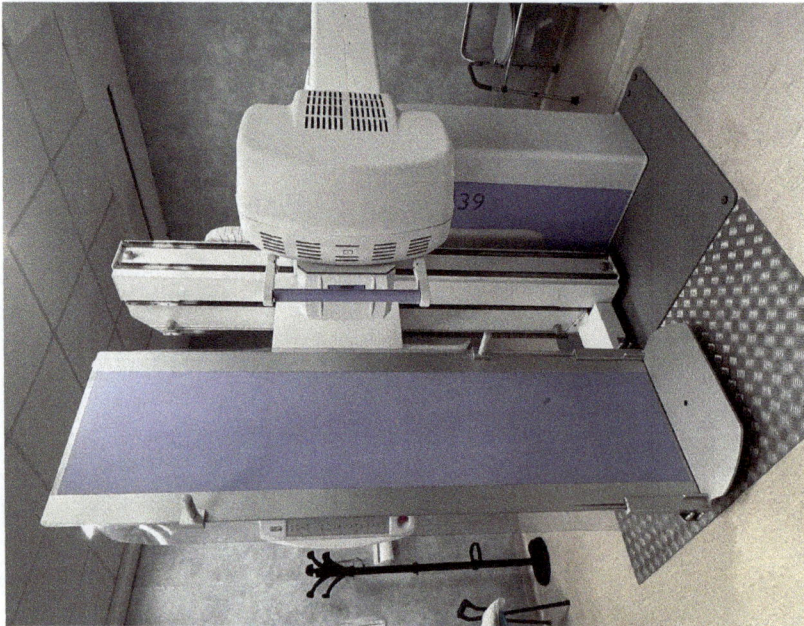

Figure 6.5 Our radiography-fluoroscopy unit.

REFERENCES

1. Levine MS, Rubesin SE, Laufer I. Barium esophagography: a study for all seasons. *Clin Gastroenterol Hepatol*. 2008;6:11–25.
2. Schueler BA. The AAPM/RSNA physics tutorial for residents: general overview of fluoroscopic imaging. *RadioGraphics*. 2000;20:1115–26.
3. Nickoloff EL, Lu, ZF, Newhouse JH, Van Heertum R. RSNA physics modules. *Fluoroscopy*. https://www.rsna.org/Physics-Modules.
4. Levine MS, Laufer I. The gastrointestinal tract: dos and don'ts of digital imaging. *Radiology*. 1998;207:311.
5. Nickoloff EL. AAPM/RSNA physics tutorial for residents: physics of flat-panel fluoroscopy systems survey of modern fluoroscopy imaging: flat-panel detectors versus image intensifiers and more. *RadioGraphics*. 2011;31:591–602.
6. Carman RD, Miller A. *The Roentgen diagnosis of diseases of the alimentary tract*. Philadelphia: WB Saunders; 1917.
7. Rumpel T. Visualization of esophagus of patient with dysphagia with bismuth. *Muench Med Wochenschr*. 1897;44:420; Cannon WB. The passage of different food stuffs from the stomach and through the small intestines. *Am J Physiol*. 1904;12:387–418.
8. Bachem C, Gunther H. Barium sulfate as a shadow-forming contrast agent in Roentgenologic examinations. *Zeitschrift f Röntg*. 1910;12:369–76.
9. Skucas J. Contrast media. In: Gore RM, Levine MS, Laufer I, editors. *Textbook of gastrointestinal radiology*. Philadelphia: WB Saunders; 1994. p. 17–30.
10. Levine MS, Ott DJ, Laufer I. Barium studies: single and double contrast. In: Gore RM, Levine MS, editors. *Textbook of gastrointestinal radiology*. 4th ed. Philadelphia: Elsevier; 2015. p. 23–40.
11. Leonard CL. The radiography of the stomach and intestines. *AJR*. 1913;1:1–42.
12. Shirakabe H. *Double contrast studies of the stomach*. Stuttgart: Georg Thieme Verlag; 1972.
13. Laufer I, Hamilton J, Mullens JE. Demonstration of superficial gastric erosions by double contrast radiology. *Gastroenterology*. 1975;68:387–91.
14. Gelfand DW. High density, low viscosity barium for fine mucosal detail on double-contrast upper gastrointestinal examinations. *AJR*. 1970;130:831–3.
15. Rubesin SE, Jessurun J, Robertson D, Jones B, Bosma JF, Donner MW. Lines of the pharynx. *RadioGraphics*. 1987;7:217–37; Rubesin SE, Laufer I. Pictorial review: principles of double-contrast pharyngography. *Dysphagia*. 1991;6:170–8.
16. Laufer I. *Double contrast gastrointestinal radiology with endoscopic correlation*. Philadelphia: WB Saunders; 1977.
17. Ott DJ, Gelfand DW, Lane TG, et al. Radiologic detection and spectrum of appearances of peptic esophageal strictures. *J Clin Gastroenterol*. 1982;4:11.
18. Chen YM, Ott DJ, Gelfand DW, Munitz HA. Multiphasic examination of the esophagogastric region for strictures, rings, and hiatal hernia: evaluation of the individual techniques. *Gastrointest Radiol*. 1985;10:311.
19. Ott DJ, Chen YM, Wu WC, Gelfand DW. Endoscopic sensitivity in the detection of esophageal strictures. *J Clin Gastroenterol*. 1985;7:121.
20. Ott DJ, Chen YM, Wu WC, Gelfand DW, Munitz HA. Radiographic and endoscopic sensitivity in detecting lower esophageal mucosal ring. *AJR*. 1986;147:261.
21. Levine MS, Rubesin SE, Herlinger H, Laufer I. Double-contrast upper gastrointestinal examination: technique and interpretation. *Radiology*. 1988;168:593–602.
22. DuBrul EL. *Sicher's oral anatomy*. 7th ed. St. Louis: CV Mosby; 1980. p. 319.

7 Imaging Technique

7.1 INTRODUCTION

The techniques, or rather protocols, we are going to describe in the next few pages have all been developed by our group through extensive practice, with daily and tailored modifications, then used in clinical practice. Although many of the things we will discuss will be mainly based on dynamic or, as we prefer to define it, morphodynamical imaging, we do understand that direct digital devices with cine modality are still not the norm and not equally available anywhere; that is why we will present a static acquisition protocol as well. The timed barium esophagogram will be considered, too, a static, quick and easy-to-perform technique that is very useful for post-therapeutic assessment. Even though our approach to the matter of barium swallow is rather one of moving forward, aimed at producing images that are more useful than just "beautiful" to watch, we do not underestimate the value of the classic barium esophagogram and its use in routine studies. Our morphodynamical protocol should not be mistaken for something to be used routinely in all patients, but rather it should be performed only in patients with certified motility disorders, considering the higher radiation dose and exposure times dynamic imaging determines. We strongly advise, though, using morphodynamical imaging whenever possible in patients with certain motility disorders, not exclusively achalasia. The analysis of the upper gastrointestinal (GI) tract should ideally be complete, from pharynx to duodenum, but generally and especially in patients with achalasia or motility disorders, we include the stomach only when evident anomalies are present, focusing our evaluation on swallowing, esophageal emptying, esophageal morphology and motility, evaluation of the gastroesophageal (GE) junction, and assessment for gastroesophageal reflux (GER). Patients who have undergone recent esophageal or gastric surgery or recent trauma, or who are unable to cooperate with the examination are, however, not candidates for this kind of evaluation. Relevant patient history should be obtained prior to the procedure to determine the appropriate type of procedure and contrast medium. In these instances, assuming that the patient can cooperate, a single-contrast examination should be performed [1].

7.2 TECHNIQUE

For much of the 20th century, the barium swallow was performed as a single-contrast study in which the patient swallowed low-density barium to distend the pharyngeal and esophageal lumen with a continuous column of thin barium. The single-contrast technique enabled the detection of pharyngeal and esophageal strictures, contour abnormalities (i.e., ulcers or masses), and large protruded lesions seen *en face* as radiolucent defects in the barium column. However, this technique did not permit visualization of small protruded or depressed mucosal lesions and therefore had a low sensitivity for detecting inflammatory or neoplastic conditions. The concept of using a combination of air and barium to visualize the mucosal surface of the GI tract was first suggested in the early part of the 20th century. High-density, low-viscosity barium products were developed for optimal coating of the mucosa on double-contrast GI studies, particularly in the stomach and the colon. However, these double-contrast studies were subsequently shown to markedly improve the detection of subtle mucosal abnormalities in the pharynx and esophagus. In the 1970s, Igor Laufer at the University of Pennsylvania became a leading proponent of the double-contrast technique for improving the detection of mucosal lesions in the esophagus. In his classic text, *Double Contrast Gastrointestinal Radiology with Endoscopic Correlation*, first published in 1977, he presented a simplified technique for performing double-contrast esophagrams in which the patient ingested an effervescent agent that released carbon dioxide gas into the gastric lumen and then continuously swallowed a high-density barium suspension to coat the mucosa for double-contrast views of the esophagus. This technique greatly improved the detection of reflux esophagitis, infectious esophagitis, other esophagitides, and esophageal cancer and also facilitated the differentiation of benign and malignant strictures (see later sections). Despite the advantages of the double-contrast technique for visualizing the mucosa, it was recognized that continuous swallowing of a low-density barium suspension in the prone, right anterior oblique (RAO) position produced better esophageal distention for visualization of rings and strictures, especially in the distal esophagus. Between 1982 and 1986, Ott et al. published a series of articles showing that prone, single-contrast views markedly improved the detection of distal esophageal rings and strictures, including those missed on upright double-contrast views or even endoscopy. As a result, the barium study is now performed as a biphasic examination that includes both upright double-contrast and prone single-contrast views of the esophagus. Although anatomic structures are best demonstrated with high-density barium,

DOI: 10.1201/9781003508113-7

the swallowing function is evaluated by having the patient ingest barium of varying viscosities and foodstuffs of varying flavors, textures, and consistencies. In the 1980s, better-tasting barium products of varying viscosities were developed by E-Z-EM, Inc., in response to intensive lobbying from speech pathologists. It was not practical to have pre-packaged foods impregnated with barium, so E-Z-EM created barium products of uniform texture, mimicking homogeneous liquids and solids of varying viscosities (including liquid, nectar, honey, and pudding) to facilitate the assessment of swallowing.

7.3 DYNAMIC BARIUM SWALLOW PROTOCOL

Many years ago, in 2003, in his seminal book on dysphagia, Prof. Olle Ekberg advocated the use of video recorders to tape fluoroscopy sessions during barium swallows, to allow a morphodynamical analysis of the upper GI tract and avoid acquiring "pointless" static images. Almost 20 years ago, he was already aware of the impending manometry revolution and of the fact that classic barium radiography was to become of little or no need to the diagnosis. Now, barium swallow exam techniques can differ greatly between institutions. What does not change, though, are the two components of the examination, the first involving the evaluation of the hypopharynx with the cervical esophagus and, subsequently, the assessment of the thoracic esophagus using fluoroscopy or, as in our case, acquisition of frames in cine-modality. Our protocol starts where all protocols should start, no matter what will happen next: history taking and control films. We advise radiologists to carefully take each patient's clinical history before the examination takes place; in our own experience, patients referred to barium swallow for many reasons actually ended up with a suspect diagnosis of achalasia. Taking the clinical history should obviously focus on dysphagia, its duration and onset, asking whether it refers to solids and/or liquids and asking for other symptoms, mainly regurgitation, heartburn, and chest pain. Heartfelt advice is to let the patients talk, only interrupting them when their talk goes astray; they usually point out very clearly what is going on with them, and this is of invaluable help concerning the execution and reporting of barium swallows. Also before the actual morphodynamical assessment begins it is important to acquire control films, especially in patients with a history of cervical and thoracic surgery. Good practice requires acquisition of anteroposterior and lateral films of the neck and just anteroposterior of the thorax, which includes the upper abdomen, the latter allowing the assessment of eventual bowel perforations. In patients with dysphagia, we perform the complete dynamic barium swallow, first examining the pharynx and upper esophagus, then mid- and lower esophagus, in double contrast. The single-contrast evaluation of the pharynx and esophagus starts by positioning the patient in the right lateral (RL) position, with the patient's right shoulder close to the detector. The lateral view of the upper esophagus and pharynx should include the top of the palate. We advise setting the magnification to medium, acquiring at 6 frames per second. Timing is very important: you should start acquiring just as you ask the patient to swallow or just before, stopping as soon as there is maximal distension of the most distal part of the visible esophagus. The AP view of the upper esophagus and pharynx should be taken at the same level craniocaudally as the lateral view, but with tighter coning to produce a narrower image, if you prefer. No change in machine position is required. Magnification should be kept to medium, acquiring at 3–4 frames per second. Just as before, you should start acquiring just as you ask the patient to swallow or just before, stopping as soon as there is maximal distension of the most distal part of the visible esophagus. The middle part of the esophagus is acquired in the right anterior oblique (RAO, Figure 7.1) position, with the patient's right shoulder closer to the detector and facing it, or in the left posterior oblique (LPO, Figure 7.2) position, which is the one we prefer routinely, with the patient giving the back to the detector, left shoulder closer to it. At this point, effervescent tablets or granules should be administered to the patient to obtain double-contrast images. Coning should be used laterally to narrow the image as much as possible, without obscuring any of the esophagus, with magnification set at low, acquiring at 3 frames per second, from the moment the patient is invited to swallow until as soon as there is maximal distension of the most distal part of the visible esophagus. The distal esophagus can also be acquired either in the RAO or LPO positions, our group preferring the latter in clinical practice. We also prefer to acquire the distal esophagus separately and not in a single run with the middle esophagus, using medium magnification and a number of frames variable from 1 to 3; we tend to use more frames when in need to demonstrate spasm. Start acquiring 2 seconds after inviting the patient to swallow, stopping just as soon as there is maximal distension of the gastroesophageal junction (GEJ) (Figure 7.3). Optional frontal acquisition of the lower esophagus may be added. This protocol should be considered just like some solid foundations on which we can work, but very

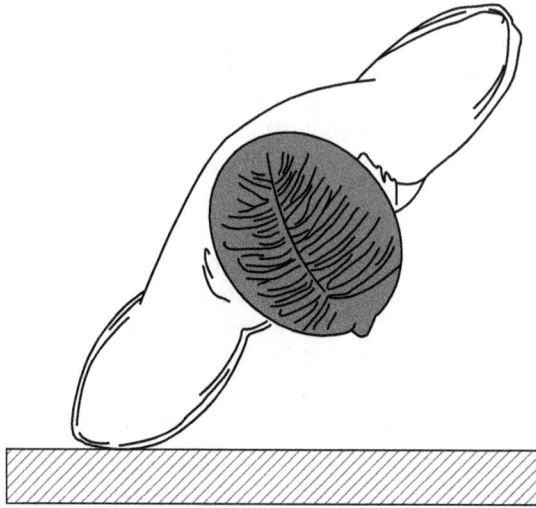

Figure 7.1   Right anterior oblique projection.

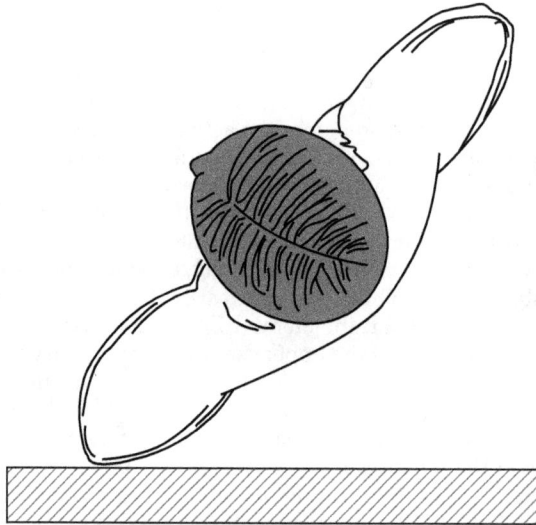

Figure 7.2   Left posterior oblique projection.

often it cannot, or should not, be carried out exactly as explained, every time. Each patient is different from one another and we have clearly seen in the previous chapter how especially patients with achalasia tend to fall in one of three phenotypes. The morphodynamical analysis we propose here is something that requires constant attention from the radiologist, who must be present and may even lead the examination in first person. Only by doing this, one might be able to "tailor" the examination on the single patient, with his own peculiar disease. Even during the execution of the exam, the radiologist has to focus the attention on the presence of the five main findings that, as we will see in the next chapter, form the basis of our FBF scoring system: bird-beak sign, endoluminal stasis, esophageal dilatation, hypotonia, and spasm. Keeping in mind the manometric considerations of the Chicago classification, one might be able to recognize, even at first glance, the achalasia phenotype that is being studied, forcing a "tailored" examination. For example, in a patient that clearly shows a "classic," hypotonic subtype 1 pattern, with the presence of bird-beak sign, hypotonia, endoluminal stasis with esophageal dilatation of varying degrees, there is little need of acquiring multiple frames per second, when 1 or 2 per second might just be enough; what

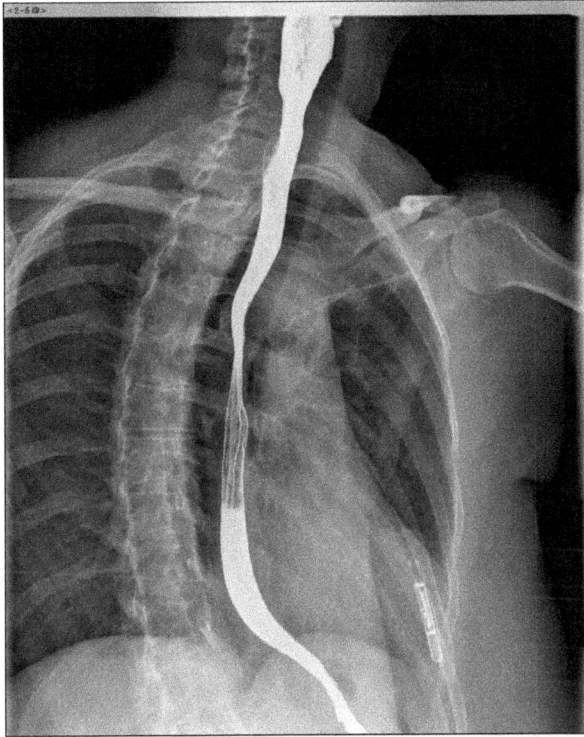

Figure 7.3 Maximal distension of the GEJ in an unremarkable study.

could be truly helpful in such a case would be to add, or incorporate, a timed barium esophago-gram in the protocol, to assess the degree of esophageal emptying at the moment of the diagnosis and, hopefully, to monitor the patient's progress after therapy. When, instead, we recognize sub-type 2 or 3 patterns and, more specifically, when there is the need to demonstrate the presence of spasm, one may acquire the mid- and lower esophagus using 3–6 frames per second. This kind of fluid adapting of the protocol has to become second nature for those practicing barium swallow on a daily basis; moreover, it allows you to have a clear idea of the case and mentally "report" the examination, making the actual reporting process faster and a mere formality. It is not difficult nor impossible to attain, but it requires study and practice.

7.4 TIMED BARIUM ESOPHAGRAM

Barium esophagography and dynamic barium swallow are usually performed to assess the esopha-gus in a detailed way, both from a morphological and a functional way [2]. The need for a timed barium esophagogram (TBE) (Figure 7.4) arises when we specifically have to study the esophageal emptying, both initially at the moment of the diagnosis and, especially, after therapy. TBE allows the quantification of the esophageal emptying in an easy and very accurate way. The technique used to obtain TBE is substantially similar to other barium swallow protocols, even though many differ-ent techniques to perform TBE have been described in the literature, by various authors and with some variations. The protocol we adopt requires using a standard radiography device, not necessar-ily with cine-acquisition, with the patient, advised to fast overnight before the examination, in the erect posture and in the LPO or, as we prefer doing, in the frontal view. Multiple films are acquired at fixed time intervals after a single swallow of a specific volume of diluted barium suspension, generally of a specific density. We tend to use low-density barium suspensions (45% w/v), asking the patients to ingest a variable volume, generally 100–250 mL, in 15–20 seconds. Even though we prefer to use 200 mL as a fixed standard volume in our protocol, to allow a standardized evaluation, especially if the same patient is then reevaluated after therapy, the volume of suspension we may use has to be able to fill the dilated esophagus adequately and not harm the patient, causing regur-gitation or aspiration. After ingestion is complete, considering barium completely empties from the

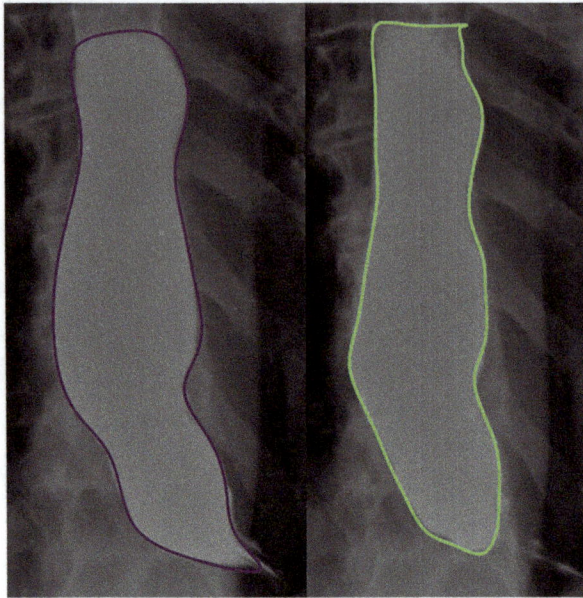

Figure 7.4 Timed barium esophagogram, area measurement type.

esophagus in 1 minute in most and in 5 minutes in all healthy individuals, images are acquired in the LPO at 1, 2, and 5 minutes, generally using three-on-one spot radiographs, or two-on-one spot radiographs when the esophagus is so dilated it would not fit on a smaller radiogram. It is important to keep the distance between the patient and the fluoroscope carriage constant throughout the examination. While some argue that the 2-minute radiograph may be optional, at 2 minutes we perform fluoroscopy and acquire a short sequence at a rate of 3 images per second, to check on the state of esophageal emptying. What can be omitted is the 5-minute acquisition, but only when barium has completely cleared from the esophagus on the 2-minute film. As we pointed out before, considering TBE usually is performed in sequential studies, before and after treatment for achalasia, to obtain consistent results one should ideally use the same volume of barium in every patient or, at least, in the same patient. It is, therefore, of utmost importance to state the precise amount of barium consumed on the report. By performing the examination in such a fashion, it is possible to assess the degree of esophageal emptying, both qualitatively and quantitatively. To perform a quantitative assessment, one should measure the height of the barium column from its distinct superior level to the gastroesophageal junction, the latter being identified by the classic bird-beak sign in patients with achalasia. The height is quantified by tracing two horizontal parallel lines both at the lowest and at the highest barium level, measuring the distance between them. It is also possible to measure the diameter of the esophagus at the widest point of the barium column found perpendicularly to the long axis of the esophagus. Emptying assessment may be performed by using height and width in sequential images, and eventual post-therapy improvements may be recognized by doing the very same thing on sequential studies. Another method that can be used to assess esophageal emptying, something we prefer doing in our practice, is to calculate the area of the endoluminal barium column at 1, 2, and 5 minutes, making a much more precise assessment (Figure 7.4). This is what makes TBE a highly reproducible technique to estimate esophageal emptying, with an almost perfect inter-observer agreement. There are, however, some small pitfalls to be carefully avoided. Sometimes, the height of the barium column may not fit lengthwise on one film; in this case a spot film should be acquired centered over the lower portion of the esophagus and another image acquired centered over the upper portion of the esophagus. Afterward, a fixed point should be located on each film, generally a vertebral body, serving as a reference point for both images. The barium column shall now be measured both above and below the reference point, on the respective films, and the height of the entire barium column obtained by adding the two measurements. The presence of prominent tertiary esophageal contractions in patients with subtype 2 or, especially, subtype 3 achalasia makes it really difficult to acquire images and obtain a continuous barium column. When in this situation, images should be acquired only when the esophagus is relaxed. Retained food material and secretions are often found in achalasia, and these may form a barium-foam interface after barium ingestion and the height of the barium column may be difficult objectively difficult to measure. When in presence of a barium-foam interface, the superior aspect of the barium column should be measured at a point where the margin is well defined and consistent.

7.5 CLASSIC BARIUM SWALLOW

Of course, it is not possible to carry out the morphodynamical analysis we advocate so strongly in this book, exactly as it should be performed, without the right equipment. Digital direct devices are progressively being implemented, but we are aware that technology improvements, due to costs or "cultural" problems, often take time to enter routine clinical practice. One way of solving this problem would be, as already stated before and suggested by Prof. Ekberg in his seminal work on dysphagia, to equip fluoroscopy with a videotape recorder, or similar digital recording device, allowing fluoroscopy to be recorded every time the pedal is pushed down. This requires very little cost and would allow a morphodynamic examination of the esophagus to be carried out. However, we do understand this cannot be easy to do and for many different reasons. If there is no way of recording fluoroscopy, all that can be done is a cautious classic "static" examination, making use of in-vivo fluoroscopy for dynamical considerations. The protocol we suggest to adopt in these circumstances is a slightly modified version of our morphodynamical evaluation. After control films, lateral and frontal for pharynx and cervical esophagus, just frontal for the thorax, the exam should start in the right lateral position, with a spot film acquired when dilatation of cervical esophagus is obtained; fluoroscopy should be used here to assess eventual penetration/aspiration or problems related to "high" dysphagia. The evaluation of the mid- and lower esophagus should be carried out by acquiring each, on three-on-one radiographs, in the RPO, frontal, and LPO views.

7.6 SPECIAL MANEUVERS AND POSITIONS

7.6.1 Trendelenburg

According to the initial description, the Trendelenburg position involved the patient lying supine on his or her back with the table plane angled 30–40 degrees cephaladically [1,3]. The patient is additionally moved to the right (right side against the table) for radiography reasons in order to distinguish the lower part of the esophagus from the spine. Additionally, to aid with lesion localization, the patient may be moved from side to side throughout the investigation. Rotating the patient to the left while they are supine is the original modification and a more widely utilized form. This is typically done in conjunction with applying physical pressure to the abdomen.

7.6.2 Wolf

In order to demonstrate a hiatal hernia or reflux, Wolf's maneuver is employed to raise intra-abdominal pressure. The patient lies on a radiolucent bolster in a prone position with his or her left side slightly raised. The central ray is at right angles to the spine and inclined cephalad. The patient is exposed either after swallowing to visualize reflux or during swallowing to show a hiatal hernia. It is also possible to combine Wolf's position with a modified Trendelenburg technique. A straight leg raising test, in which the patient is positioned supine and both heels are raised off the table with legs fully extended while breathing normally, can also be used to increase intraabdominal pressure.

7.6.3 Johnston

When demonstrating a hiatal hernia or reflux, Johnston's bending-over position, also known as the toe-touch position, may be useful. With their arms drooping and their knees straight, the patient stands lateral to the table and bends forward as much as they can. Additionally, this position is employed in conjunction with the Müller or Valsalva maneuvers.

7.6.4 Valsalva

The patient strains against a closed glottis in order to perform the Valsalva maneuver. The modified Valsalva maneuver involves the patient tightly closing their lips and blowing forcefully across their cheeks.

7.6.5 Müller

By forcibly inhaling against a closed glottis, the Müller technique raises intraabdominal pressure.

7.7 PARTICULAR EXAMINATIONS

7.7.1 Water Siphonage

The main purpose of the water siphonage test is to illustrate gastroesophageal reflux [1,3]. The patient is laid on his or her back (supine) and rotated to the right at a 45-degree angle (left side elevated) following the consumption of barium. The patient's left arm is flexed above his or her head, out of the way of the examination area, while the right hand holds a container of cold water. The patient quickly consumes the water through a straw or tube while being seen under a microscope. When barium exits the stomach and enters the esophagus, reflux is evident.

7.7.2 Captured Bolus

A hiatal hernia can be found with the captured bolus test. The RAO position is applied to the patient while they are prone. Immediately after swallowing barium, the patient takes a deep breath and holds it while performing a prolonged straining effort (modified Valsalva maneuver) to obtain films. At the esophageal hiatus, some "tenting" or "funneling" typically occurs. The "captured bolus" is the bolus that becomes stuck between the diaphragm and the distal end of the sphincter when there is a hernia.

7.7.3 Double-Lumen Tube-Balloon

Esophageal varices can be seen using the double-lumen tube with inflatable distal balloon test. The tube is sent down the esophagus to a level just above the point where the middle and lower thirds of the esophagus meet to perform the test. Venous dilation occurs distal to this location when the lower balloon is inflated to a pressure of 650 mm of water, compressing the veins in this region. If there are varices in the lower esophagus, they can be seen by injecting barium via the second lumen of the tube opening beneath the balloon.

7.7.4 Acid Barium

Acid barium is a straightforward test that can be used to induce substernal pain associated with the reduced esophageal sensitivity to acid perfusion. One milliliter of strong hydrochloric acid and 10 mL of conventional barium sulfate suspension are combined to create acid barium, which has a pH of 1.7. First, a nonacidic barium mixture is used for a fluoroscopic examination of the esophagus. After that, acid barium is consumed. Peptic esophagitis is typically seen when aberrant esophageal contraction and reflux appear, which is a positive test result. The esophagus motility returns to normal after an alkali medication is used to offset the effects of the acid. The original Bernstein's test involved intubation and up to 15 minutes of perfusion with a hydrochloric acid solution. A negative test suggests that the patient's pain is due to angina or another heart condition rather than esophagitis.

7.7.5 Mecholyl

Mecholyl is utilized to differentiate early achalasia from benign stricture, scleroderma, and cancer. Mecholyl is a parasympathetic medication that improves esophageal tone and peristalsis. It is a synthetic choline derivative. After filling the esophagus with a barium paste, 2.5 mg of mecholyl is administered subcutaneously. An increase in disorganized esophageal contractions within 2–3 minutes indicates a good reaction. Five minutes later, another dose is administered if there is no reaction; the total dose cannot be more than 10 mg. The dosage required will increase with the degree of esophageal dilation. The stimulating dose is neutralized by a subcutaneous injection of 1 mg of atropine sulfate.

7.8 ADJUSTMENTS TO PECULIAR DISEASES

7.8.1 Hiatal Hernia

Sometimes careful methodology is needed to demonstrate an esophageal hiatal hernia radiologically [4]. If the hernia is not seen in earlier, more conventional examinations, it is typically discovered by increased abdominal pressure on a filled gastric cardia and fundus in the Trendelenburg position. Nonetheless, the recorded bolus test, films following the Valsalva or Müller's maneuvers, films on continuous inspiration, films with straight leg-raising, the Wolf position, the Johnston position, and others may all be tried. If a hiatal hernia or insufficiency is present, it can be easily observed during a fluoroscopic examination while the patient is continuously consuming the regular barium mixture or while ingesting a thick barium bolus. Instead of using multiple recording or serial "spot filming," cineradiography can be useful in identifying a hiatal hernia that was previously undetectable. A minor hiatal hernia may not always be visible due to a variety of dynamic factors involving abdominal pressure and muscle tone. When the esophagus is fully filled and the swallowing motion is active, the RAO posture is the best way to visualize a hiatal hernia in infants and children.

7.8.2 Gastroesophageal Reflux

It can be challenging to show gastroesophageal reflux radiologically. When barium is added to the formula and the newborn is fluoroscopically examined in the prone right anterior oblique position while sucking from the bottle, it is possible to observe the frequent regurgitation that occurs in infants. However, abdominal palpation is typically necessary to demonstrate aberrant regurgitation, with pressure given to the full stomach following the barium meal ingestion. The Trendelenburg position is one of the supine positions used for this. It is also possible to try the water siphon test, especially on adults. First, dry swallows are attempted, then water sips are taken while applying regular pressure to the full stomach. If the barium is seen to regurgitate and refill the lower esophagus, reflux is diagnosed. The degree of lower sphincter incompetence is indicated by the ease and extent of this regurgitation.

7.8.3 Foreign Bodies

It is not unusual for children and newborns to inadvertently consume alien objects. There are other options, though, if the object is not opaque. A lateral cervical film and films of the chest and belly are often obtained as a starting point. To reveal the sphincter zone, the lateral cervical film should be exposed at the height of a dry swallow. A thin barium mixture should be consumed in order to check the hypopharynx and esophagus if no opaque foreign body is found and symptoms are present, or if the history of ingestion is initially uncontested. To check for esophageal blockage at the location of a nonopaque foreign body, barium-filled capsules or tablets should be given if no foreign body is visible. When a fish bone becomes stuck to the "back of the throat" (often the oropharynx), a cotton pledget soaked in an aqueous contrast agent might be swallowed in the hopes that the foreign body will prevent the cotton pledget from descending. Inducing hyperperistalsis carries some risk because it may make perforation easier. With the use of a barium combination, a solid marshmallow can be ingested under fluoroscopic surveillance in order to identify the obstruction site if it is farther down the esophagus. There are no further issues because the marshmallow dissolves gradually. You can also use a marshmallow that has been impregnated with barium.

7.8.4 Webs

During fluoroscopic inspection, webs, strictures, and rings are best seen in an esophagus that is completely dilated. The Valsalva maneuver is another way to see them. Ingestion of pills, capsules, or a marshmallow impregnated with barium can also demonstrate the presence of lower esophageal rings.

7.8.5 Atresia

A specific method is needed to identify infants with atresia and/or tracheoesophageal fistulae. A tiny polyethylene catheter is inserted via the nose and down to the blockage site in cases when atresia, with or without tracheoesophageal fistula, is suspected. Under fluoroscopic supervision, a thin barium mixture is consumed. To avoid aspirating the contrast, the patient is put in the prone position. When fistulae are present, they are typically seen in the esophageal anterior wall. To find fistulae that are proximally placed, an examination in the Trendelenburg (prone) posture is also necessary. When there is no obstruction, the catheter tip should be inserted in the middle of the esophagus, and the contrast should be administered during the fluoroscopy. The examination may be hampered if the contrast is aspirated into the larynx due to overflow.

7.8.6 Acute Esophagitis

Clinical suspicions are typically used to diagnose acute esophagitis. The acute inflammatory alterations are typically followed by radiologic findings. Nonetheless, esophagitis can be identified with the acid barium test, which is typically overlooked during a standard esophageal examination.

REFERENCES

1. Levine MS, Rubesin SE. Radiologic investigation of dysphagia. *AJR Am J Roentgenol*. 1990;154(6): 1157–63. doi:10.2214/ajr.154.6.2110721.
2. Levine MS, Rubesin SE, Ott DJ. Update on esophageal radiology. *AJR Am J Roentgenol*. 1990;155(5): 933–41. doi:10.2214/ajr.155.5.2120962.
3. Anatomy for Diagnostic Imaging. Saunders Ltd. Google Books.
4. Semenkovich J, Balfe D, Weyman P, Heiken J, Lee J. Barium pharyngography: comparison of single and double contrast. *AJR Am J Roentgenol*. 1985;144(4):715–20. doi:10.2214/ajr.144.4.715.

8 Contrast Media

8.1 BARIUM SULFATE-BASED CONTRAST

Barium (Ba) is an alkaline earth metal located in the second column of the periodic table. When in its pure state, it is a malleable and bright metal with a faint golden tint. Barium, with an atomic number of 56, is highly effective at blocking X-rays with the specific energy employed in medical imaging. Barium, due to its high reactivity, cannot naturally exist as a pure metal and hence cannot be used in its pure form for medical imaging. Barium sulfate ($BaSO_4$, Figure 8.1) is a widely used inorganic mineral salt that is stable and insoluble (Figure 8.2). It is commonly employed in industries as a filler for rubber, plastics, and resins. Despite its limited solubility in water, $BaSO_4$ can be effectively dispersed in water by using additives. This dispersion enhances the radiodensity (i.e., radio-opacity) and physical density (measured in g/mL) of the suspension. Suspensions with high concentrations, ranging from 40% to 240% weight-to-volume (w/v), can be used in fluoroscopy and radiography for various clinical purposes (Figure 8.3). In order to use $BaSO_4$ for computed tomography (CT), it is necessary to dilute the suspension significantly, to approximately a concentration of 2% w/v. Preparations with a low concentration are produced and marketed for certain specific abdominal CT imaging techniques. Barium-containing contrast media, such as $BaSO_4$, have many additional components, most of which are common food additives. These substances play a crucial role in determining the physicochemical properties of each product. In this document, we provide an explanation for the function of each ingredient or additive present in $BaSO_4$ contrast media

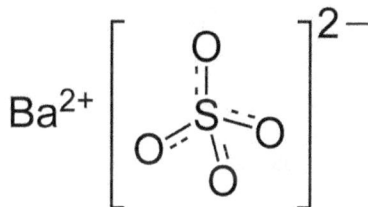

Figure 8.1 Barium sulfate chemical formula.

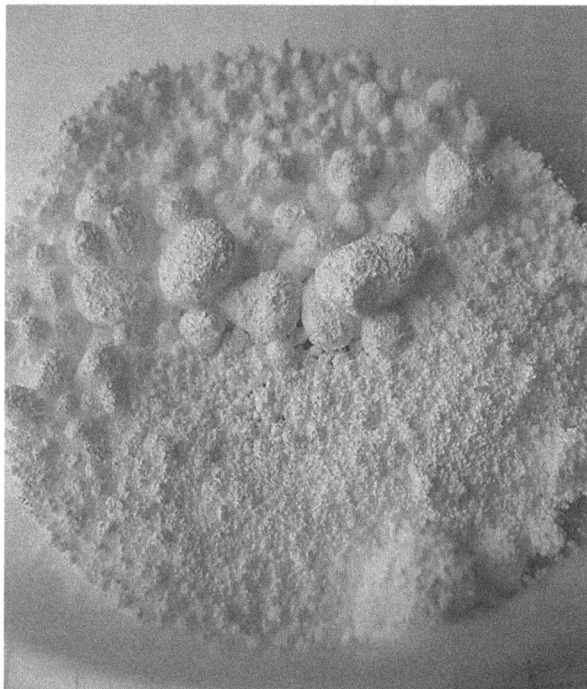

Figure 8.2 Barium sulfate powder.

DOI: 10.1201/9781003508113-8

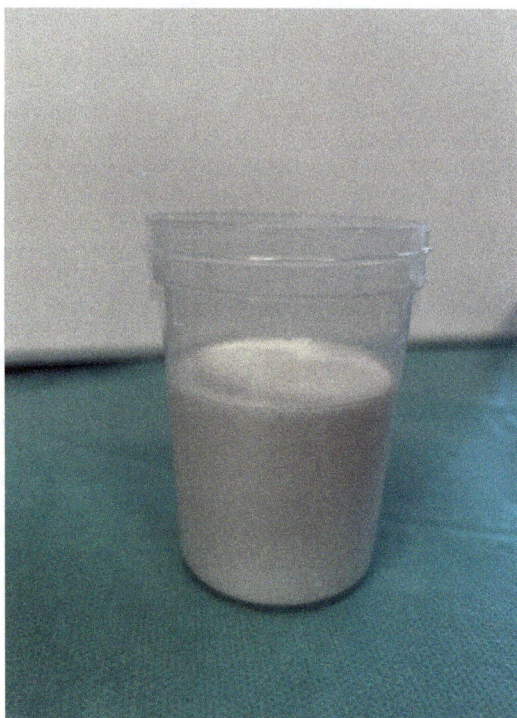

Figure 8.3 Barium sulfate intermediate density suspension.

products that are currently used for fluoroscopic and radiographic exams. Furthermore, we examine the function of these barium products in both the anatomical radiography assessment of the gastrointestinal (GI) tract and the evaluation of swallowing physiology. Lastly, we examine barium preparations utilized in CT applications [1–12].

8.1.1 Usage in Radiographic Procedures

Since $BaSO_4$ is inert, the GI tract does not absorb it. It is present in contrast media to provide physical density and radio-opacity, which are based on the concentration of $BaSO_4$. It cannot result in an allergic reaction and has no pharmacologic effects. On the other hand, retroperitonitis, peritonitis, or mediastinitis may result from $BaSO_4$ leakage from the GI lumen. Crucially, these unfavorable clinical outcomes stem from a strong granulomatous response, making them separate from the ideas of "hypersensitivity" and "toxicity." $BaSO_4$ contrast media formulations contain additives such as dispersants, stabilizers, and emulsifiers to maintain the $BaSO_4$ particles' smooth suspension in water; otherwise, the $BaSO_4$ particles would clump and sink to the bottom. Stickiness is produced by mucosal-coating thickeners, whereas viscosity is increased by non-coating thickeners. The use of these thickeners must be considered carefully because, while mucosal coating is beneficial in some applications (such as double-contrast GI imaging), it can be harmful in others (such as the modified barium swallow study [MBSS], which assesses swallowing physiology and requires exact viscosities). In order to make $BaSO_4$ products appetizing, easily removed, non-foaming, and long-lasting, additives are finally added. Here, we discuss the additives that offer each of these characteristics to help you better understand how they affect the various barium-containing contrast media's clinical value.

8.1.2 Dispersants, Stabilizers, and Emulsifiers

Since $BaSO_4$ is not soluble in water, emulsifiers, stabilizers, and dispersants must be added to maintain a smooth suspension of $BaSO_4$ particles, as well as pH regulators to ensure the effectiveness of the suspension. Among these is carboxymethylcellulose sodium, a polymer with a negative charge that covers the particles of $BaSO_4$. Through electrostatic repulsion, carboxymethylcellulose sodium aids in the suspension of the particles in water at low concentrations. Additional emulsifiers, stabilizers, and dispersants include polysorbate 80, a surfactant with anti-foaming properties, and sodium citrate, a dispersant that also aids in pH regulation. Several $BaSO_4$ formulations contain these three multifunctional ingredients.

8.1.3 Mucosal Coating and Non-Coating Thickeners

The goal of mucosal coating is to make the barium product stickier. Acacia gum (also known as gum arabic, the sap of the acacia tree) and, to a lesser extent, tragacanth gum (the sap of the astragalus gummifer shrub) are examples of additives that promote stickiness. Mucosal coating can also be produced by electrostatic forces, and this is accomplished by adding large amounts of sodium carboxymethylcellulose. These additives also have multiple functions: acacia gum and carboxymethylcellulose assist in suspending the $BaSO_4$ particles, while all three act as thickeners by raising viscosity. Non-coating thickeners cause the barium product to become more viscous rather than stickier, which prevents mucosal coating. Products with non-coating thickeners are appropriate for single-contrast anatomic imaging and the MBSS, where mucosal coating is not desired. Xanthan gum is a bacterial polysaccharide; carrageenan is a sulfated polysaccharide from red seaweed; pectin is a heteropolysaccharide from plant cell walls; modified cornstarch is also an anti-sticking/anti-caking agent; and methylcellulose is a plant fiber molecule bound to –CH3 moieties. These are examples of non-coating thickeners. The viscosities of the barium products used in the MBSS are strictly regulated and highly standardized, with increasing levels of non-sticky thickeners included in proportionately more viscous preparations. This is in contrast to the wider ranges of viscosity permitted in GI tract anatomic imaging.

8.1.4 Laxatives, Sweeteners, and Moisturizers

$BaSO_4$ contrast agents need sweeteners, like glycerin (also known as glycerol, a polyol), maltodextrin (a variable short-chain polysaccharide of glucose), and sorbitol and xylitol (poorly digested sugar alcohols), in order for them to be pleasant. Notably, some sweeteners have other crucial functions. All $BaSO_4$ preparations contain xylitol or sorbitol, two additional osmotic laxatives that retain water in the colon, preserving suspension and accelerating transit time through the GI tract. Additionally, sweeteners can thicken and/or texturize, giving food-like texture (also known as "mouthfeel") and raising viscosity. Moreover, glycerol has surfactant properties.

8.1.5 Others

Other crucial additions are pH regulators, such as citric acid, sodium citrate, HCl, and KCl, to maintain the right acid/base balance for a successful suspension; anti-foaming agents, like simethicone and polysorbate 80, to guarantee that the product doesn't become bubbly when shaken; and preservatives, like sodium benzoate, potassium sorbate, methylparaben, and propylparaben, to lengthen the shelf life of liquid $BaSO_4$ preparations. Powdered $BaSO_4$ preparations don't have preservatives added to them; according to manufacturer recommendations, they should be used soon after reconstitution. Additional ingredients include natural or artificial fruit flavors, saccharin, ethyl maltol, ethyl vanillin, and nontoxic solvent propylene glycol, which is used to facilitate the mixing of a powdered mixture with water.

8.2 EXPLORING BaSO$_4$ PREPARATIONS FOR GI IMAGING

Barium preparations may be used to assess each segment of the GI tract. In the next few paragraphs, we will be exploring its potentialities and different modalities of use, both for fluoroscopy and the remaining types of examinations (enemas, defecating proctograms, CT). While this book focuses on fluoroscopy, a thorough assessment of barium products is, in our opinion, mandatory in order to understand the differences, advantages, and potential disadvantages of using liquids with varying degrees of inherent radio and physical density.

8.2.1 Examining the GI Tract through Radiographic Imaging

Examining the GI tract using barium products involves assessing the anatomy of various parts, such as the esophagus, stomach, duodenum, small bowel, colon, and rectum. These exams aim to detect and describe anatomical abnormalities such as tumors, inflammation, obstructions, malformations, and more using a contrast agent that can either coat or fill the affected area. Products used for all these applications must have a high density, both physically and radiographically, ranging from 24% to 240% w/v. Double-contrast upper gastrointestinal imaging is employed to uncover intricate details of the GI tract's mucosal inner lining, exposing ulcers, polyps, inflammatory patterns, and more. To visualize these structures, a thin and uniform layer of a dense and adhesive $BaSO_4$ preparation needs to be applied to the mucosal lining, while the lumen is filled with air or gas. Thus, the $BaSO_4$ contrast agent should include a viscous gum (such as acacia gum) to provide a protective coating for the mucosa, and it should have a high radiodensity (100–240% w/v). However, single-contrast upper GI imaging is utilized to observe overall anatomy and anatomical lesions. When it comes to filling the GI structures with contrast, there usually aren't any issues in AP or mildly oblique projections. This is because there is minimal overlapping of the upper GI structures in those projections. For this examination, it is important to fill the lumen with a well-mixed solution of $BaSO_4$ preparation [13]. The solution should have a moderate density, ranging from 60% to 120% w/v, and should not contain any sticky gums. Small bowel follow-through (SBFT) examination or enteroclysis (direct contrast administration into the small bowel) can be performed as either a single- or double-contrast procedure. One of the primary obstacles is to effectively visualize a lengthy section of densely inter-twined intestinal loops. Therefore, it is crucial that the barium contrast solution is substantial and has a relatively low concentration. Furthermore, the application of certain mucosal coatings can potentially provide assistance. Thus, the formulation should include non-sticky thickeners/fillers like methylcellulose, xanthan, or carrageenan, along with a small quantity of sticky gum, and have a low radiodensity of less than 25% w/v. One must take into account the presence of spacious bowel loops that may overlap, particularly when examining oblique views of the sigmoid and splenic flexures during a double-contrast barium enema. Ensuring proper mucosal coating is crucial for effective barium contrast imaging. Achieving the desired filling is accomplished by introducing insufflated air. However, excessive stickiness can pose challenges when attempting to apply the coating throughout the entire length of the cecum. Thus, the barium preparation contains a moderate concentration of sticky gum and has a moderate radiodensity (100% w/v). In the case of a single-contrast barium enema, the main focus is on achieving proper filling, while the presence of overlapping loops can pose a significant challenge. The barium preparation should contain non-adhesive thickeners and fillers, such as xanthan or carrageenan, with a radiodensity of 50% w/v. During defecography, it is important to note that the rectum can hold a large amount of material; hence, the radiodensity should be relatively modest. The contrast, in addition, should replicate the texture of regular feces in order to be held within the rectum. Therefore, the barium preparation should be in the form of a paste, achieved by using a high concentration of carboxymethylcellulose, and have a relatively low radiodensity of 60% w/v [14].

8.2.2 Barium in the Assessment of the Swallowing Function

The MBSS, or videofluoroscopic swallow study (VFSS), is, as we already should know, a dynamic radiologic examination that provides real-time imaging to evaluate the physiological aspects of swallowing. The objective of this examination is to gain a methodical and replicable evaluation of the structure and function of the swallowing mechanism, as well as to identify compensation measures for any abnormalities. This is a single-contrast examination, so the $BaSO_4$ preparations must have a radiodensity that is low to moderate (40% w/v). It is crucial to have a reliable range of standardized viscosities for $BaSO_4$ preparations used in MBSS/VFSS. Common consistencies range from a watery liquid to a thick nectar, from a thin honey to a dense puree or pudding, and finally to a solid state. In addition, it is necessary to attain certain viscosities using starches and sugars that do not have a sticky consistency, namely without the use of acacia or tragacanth gum, in order to prevent the formation of a mucosal coating. Ultimately, they should be both palatable and resemble food, offering a satisfactory texture and incorporating sweetness and flavoring. It is important to be aware that carboxymethylcellulose is included in all liquid $BaSO_4$ preparations used for the MBSS as a substance that thickens the mixture. Nevertheless, the small amounts present in these liquid formulations are inadequate to generate a significant electrostatic force that would enable $BaSO_4$ particles to stick to the inner surface of the GI tract, resulting in the absence of any coating effect. When carboxymethylcellulose is added to MBSS in a concentration that is enough to form a pudding-like consistency, it counteracts the electrostatic attraction to the GI inner lining with the help of additional additives [15–20]. What is the reason behind why we cannot use "regular" GI barium products that are appropriate for single-contrast imaging in the MBSS? The reason for this is that these items do not have the exact and uniform thicknesses that the MBSS products have. During the development process, the viscosity of each MBSS barium product was carefully chosen to effectively highlight any physiological abnormalities in the swallowing mechanism. The viscosity ranged from a thin liquid consistency to that of pudding. Utilizing these products is essential for conducting a precise and consistent MBSS. Additionally, they enhance patient safety, optimize efficiency, and minimize waste. Merely diluting typical $BaSO_4$ preparations for the MBSS does not completely remove the mucosal coating. It also results in varying and potentially overly low radiodensities, as well as unknown viscosities. Moreover, this dilution undermines the effectiveness of the additives in unforeseen and likely undesirable manners. A commonly expressed issue regarding the MBSS is the inhalation of $BaSO_4$ preparations. According to the *ACR Manual on Contrast Media*, it is common for aspirated barium contrast agent to be moved in the proximal direction by the ciliary action of normal bronchial epithelium. Nevertheless, the presence of impaired epithelium resulting from bronchial illness causes a delay in this physiological process. If not fully expelled, $BaSO_4$ particles can persist indefinitely and can induce inflammation. Like any liquid, the excessive suction of barium-containing contrast can cause sudden respiratory distress or pneumonia. In order to reduce the likelihood of harm, the preparations authorized for the MBSS have a comparatively low concentration of $BaSO_4$ (40% w/v) and do not contain any adhesive substances, both of which aid in the removal of obstructions. Iodinated contrast medium should not be used for the MBSS. If ionic high-osmolar contrast media (HOCM) is inhaled, it can lead to potentially fatal pulmonary edema. Nonionic low-osmolar contrast media (LOCM), although less risky to aspirate alone, are all classified as "thin liquids." Consequently, in order to conduct a comprehensive swallowing assessment, they would need to be combined with different types of foods or food additives, which do not have standardized viscosities and may be nonsterile and potentially hazardous if aspirated [21].

8.2.3 Barium Preparations Used for Computed Tomography

There are three applications of CT that use barium contrast. The first is bowel marking, which is used for routine CT of the abdomen/pelvis. The second is tagging residual solid stool, which is used for CT colonography (CTC). Residual liquid stool is tagged with iodinated contrast media. The third use is bowel distention at near-water density, which is used for CT enterography (CTE). Barium preparations are used in normal CT scans of the abdomen/pelvis to differentiate bowel loops from nearby structures such as arteries, tumors, and nodes. The preparations for routine CT should have a concentration of 2% w/v of $BaSO_4$, which is enough to show improvement. They should also be very appetizing to ensure patient compliance. Additionally, the preparations should contain sorbitol to maintain filling and facilitate intestinal transit. Barium preparations are utilized in CTC to label remaining solid stool particles in order to differentiate them from polyps. The preparations for this use should have a concentration of 40% w/v. They should contain carboxymethylcellulose for tagging purposes. They should also be extremely palatable and come packed and labeled for home use. Barium-based contrast material is utilized in CTE to inflate intestinal loops to a density similar to water. This aids in the evaluation of the gut wall, specifically looking for signs of inflammation associated with inflammatory bowel disease. In this application, the $BaSO_4$ preparations should have a concentration of no more than 0.1% w/v. They should also comprise natural gum to provide substance and contain sorbitol to maintain filling and promote intestinal transit [22].

8.2.4 Considerations on Barium-Based Products and Complications

Barium sulfate offers barium-containing contrast compounds with two distinct characteristics: radiodensity and physical density. The radiodensity, which is influenced by the concentration of $BaSO_4$, is modified to account for the specific imaging equipment, technique, and structures being examined. All remaining ingredients contribute to the additional beneficial characteristics seen in $BaSO_4$ products: the $BaSO_4$ particle suspension is utilized for its mucosal coating properties, as well as its ability to enhance viscosity and texture in MBSS preparations. Additionally, it provides sweetness, acts as a filling agent and laxative, aids in preservation, prevents foaming, and adds flavor. To choose the appropriate $BaSO_4$ product for a certain examination, one must have a comprehensive awareness of the anatomical structures being visualized and the disorders being assessed. Every imaging technology and clinical application has its own specific and ideal concentration or range of $BaSO_4$, as well as a specific mix of additives that allows for the assessment of the desired anatomy and/or function. The oral administration of barium sulfate for diagnostic purposes carries risks that are primarily associated with the disease process in the patient being examined. Hazards include perforation, obstruction, impaction, aspiration, and embolization [23].

8.2.5 Perforation and Barium

The perforation of the upper GI tract or small bowel is a relatively common occurrence; this carries a constant, albeit small risk, when introducing particulate barium sulfate into bodily cavities. The impact of barium outside the GI tract is consistently harmful, but it significantly differs depending on the location and circumstances of the perforation. Esophageal perforations commonly occur as a consequence of vigorous and protracted vomiting, or Boerhaave's syndrome. Esophageal perforation can occur due to various factors, including medical procedures such as endoscopy, ingestion of sharp objects, and physical injury. Using barium sulfate to examine a perforated or lacerated esophagus can lead to mediastinitis or empyema, especially if there is a bacterial infection present. Radiologists typically choose to evaluate a possibly torn esophagus using a water-soluble contrast media. The most common cause of stomach perforation is peptic ulcer disease. Administering barium sulfate suspensions in these circumstances greatly complicates the clinical scenario, although most patients do recover after undergoing the necessary laparotomy. Fortunately, the majority of perforations are typically detected through clinical suspicion prior to ordering a contrast examination. In such cases, plain films of the abdomen are usually sufficient to identify the presence of free air in the peritoneal cavity. If there is suspicion of stomach or duodenal perforation caused by ulcer disease, it is recommended to use water-soluble contrast material for the examination. Reports indicate that perforation of gastric and duodenal ulcers can occur during X-ray examinations, accounting for up to 1% of all peptic ulcer perforations [24]. The majority of reports ascribe the occurrence of perforation during inspection to either compression or the weakening of the viscus wall caused by medicinal drugs like steroids. Perforation of the small intestine, with the exception of duodenal ulcers, is rare. Nevertheless, there is a possibility of barium entering the peritoneal cavity in situations when the small bowel is weakened due to conditions such as small bowel ischemia, scleroderma, systemic lupus erythematosus, polyarteritis, or rupture caused by a foreign object.

8.2.6 Barium Obstruction and Impaction

It is widely recognized that orally administered barium sulfate may accumulate near a narrowing of the bowel, causing obstruction or impaction [25]. This rarely occurs in the upper GI tract and small bowel because the fluidity of the barium suspension is maintained. In the colon, progressive dehydration of the barium may cause impaction proximal to even an incomplete obstruction. The typical causes of these obstructions are carcinomas and diverticulitis. The primary complication of barium impaction in the colon is perforation. Barium can have an impact on the colon due to prolonged stasis, even without an underlying obstructing lesion. This, however, is rather rare. Barium appendicitis has also been reported following barium meal examination. In a report consisting of three cases, appendicitis occurred as early as the ninth day after the examination and as late as three months afterward. The mechanism was believed to involve an obstructing barium-fecolith causing acute appendicitis. The probability of barium impaction can be reduced by various measures. The use of well-suspended, isosmotic barium suspensions reduces the likelihood of severe dehydration of the barium in the distal small intestine, bowel, or colon and enhances the probability that the suspension will remain fluid. Maintaining adequate hydration of the patient further reduces the absorption of water from the barium suspension in the distal colon. Using the concept of catharsis, namely through the use of saline, cathartics significantly reduce the likelihood of barium becoming dehydrated in the distal bowel. It is important to be aware that drugs that inhibit peristalsis may contribute to impaction, and this awareness is also important in preventing it.

8.2.7 Barium Aspiration

Introducing pure barium sulfate into the bronchial tree is generally innocuous, as long as the barium does not block important bronchial passages or certain regurgitated stomach contents [26]. Typically, a combination of coughing and the movement of cilia helps to expel most of the inhaled barium within a day or two. Barium's generally harmless properties in the tracheobronchial tree have led several authors to recommend it as a contrast medium for bronchography. Ingesting high amounts of barium sulfate suspension may lead to complications. Due to its large quantity and thick consistency, barium sulfate suspension can effectively block small peripheral bronchi, and even larger bronchi. If barium is aspirated due to vomiting or regurgitation, and there is a large amount of gastric contents also aspirated, it can lead to the development of severe chemical bronchitis and pneumonia. If a sufficient amount of barium is inhaled, it can enter the alveolar gaps and become lodged in the outer parts of the lungs permanently. While ciliary activity and phagocytosis can remove some of the trapped barium, any residual barium particles are likely to trigger a granulomatous foreign-body reaction. Radiologists frequently receive requests to conduct contrast exams of the upper GI system using iodinated water-soluble substances in cases when patients are known to be aspirating or vomiting, or when there is suspected obstruction before the ligament of Treitz. Referring physicians erroneously believe that the act of inhaling water-soluble substances is less detrimental than inhaling barium sulfate suspension. Indeed, the inhalation of hyperosmotic iodinated contrast materials leads to the development of acute pulmonary edema. It is recommended to utilize barium suspension in this situation due to its generally harmless impact on the lung. However, caution must be taken to prevent the patient from inhaling significant amounts of it. Particular conditions enhance the likelihood of inhaling a contrast agent. The potential risks of aspiration, such as chemical pneumonitis and foreign-body response, have already been mentioned in relation to vomiting or regurgitation. Due to laryngeal issues, a patient may also inhale barium suspension during an examination. This typically occurs in geriatric patients or individuals who are exceptionally frail, as well as in patients with neurological disorders. Another factor that can lead to inhalation, both into the nasal cavity and the lungs, is the incorrect delivery of barium to patients, particularly when they are lying flat on their back. Contrast material may potentially enter the lungs as a result of a fistula. Two common examples include the introduction of barium through a tracheoesophageal fistula caused by necrotic cancer or during the examination of esophageal atresia and tracheoesophageal fistula. Tracheoesophageal fistulas can also occur due to trauma, as a complication of tracheostomy and after surgical procedures or radiotherapy involving the esophagus or mediastinum. It is recommended that the fistula is examined using barium sulfate suspension instead of a water-soluble contrast material in all of these cases [27].

8.2.8 Barium Embolization

A single case of barium embolization following an upper GI examination was reported in a patient with Hodgkin's disease who was experiencing massive upper GI bleeding. The authors postulated that extensive mucosal ulcerations of the duodenum and upper small bowel in this patient allowed barium to enter the portal venous circulation [28].

8.3 WATER-SOLUBLE HIGH-OSMOLALITY IODINATED CONTRAST MEDIA (HOCM)

The capacity to differentiate between tissues with varying X-ray attenuation relies on two types of interactions between photons and matter: Compton scattering and photoelectric absorption. Both of these interactions are influenced by the physical density of the matter, while the latter is additionally influenced by the atomic number of the matter. Due to its high atomic number of 53, iodine creates visual contrast when administered as iodinated material, as it is more readily absorbed through photoelectric absorption compared to most tissues in the body. Iodine possesses a distinct advantage as a contrast agent due to its k-shell binding energy (k-edge) of 33.2 keV, which closely matches the average energy of X-rays employed in diagnostic radiography. When the incident X-ray energy approaches the k-edge of the atom it interacts with, the likelihood of photoelectric absorption increases. Iodinated contrast media are contrast agents that consist of iodine atoms and are used in X-ray-based imaging techniques such as fluoroscopy and CT. They can either be water-insoluble or water-soluble, the latter subsequently divided into two main categories: high- (HOCM) and low-osmolality (LOCM). Water-soluble high-osmolality iodinated contrast agents, substantially diatrizoate sodium/meglumine, are those we use in clinical practice for upper- and lower-GI studies, after oral administration, both in fluoroscopy and CT. HOCM have an osmolality that is approximately five to eight times higher than that of serum. Generally, HOCM refers to ionic compounds composed of a benzene ring with three iodine atoms and a side chain that contains a carboxylic acid (–COOH) group. Due to their high occurrence of negative effects, HOCM, which were the initial kind of iodinated contrast agents, lost popularity in the 1990s for use in blood vessels and the spinal canal. HOCM are still utilized for GI and cystourethral administration. An important benefit of iodinated water-soluble contrast materials is their easy absorption from the peritoneal cavity, pleural cavities, and interstitial tissues. This makes them valuable for examining patients who are suspected of having a perforation in an organ. Studies have shown no residual effects from the transient presence of liquid contrast materials in the peritoneum [29].

8.3.1 Complications Due to HOCM Usage

The significant and constant hazards of water-soluble high-osmolality media essentially stem from two specific physical traits: high osmolality, obviously, and the possibility of precipitation under particular conditions [30].

8.3.2 HOCM Aspiration

Aspiration is a common and significant outcome that often occurs when aqueous contrast materials are used orally. As previously stated, these drugs are hyperosmolar, with a concentration of 1900 mOsm/L, which is approximately six times higher than that of normal serum. The hyperosmolarity within the lungs attracts fluid into the alveoli, resulting in pulmonary edema that is similar to the edema caused by drowning in seawater. Injecting an aqueous contrast medium into a bronchopleural or bronchocutaneous fistula results in comparable effects when a significant volume of contrast material reaches the bronchi. When this event takes place, it typically leads to abrupt and intense respiratory discomfort. In animal experiments, the administration of diatrizoate into the trachea has been demonstrated to induce pulmonary edema. Nevertheless, animals that managed to survive the pulmonary edema did not exhibit any signs of enduring lung injury. HOCM is also recognized for its irritative effects on several tissues, potentially leading to reflex bronchospasm. As previously stated, it is generally not advisable to request oral investigations that involve the use of water-soluble contrast agents, especially in cases where there is a significant likelihood of tracheo-esophageal fistula, severe vomiting, high blockage, or similar conditions. Many referring physicians are unaware that the aspiration of significant amounts of water-soluble iodinated contrast chemicals can be lethal due to the subsequent pulmonary edema. These investigations should be conducted with less harmful substances, such as a suspension of barium sulfate. When there is a potential risk of perforation and aspiration, it is important to use water-soluble contrast materials sparingly to decrease the amount used and reduce the likelihood of significant aspiration [31].

8.3.3 Precipitation

Occasional precipitation of aqueous contrast materials may occur. Hydrochloric acid has the ability to cause diatrizoate meglumine 76% to form a solid substance in solutions with a concentration of 0.1 N. This kind of event is infrequent among patients. Obstruction can also lead to the precipitation of HOCM in people who have low levels of stomach acid (achlorhydric). Precipitation of HOCM was noted in the literature in a blocked gastric stump, resulting in the formation of a solid mass that led to stomach erosions and hematemesis [32].

8.3.4 Hypovolemia

Hypovolemia is an additional result of the hypertonic nature of HOCM and similar water-soluble contrast agents when administered in the GI tract. The high osmolarity of HOCM, which is six times greater than that of serum, leads to the movement of fluid into the lumen of the GI tract. This may result in a significant decrease in plasma volume. The most significant alterations have been observed in newborns who have taken HOCM orally. However, similar effects have also been observed in adults, with an increase in blood protein, uric acid, calcium, and hematocrit levels [33].

REFERENCES

1. National Center for Biotechnology Information: PubChem Periodic Table of Elements. Barium (Element). Available at: https://pubchem.ncbi.nlm.nih.gov/element/56. Accessed February 7, 2021.
2. *Miller-Keane encyclopedia & dictionary of medicine: nursing & allied health.* Revised Reprint, 7th Edition, Elsevier, Amsterdam.
3. American College of Radiology (ACR) Committee on Drugs and Contrast Media. *ACR manual on contrast media.* 2020. Available at: https://www.acr.org/-/media/ACR/files/clinical -resources/contrast_media.pdf. Accessed February 7, 2021.
4. Goldner RD, Adams DO. The structure of mononuclear phagocytes differentiating in vivo. III. The effect of particulate foreign substances. *Am J Pathol* 1977;89:335–350.
5. Hazelwood RJ, Armeson KE, Hill EG, Bonilha HS, Martin-Harris B. Identification of swal-lowing tasks from a modified barium swallow study that optimize the detection of physi-ological impairment. *J Speech Lang Hear Res* 2017;60:1855–1863.
6. Gelfand DW. Complications of gastrointestinal radiologic procedures: I. Complications of routine fluoroscopic studies. *Gastrointest Radiol* 1980;5:293–315.
7. Regan PT, Weiland LH, Glall MG: Scleroderma and intestinal perforation. *Am J Gastroenterol* 1977;68:566–571.
8. Matolo NH, Albo D: Gastrointestinal complications of collagen vascular diseases. *Am J Surg* 1971;122:678–682.
9. Wolfson JJ, Williams H: A hazard of barium enema studies in infants with small bowel atre-sia. *Radiology* 1970;95:341–343.
10. Killingback M: Acute large bowel obstruction precipitated by barium X-ray examination. *Med J Aust* 1964;2:503–508.
11. Ansell G (ed): *Complications in diagnostic radiology.* Oxford: Blackwell; 1976. p. 334.
12. Serjeant JCB, Raymond JA: Perforation of apparently normal colon after a barium meal. *Lancet* 1952;263:1245–1246.
13. Prout BJ, Datta SB, Wilson TS: Colonic retention of barium in the elderly after barium meal examination and its treatment with lactulose. *Br Med J* 1970;4:530–533.

14. Young MO: Acute appendicitis following retention of barium in the appendix. *Arch Surg* 1958;77:1011–1014.
15. Dixon GD, Ferris DO, Hodgson JR: Unusual complications of barium studies: report of a case of adherent cecal barolith. *Am J Roentgenol Radium Ther Nucl Med* 1967;99:106–111.
16. Schabel SI, Skucas J: Esophageal obstruction following administration of "aged" barium sulfate tablets—warning. *Radiology* 1977;122:835–836.
17. Fishel CR: Inhalation of barium in solution. *JAMA* 1923;80:102.
18. Willson JKV, Rubin PS, McGee TM: The effects of barium sulfate on the lungs. A clinical and experimental study. *Am J Roentgenol* 1959;82:84–94.
19. Spritzer AA, Watson JA: The measurement of ciliary clearance in the lungs of rats. *Health Phys* 1964;10:1093–1097.
20. Dunbar JS, Skinner GB, Wortzman G, Stuart JR: An investigation of effects of opaque media on the lungs with comparison of barium sulfate, lipiodol and dionosil. *Am J Roentgenol* 1959;82:902–926.
21. Teixeira LCV: Bronchography without oil and iodine. The use of barium as a contrast medium. *Dis Chest* 1959;36:256–264.
22. Nice CM, Waring WW, Killelea DE, Hurwitz L: Bronchography in infants and children. Barium sulfate as a contrast agent. *Am J Roentgenol Radium Ther Nucl Med* 1964;91:564–570.
23. Nelson SW, Christoforidis AJ, Pratt PC: Barium sulfate and bismuth subcarbonate suspensions as bronchogenic contrast media. *Radiology* 1959;72:829–839.
24. Nelson SW, Christoforidis AJ, Pratt PC: Further experience with barium sulfate as a bronchographic contrast medium. *Am J Roentgenol Radium Ther Nucl Med* 1964;92:595–614.
25. Fite F: Granuloma of the lung due to radiographic contrast medium. *Arch Pathol* 1955;59:673–676.
26. Huston J, Watlach DP, Cunningham GJ: Pulmonary reaction to barium sulfate in rats. *Arch Pathol* 1952;54:430–438.
27. Castellino RA, Verby HD, Friedland GW, Northway WH: Delayed barium aspiration following complete reflux small bowel enema. *Br J Radiol* 1968;41:937–939.
28. Nelson SW: Facts versus folklore. *Am J Surg* 1965;109:543–545.
29. Frech RS, Davie JM, Adatepe M, Feldhaus R, McAllister WH: Comparison of barium sulfate and oral 40% diatrizoate injected into the trachea of dogs. *Radiology* 1970;95:299–303.
30. Reich SB: Production of pulmonary edema by aspiration of water-soluble nonabsorbable contrast media. *Radiology* 1969;92:367–370.
31. Chiu CL, Gambach RR: Hypaque pulmonary edema. *Radiology* 1974;111:91–92.
32. Ansell G: A national survey of radiological complications: interim report. *Clin Radiol* 1968;19:175–191.
33. Mahboubi S, Gohel VK, Dalinka MK, Cho SY: Barium embolization following upper gastrointestinal examination. *Radiology* 1974;14:301–302.

9 Approach to Image Interpretation

9.1 INTRODUCTION

Swallowing, or deglutition, is one of the most intricate neuromuscular processes in the human body, involving the precisely timed coordination of over 30 pairs of muscles and multiple cranial nerves across the oral, pharyngeal, and esophageal regions. When any part of this system becomes impaired—due to stroke, neurological disorders, structural anomalies, or aging—the result is dysphagia, and this can lead to serious medical complications such as aspiration pneumonia, malnutrition, and dehydration. To assess and diagnose dysphagia effectively, the videofluoroscopic swallow study (VFSS), also known as the modified barium swallow study (MBSS), is widely recognized as the gold standard. This dynamic, real-time X-ray procedure allows clinicians to visualize bolus transit and evaluate the physiological mechanisms of swallowing in detail. However, interpretation of the VFSS has historically varied across clinicians and institutions, often lacking standardization and consistency. A transformative advancement in the field came with the work of Bonnie Martin-Harris, a leading voice in swallowing science and a pioneer in instrumental dysphagia assessment. Recognizing the need for a structured, reproducible, and objective approach to VFSS interpretation, Martin-Harris led the development of the modified barium swallow impairment profile (MBSImP). This protocol revolutionized the field by deconstructing the complex swallow into 17 discrete, observable physiological components—each systematically scored based on validated criteria. Under her leadership, the MBSImP became not only a diagnostic tool, but a clinical framework for standardization, interdisciplinary communication, and evidence-based treatment planning [1,2].

9.2 OBJECTIVES AND SIGNIFICANCE OF THE MBSImP

As already mentioned, the MBSImP was established in order to accomplish many goals, its primary objectives being to [3–43]:

- *Standardize VFSS interpretation*: By providing a uniform framework, the MBSImP reduces variability and subjectivity in VFSS assessments, ensuring consistency across clinicians and institutions, making it easier for less experienced readers to achieve consistency and confidence in diagnosing.

- *Enhance diagnostic precision*: Detailed analysis of specific swallowing components allows for precise identification of dysfunctions, aiding in targeted therapeutic interventions, leaving little to no space for personal considerations that might derail from the right path.

- *Facilitate effective communication*: A common terminology and scoring system might improve interdisciplinary communication among healthcare providers, including speech-language pathologists, radiologists, and physicians, both in the same institution and around the world.

- *Support evidence-based practice*: The protocol is grounded in empirical research, promoting interventions that are scientifically validated and tailored to individual patient needs.

9.3 THE MBSImP PROTOCOL OVERVIEW

The MBSImP protocol is a standardized checklist that evaluates the act of swallowing, breaking it down into 17 physiological components, categorized into 3 domains:

1. Oral Phase (6 components).

2. Pharyngeal Phase (9 components).

3. Esophageal Phase (2 components).

Each swallow is analyzed based on 17 components divided across 3 phases as follows.

ORAL PHASE (6 COMPONENTS)

1. Lip closure.
2. Tongue control during bolus hold.
3. Bolus preparation/mastication.
4. Bolus transport/lingual motion.
5. Oral residue.
6. Initiation of pharyngeal swallow.

DOI: 10.1201/9781003508113-9

PHARYNGEAL PHASE (9 COMPONENTS)

7. Soft palate elevation.
8. Laryngeal elevation.
9. Anterior hyoid excursion.
10. Epiglottic movement.
11. Laryngeal vestibular closure.
12. Pharyngeal stripping wave.
13. Pharyngeal contraction.
14. Pharyngoesophageal segment opening (PESO).
15. Tongue base retraction.

ESOPHAGEAL PHASE (2 COMPONENTS)

16. Pharyngeal residue.
17. Esophageal clearance.

Each component is assessed using an ordinal scale, with scores reflecting the severity of impairment. The worst observed performance across trials is documented to guide clinical decision-making. This systematic scoring method enhances reliability and facilitates comparison over time, in each component and in the same patient, making it easier to monitor and assess if and how therapeutic approaches are working.

9.4 PATIENT PREPARATION AND POSITIONING

Of course, proper preparation and positioning are crucial for the accuracy of the MBSImP:

- *Patient history*: As we have already extensively discussed in a previous chapter, a thorough history intake is needed on conditions affecting swallowing, such as stroke, neurological diseases, head and neck cancers, or reflux.

- *Positioning*: The patient is seated upright at a 90-degree angle, typically in a lateral view to visualize oral, pharyngeal, and cervical esophageal phases. Anteroposterior (AP) views may be added to assess symmetry and pharyngeal contraction. For the esophageal evaluation, please see Chapter 7 on imaging technique.

- *Safety measures*: Use of protective shielding is essential to minimize radiation exposure. Clinical staff should monitor patients for fatigue or distress during the study.

9.5 STANDARDIZED BOLUS ADMINISTRATION

The MBSImP employs a standardized sequence of bolus types and volumes to ensure consistency and reproducibility across patients and facilities. The typical sequence includes:

- *Thin liquids*: 5 mL via teaspoon, 10 mL via teaspoon, cup sip, and sequential swallows

- *Nectar-thick liquids*: 5 mL via teaspoon

- *Honey-thick liquids*: 5 mL via teaspoon

- *Puree (pudding-thick)*: 5 mL via teaspoon

- *Solid*: 1/4 of a Lorna Doone cookie coated with barium

Each bolus is mixed with a standardized barium sulfate contrast agent to enhance visibility under fluoroscopy. The order of administration is designed to progress from least to most challenging, enabling the identification of fatigue or consistency-specific deficits.

9.6 DETAILED ANALYSIS OF THE 17 PHYSIOLOGICAL COMPONENTS

9.6.1 Lip Closure

Lip closure assesses the ability to maintain an anterior seal during bolus intake and transport. Adequate lip closure is essential to prevent anterior spillage and maintain intraoral pressure necessary for effective bolus manipulation and transport. Impaired lip closure may result in drooling, reduced oral intake, and a heightened risk of aspiration. Score, at any point during the swallow, the presence and location of contrast material seen between or outside the lips on the lateral view. If lips are not completely in frame, score what can be seen and note that the exam was limited (Figure 9.1a–f).

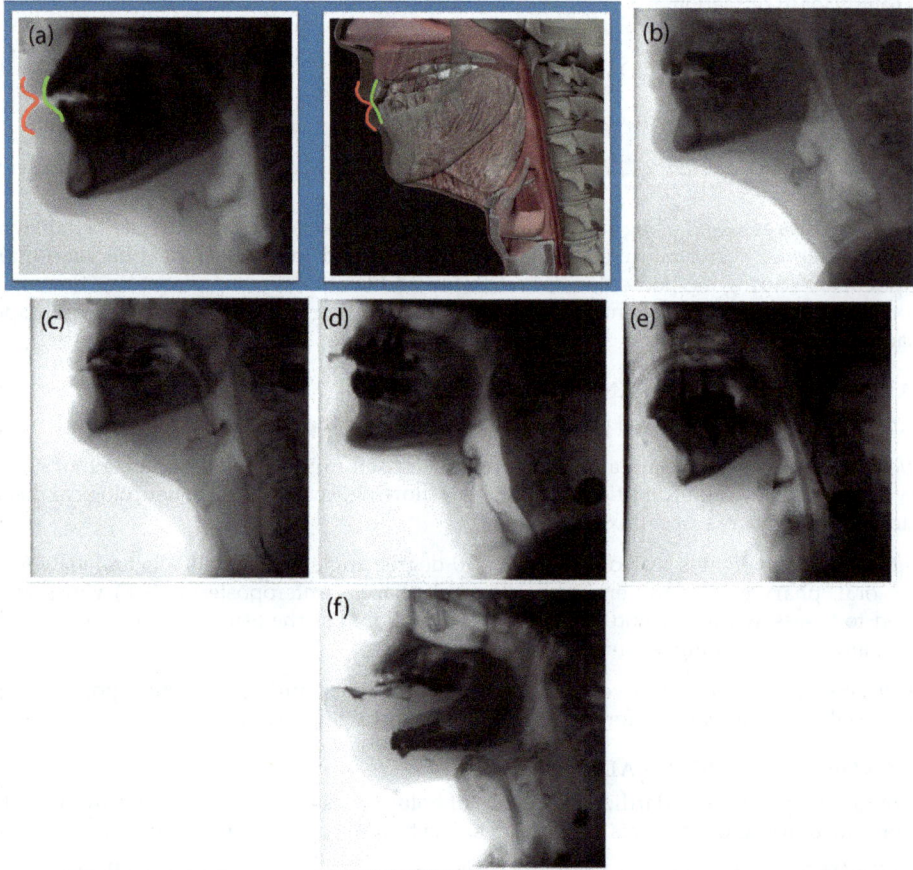

Figure 9.1 Component 1: Lip Closure. 0 = No labial escape. Contrast is contained within the oral cavity; there is no evidence of escape beyond the oral mucosa. 1 = Interlabial escape; no progression to anterior lip. Trace amounts of contrast outline the interlabial space. No progression to the anterior lip. 2 = Escape from interlabial space or lateral juncture; no extension to vermilion border. Progression of contrast onto but not beyond the vermilion border of the lower lip. 3 = Escape progressing to mid-chin. Contrast progresses beyond the vermilion border to the mid-chin but not beyond. 4 = Escape through open lips. Profuse escape between open lips progresses beyond the chin regardless of bolus consistency or swallow task.

- 0: No labial escape.
- 1: Interlabial escape; no progression to anterior lip.
- 2: Escape from interlabial space or lateral juncture; no extension beyond vermilion border.
- 3: Escape progressing to mid-chin.
- 4: Escape beyond mid-chin.

9.6.2 Tongue Control during Bolus Hold

This component evaluates the ability to hold a cohesive bolus in the oral cavity before initiating the swallow. Impaired control can result in premature spillage into the pharynx, increasing the risk of penetration or aspiration before protective reflexes are triggered. Score during swallowing tasks that require the patient to perform a bolus hold, so essentially with 5 mL thin, cup sip thin, 5 mL nectar, cup sip nectar, 5 mL honey, prior to the initiation of productive tongue movement to propel the bolus. Score even if the patient is unable to follow instructions or there is neuromuscular impairment. "Dippers," described by Jeri Dodds in the 1980s, hold the bolus on the anterior floor of the mouth prior to swallowing. If this is a customary manner of holding the bolus, score 0 (Figure 9.2a–f).

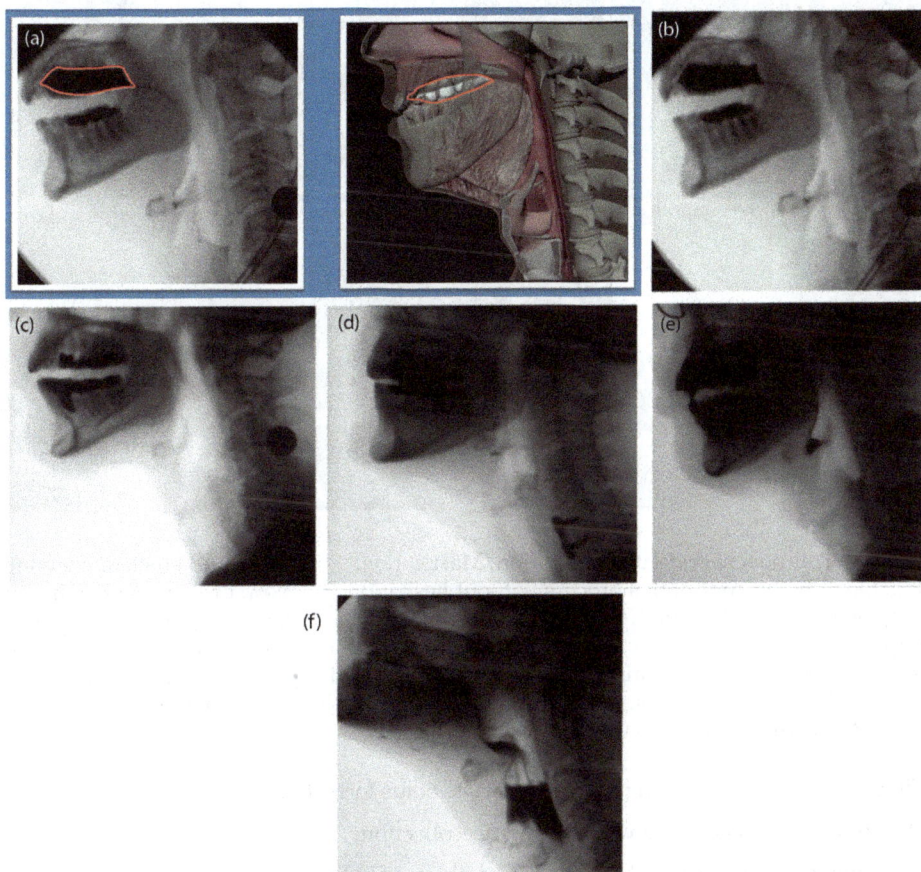

Figure 9.2 Component 2: Tongue Control. 0 = Cohesive bolus between tongue and palatal seal. Contrast is contained between the tongue and palatal seal, anteriorly, posteriorly, and laterally. No escape to the lateral sulci, floor of mouth, or pharynx "dippers/tippers." The bolus is held on the anterior floor of the mouth prior to swallowing; if the customary manner of holding is not impaired, score 0. 1 = Escape to lateral buccal cavity/floor of mouth (FOM). Bolus escapes to either or both of the lateral sulci or the floor of the mouth or is spread diffusely throughout the oral cavity. 2 = Posterior escape of less than half of the bolus. Less than half of the bolus (relative to the amount given) passes through the tongue to the palatal seal posteriorly. 3 = Posterior escape of greater than half of the bolus. Greater than half of the bolus (relative to the amount given) enters the pharynx.

- 0: Bolus held cohesively with no escape, between tongue and palate.

- 1: Escape to lateral sulci or floor of the mouth.

- 2: Posterior escape of less than half the bolus.

- 3: Posterior escape of more than half the bolus.

9.6.3 Bolus Preparation/Mastication

This component assesses the ability to manipulate and chew solid textures, forming a cohesive bolus ready for swallowing. Effective mastication is critical for reducing food to a safe-to-swallow consistency. Inadequate preparation may result in unchewed food entering the pharynx, leading to increased aspiration and choking risks (Figure 9.3a–e).

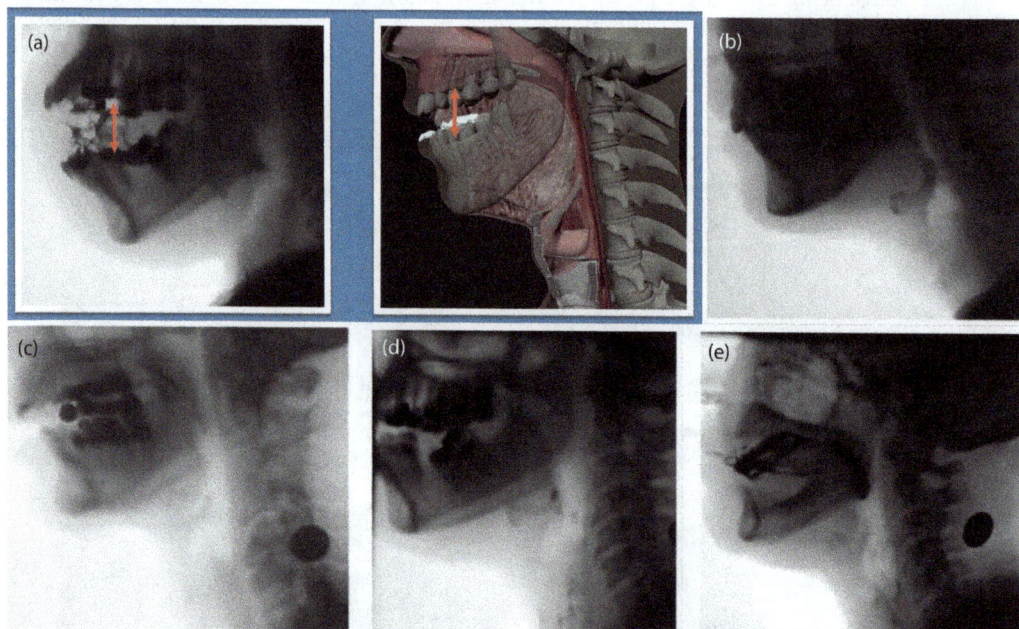

Figure 9.3 Component 3: Bolus Preparation/Mastication. 0 = Timely and efficient chewing and mashing. Smooth and continuous process without hesitation. 1 = Slow, prolonged chewing/mashing with complete recollection. Complete recollection prior to bolus transport. 2 = Disorganized chewing/mashing with solid pieces of bolus unchewed. Unchewed pieces of food are swallowed/remaining in the oral cavity, continuing to chew after the initial swallow. Many times depicted as vertical munching-type behavior. 3 = Minimal chewing/mashing with the majority of the bolus unchewed. Many times the bolus warrants expectoration.

- 0: Timely and efficient chewing with appropriate bolus formation.
- 1: Slow or prolonged chewing with complete recollection.
- 2: Disorganized chewing/mashing with solid pieces of bolus unchewed.
- 3: Minimal chewing with incomplete bolus formation.

9.6.4 Bolus Transport/Lingual Motion

This component assesses the effectiveness of the tongue in transporting the bolus from the oral cavity to the oropharynx. Inadequate lingual motion can result in oral residue, delayed swallow initiation, and compromised bolus clearance. It has to be scored after the initial gesture toward a productive tongue movement for oral bolus transport. Take care not to base your score on oral residue (Figure 9.4a–f).

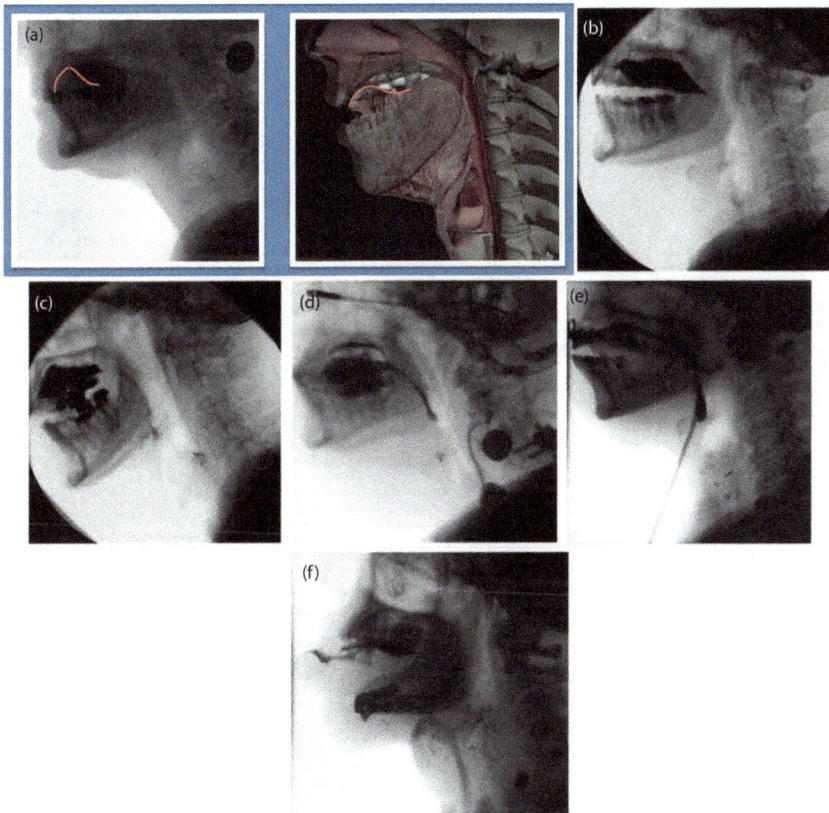

Figure 9.4 Component 4: Bolus Transport/Lingual Motion. 0 = Brisk tongue motion. Quick and efficient anteroposterior transition of the bolus through the oral cavity. 1 = Delayed initiation of tongue motion. Patient who experiences difficulty in planning and initiating any goal-directed motor task. Patients usually require multiple cues to initiate bolus transport. Once initiated, though, tongue movement and bolus transport progress normally. 2 = Slowed tongue motion. Tongue movement progresses slowly in an anterior-to-posterior direction. Bolus is slowly manipulated but progresses through the oral cavity in a posterior direction toward the oropharynx. 3 = Repetitive/disorganized tongue motion. The tongue rocks the bolus anteriorly and posteriorly prior to productively moving the bolus through the oral cavity. Do not confuse bolus accommodating movement; you must observe at least 3 repetitions of tongue rocking. 4 = Minimal to no tongue motion. No apparent movement of the tongue despite cueing.

- 0: Complete and coordinated lingual movement with full bolus transport.
- 1: Delayed initiation of tongue motion.
- 2: Slowed tongue motion.
- 3: Repetitive/disorganized tongue motion.
- 4: Minimal to no tongue motion.

9.6.5 Oral Residue

Oral residue refers to any material remaining in the oral cavity after the swallow is completed. Residue in the oral cavity may indicate impaired bolus clearance, increasing the risk of aspiration on subsequent swallows. This can also contribute to inefficient oral intake and extended mealtimes. This has to be scored after completion of the first swallow, or following the last swallow of the sequential swallowing task. Compensatory swallows should not be considered when formulating OR score (Figure 9.5a–f).

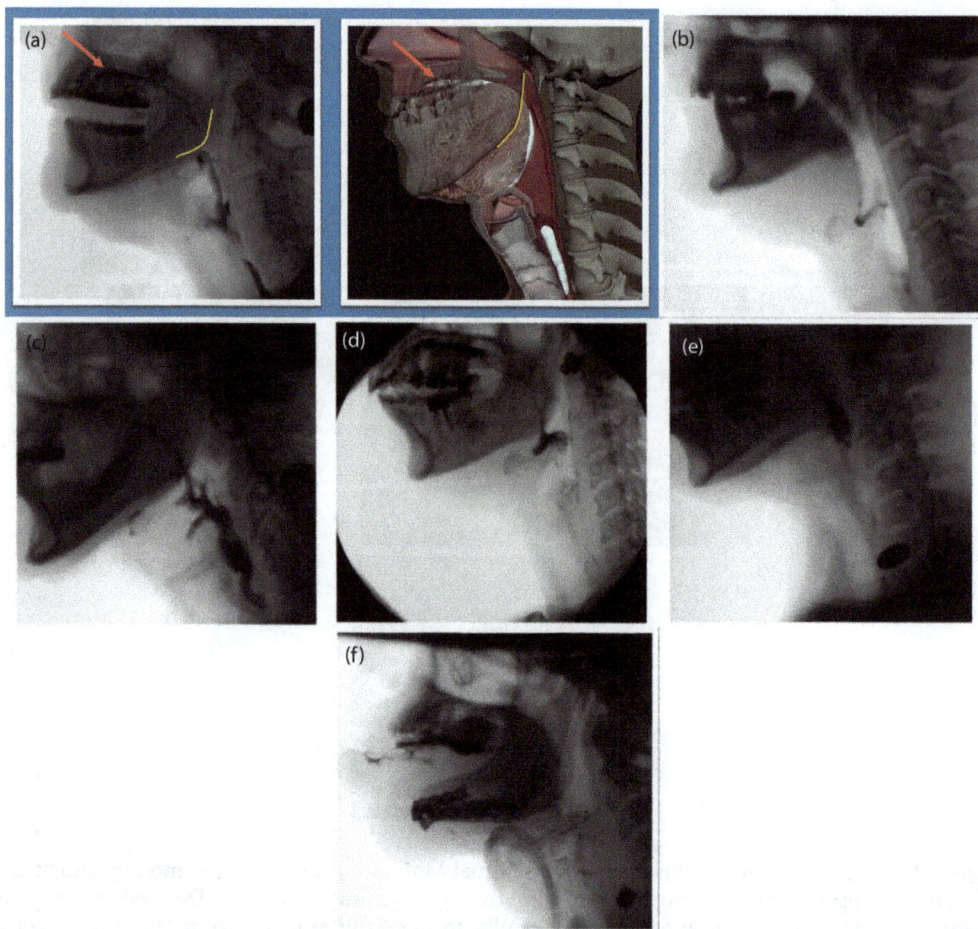

Figure 9.5 Component 5: Oral Residue. 0 = Complete oral clearance. Complete oral clearance with no contrast remaining. 1 = Trace residue lining oral structures. Trace residue that resembles an outline or coating of the structures. 2 = Residue collection on oral structures. A collection of bolus remaining on the oral structures, an amount sufficient to extract or "scoop" from the oral cavity. 3 = Majority of bolus remaining. The majority (> half) of the bolus remains in the oral cavity, relative to the bolus size. 4 = Minimal to no clearance. Generally requires expectoration; anterior escape is not considered clearance.

- 0: No residue present.
- 1: Trace residue on tongue or in sulci.
- 2: Residue collection on tongue, hard palate, or floor of the mouth.
- 3: Majority of bolus remains in the oral cavity.
- 4: Minimal to no bolus clearance.

9.6.6 Initiation of Pharyngeal Swallow

This component evaluates the location of the bolus head at the moment the pharyngeal swallow is triggered. The first initiation of the pharyngeal swallow is represented by the first movement of the brisk superior-anterior hyoid trajectory. Delayed initiation of the swallow can allow bolus material to spill into the unprotected airway before laryngeal closure, significantly increasing the risk of penetration or aspiration (Figure 9.6a–f).

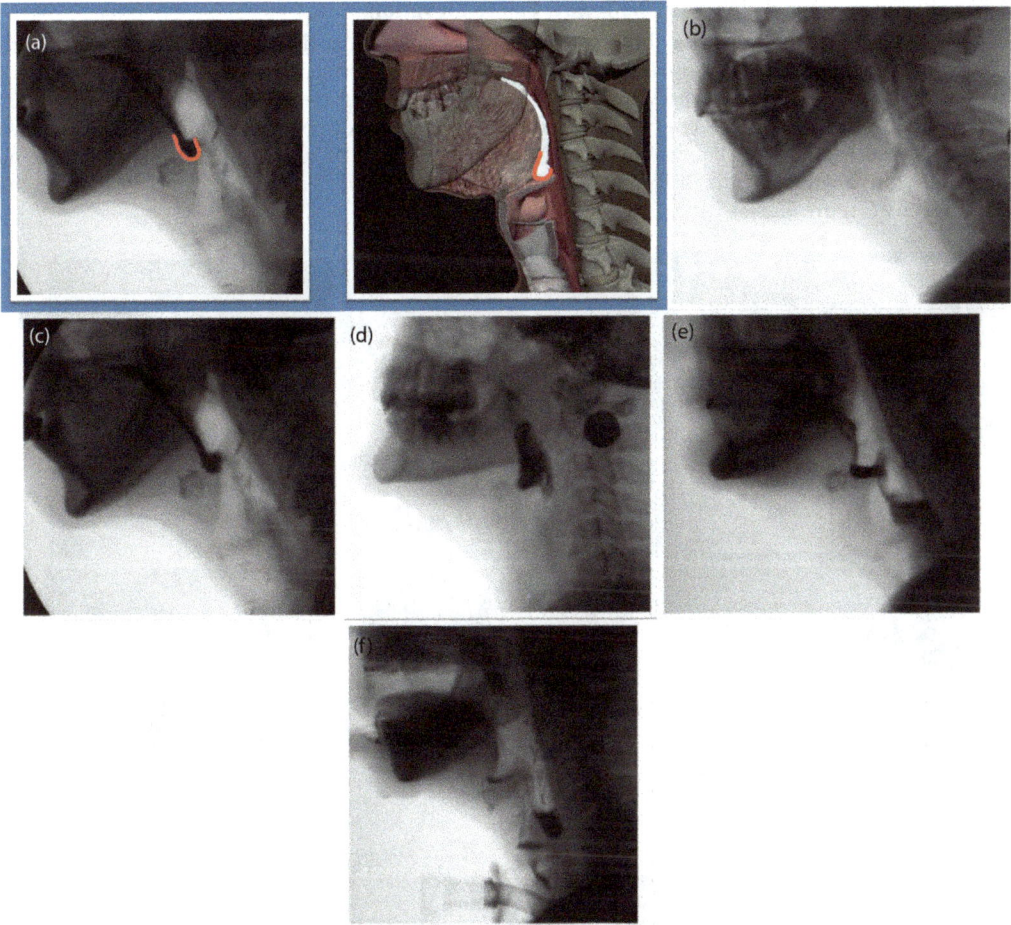

Figure 9.6 Component 6: Initiation of Pharyngeal Swallow. 0 = Bolus head at posterior angle of ramus. Bolus head at the posterior angle of the ramus of the mandible and the back of the tongue at the time of the first hyoid excursion. Do not consider residue from a previous swallow. 1 = Bolus head in valleculae. Bolus head in the region of the valleculae at the time of first hyoid excursion. 2 = Bolus head at the posterior laryngeal surface of the epiglottis, the space between the base of the valleculae and the superior surface of the pyriform sinuses. If the bolus head has exited the valleculae and has not reached the superior limit of the pyriform sinuses, score (2). 3 = Bolus head in pyriforms, at the time of first hyoid excursion. 4 = No visible initiation at any location.

- 0: Swallow initiated with bolus at posterior angle of ramus of mandible.
- 1: Bolus reaches valleculae before swallow initiates.
- 2: Bolus reaches laryngeal surface of epiglottis.
- 3: Bolus enters pyriform sinuses before swallow.
- 4: No observable initiation.

9.6.7 Soft Palate Elevation

Soft palate elevation assesses the ability of the velum to elevate and retract to make contact with the posterior pharyngeal wall during swallowing. Adequate soft palate elevation is essential for preventing nasal regurgitation and maintaining oropharyngeal pressure during bolus propulsion. Soft palate to pharyngeal wall contact is based on the presence of contrast or air between the two structures, best seen on the lateral viewing planes at the height or maximum displacement of the soft palate. Impairment can lead to nasal leakage, reduced swallow efficiency, and residue in the nasopharynx (Figure 9.7a–f).

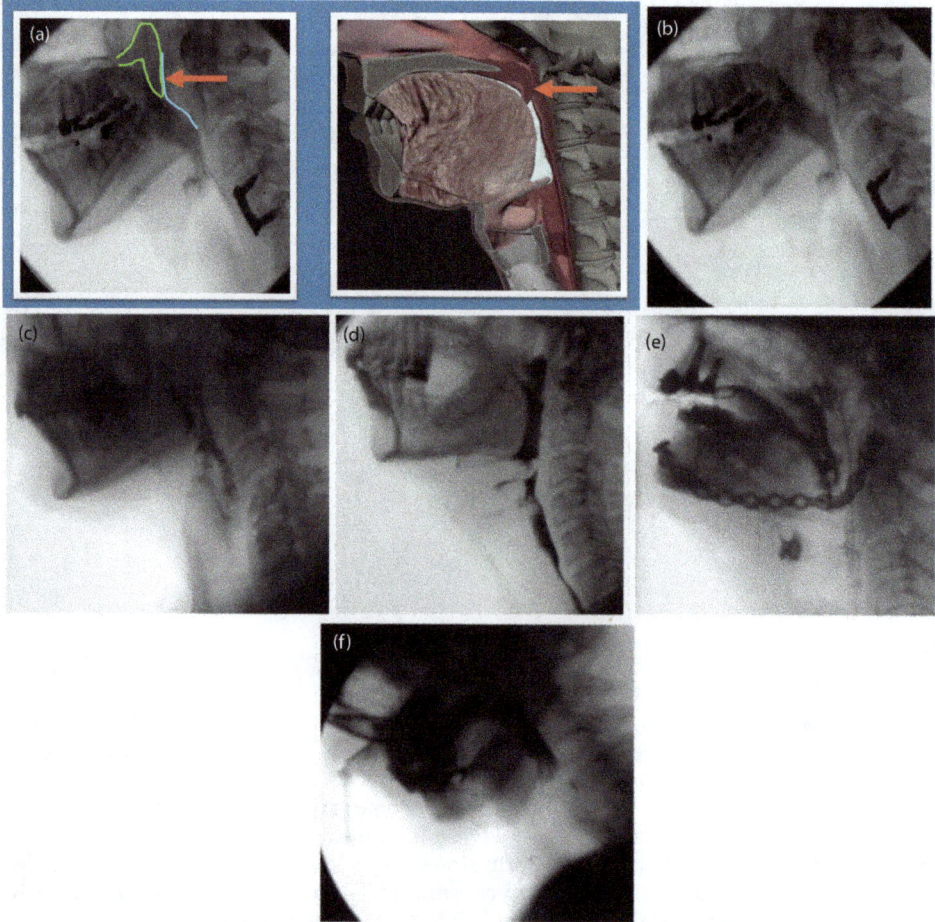

Figure 9.7 Component 7: Soft Palate Elevation. 0 = No bolus between soft palate/pharyngeal wall. 1 = Trace column of contrast or air between SP and PW, at maximum displacement of the soft palate. 2 = Escape to nasopharynx. 3 = Escape to nasal cavity, or presence of contrast material progressing to the level of the nasal cavity at the time of maximum soft palate displacement. 4 = Escape to nostril with/without emission. Escape or presence of contrast material progressing to the level of the nostril with or without nasal emission.

- 0: Complete elevation and contact with the posterior pharyngeal wall; no nasal penetration.
- 1: Trace column of contrast or air between soft palate and pharyngeal wall.
- 2: Escape of contrast into nasopharynx.
- 3: Escape of contrast into the nasal cavity.
- 4: Escape to nostril with/without emission.

9.6.8 Laryngeal Elevation

This component assesses the vertical movement of the larynx during swallowing, which is critical for airway protection and upper esophageal sphincter (UES) opening. The elevation of the larynx is accomplished by contraction of the thyrohyoid muscle and pharyngeal shortening. We evaluate the approximation of the forwardly displaced arytenoid cartilages to the posteriorly displaced epiglottic petiole, at the time the epiglottis reaches its most horizontal position. Inadequate elevation compromises airway closure and can lead to aspiration. It also impairs the mechanical opening of the UES, causing residue in the pharynx or pyriform sinuses (Figure 9.8a–e).

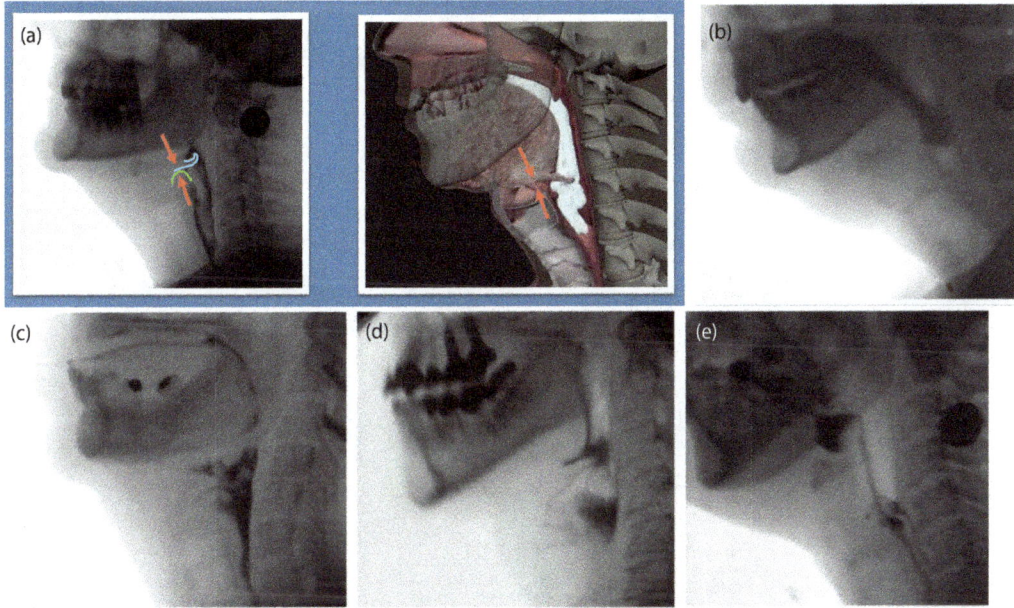

Figure 9.8 Component 8: Laryngeal Elevation. 0 = Complete superior movement of thyroid cartilage with complete approximation of arytenoids to epiglottic petiole. No visible air or contrast in the laryngeal vestibule. The arytenoids are firmly pressed into the base of the epiglottis. 1 = Partial superior movement of thyroid cartilage with partial approximation of arytenoids to epiglottic petiole. Partial approximation of the arytenoids to the epiglottic petiole with a trace or narrow column of air or contrast between the arytenoids and the epiglottic petiole. 2 = Minimal superior movement of thyroid cartilage with minimal approximation of arytenoids to epiglottic petiole, with a wide column of air or contrast between the arytenoids and epiglottic petiole. 3 = No superior movement of thyroid cartilage. No approximation of the arytenoids to the epiglottic petiole.

- 0: Complete superior movement with full approximation of arytenoids to the epiglottic base.
- 1: Partial superior movement with partial approximation.
- 2: Minimal movement with minimal approximation.
- 3: No movement or approximation.

9.6.9 Anterior Hyoid Excursion

This component evaluates the forward movement of the hyoid bone during swallowing. Anterior excursion of the hyoid is essential for effective epiglottic inversion and opening of the UES. We study the angle of the thyroid cartilage relative to the position of the hyoid bone, at the height of the pharyngeal swallow or maximal anterior displacement of the hyoid bone. Limited movement can result in pharyngeal residue and increased aspiration risk due to incomplete airway protection (Figure 9.9a–d).

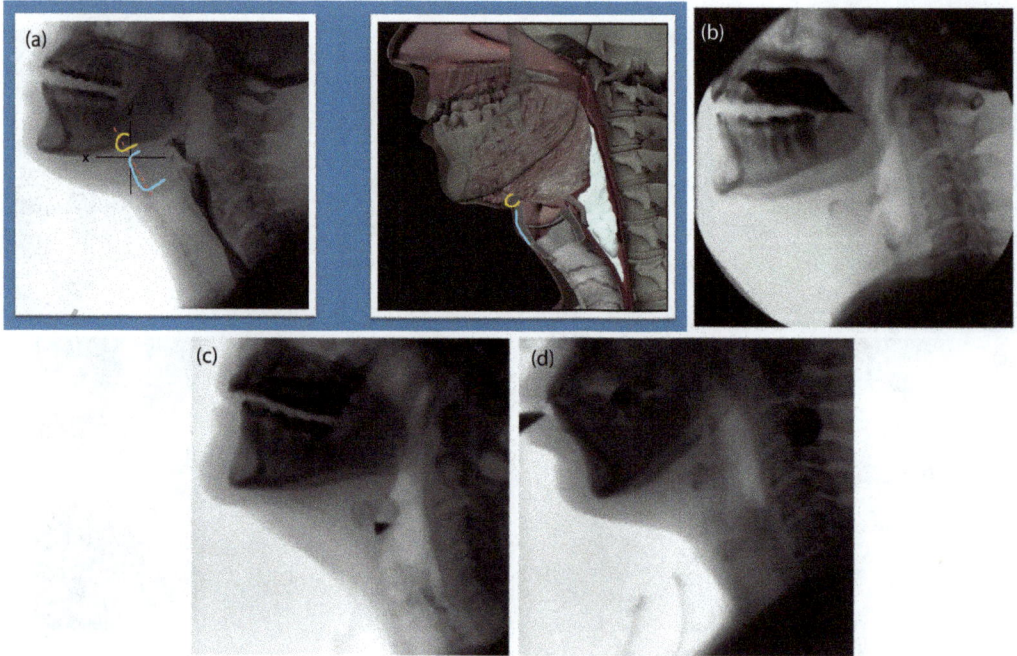

Figure 9.9 Component 9: Anterior Hyoid Excursion. 0 = Complete anterior movement. Acute angle (45° or less) between the thyroid cartilage and hyoid bone at the height of anterior hyoid movement. 1 = Partial anterior movement. Thyroid cartilage is more in a direct line (greater than 45° but less than 90°) with the hyoid at the height of anterior hyoid movement. 2 = No anterior movement. No appreciable anterior movement of the hyoid bone. The hyoid does not deviate from the 90° angle with the thyroid cartilage.

- 0: Complete anterior movement.
- 1: Partial anterior movement.
- 2: No anterior movement.

9.6.10 Epiglottic Movement

This component assesses the degree of inversion of the epiglottis over the laryngeal inlet during swallowing.

Complete epiglottic inversion provides critical protection against aspiration. Insufficient inversion exposes the airway to bolus entry during the swallow. We evaluate laryngeal elevation and anterior traction of the hyolaryngeal complex resulting in inferior displacement of the epiglottis, at the height of the pharyngeal swallow or maximal anterior displacement of the hyoid bone (Figure 9.10a–d).

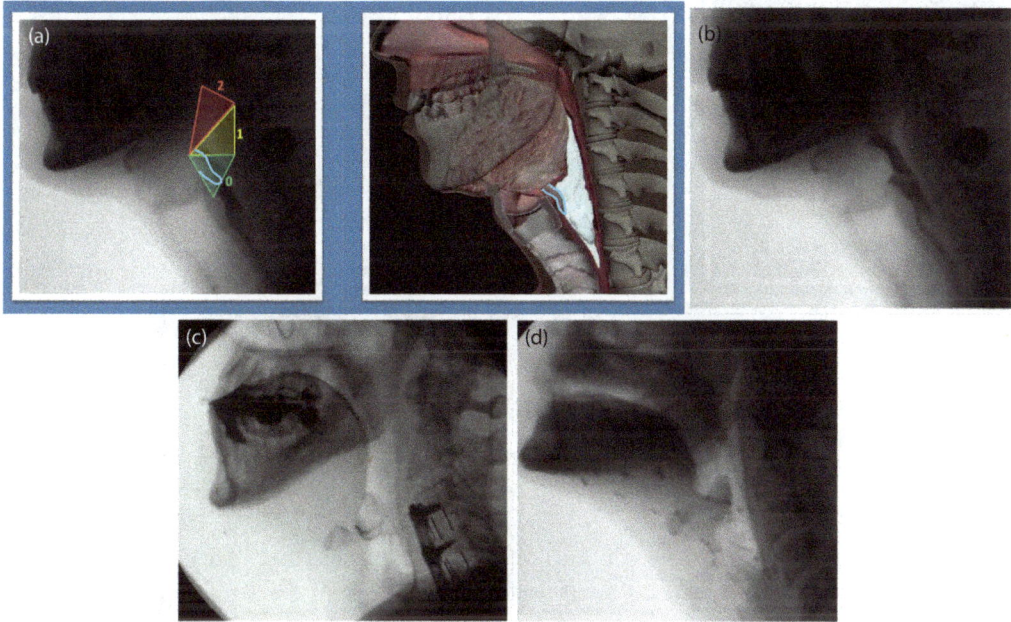

Figure 9.10 Component 10: Epiglottic Movement. 0 = Complete inversion. Complete inferior displacement of the epiglottis. 1 = Partial inversion. Movement of the epiglottis up to a horizontal position, but with no progression beyond this point. A score of (1) would also be given if the epiglottis moves inferiorly but does not reach a horizontal position. 2 = No inversion. Minimal to no movement of the epiglottis.

- 0: Full inversion over the laryngeal inlet.

- 1: Partial inversion.

- 2: No inversion.

9.6.11 Laryngeal Vestibular Closure

This component evaluates the closure of the laryngeal vestibule during swallowing, which includes the supraglottic and glottic structures that form the final protective barrier to the airway.

Effective closure of the laryngeal vestibule prevents penetration and aspiration. Incomplete closure may allow the bolus or residue to enter the airway, increasing the risk for aspiration pneumonia. This is scored during the late closure of the laryngeal vestibule, at the height of the pharyngeal swallow or maximal anterior displacement of the hyoid bone (Figure 9.11a–d).

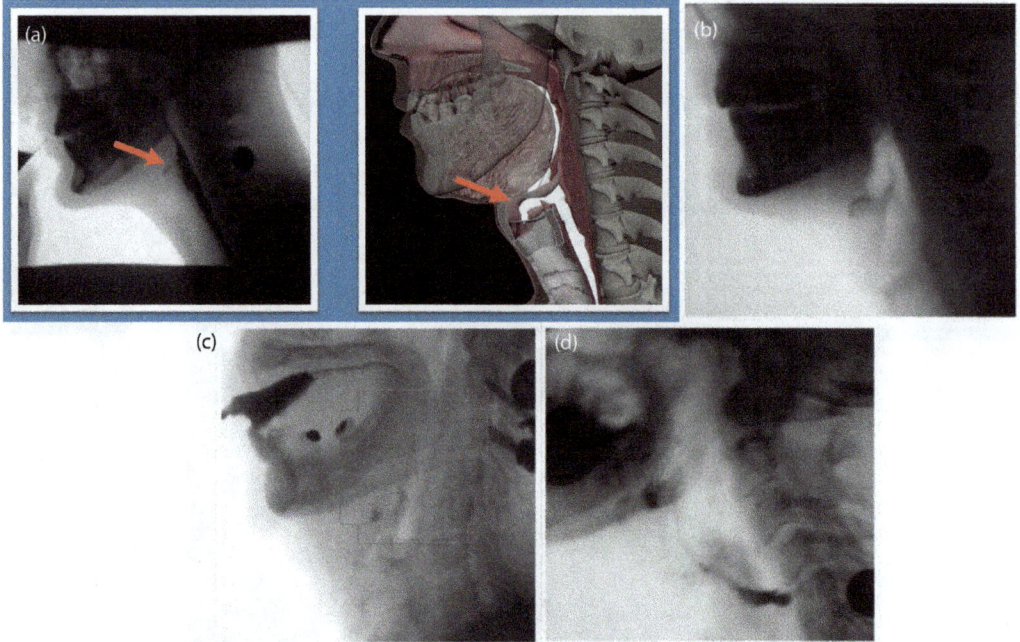

Figure 9.11 Component 11: Laryngeal Vestibule Closure. 0 = Complete; no air/contrast in laryngeal vestibule. Complete closure with no air or contrast in the laryngeal vestibule. 1 = Incomplete; narrow column of air/contrast in laryngeal vestibule. Characterized by a narrow column of air or contrast in the laryngeal vestibule. 2 = None; wide column of air/contrast in laryngeal vestibule. No closure with a wide column of air or contrast in the laryngeal vestibule.

- 0: Complete closure; no air or contrast enters the laryngeal vestibule.
- 1: Incomplete closure with a narrow column of contrast or air.
- 2: No closure; wide column of contrast or air enters the vestibule.

9.6.12 Pharyngeal Stripping Wave

The pharyngeal stripping wave refers to the sequential contraction of the pharyngeal constrictor muscles that clears the bolus through the pharynx into the esophagus.

A diminished or absent stripping wave may result in pharyngeal residue, prolonged swallow time, and secondary aspiration from pooled material. This component evaluates the progressive contraction of the pharyngeal constrictors, at the full length of the posterior pharyngeal wall from the nasopharynx to the pharyngoesophageal segment (PES), during the full duration of the pharyngeal swallow (Figure 9.12a–d).

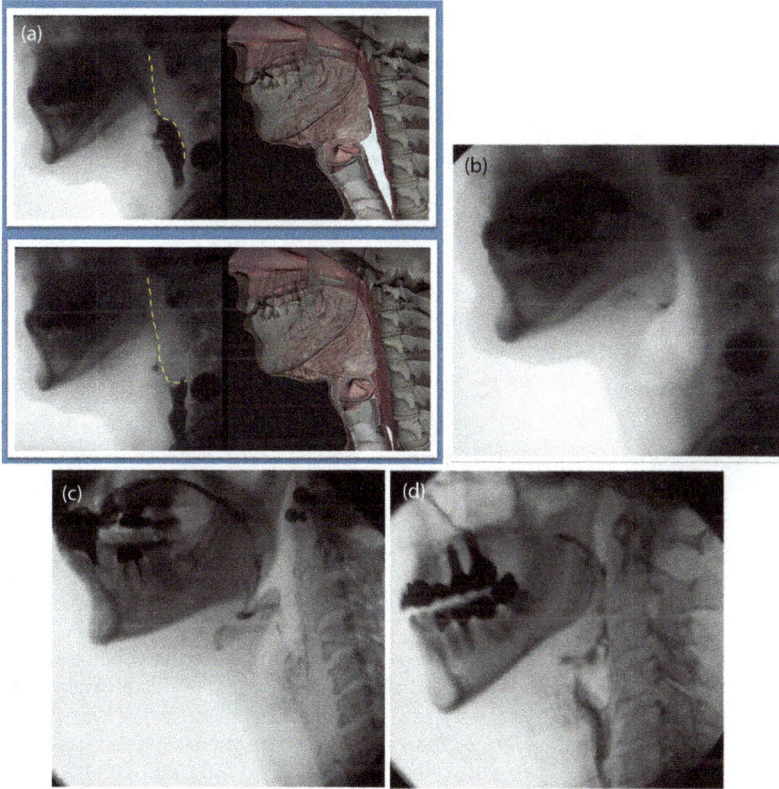

Figure 9.12 Component 12: Pharyngeal Stripping Wave. 0 = Present—complete. Full contraction from the nasopharynx to the level of the PES at the time of collapse. 1 = Present—diminished. Diminished pharyngeal stripping wave along any portion of the pharyngeal wall. 2 = Absent. Complete absence of the pharyngeal stripping wave along the entire pharyngeal wall, often represented by a straight line of the posterior pharyngeal wall throughout the swallow.

- 0: Complete and coordinated stripping wave.
- 1: Incomplete or reduced stripping wave.
- 2: Absent stripping wave.

9.6.13 Pharyngeal Contraction

This component assesses the inward and upward movement of the pharyngeal walls during swallowing. It is typically best visualized in the anteroposterior (AP) view, observing the pharyngeal walls both at rest and during maximum movement. Adequate pharyngeal contraction contributes to effective bolus clearance. Impaired contraction can lead to pharyngeal residue, inefficient swallowing, and potential post-swallow aspiration (Figure 9.13a–e).

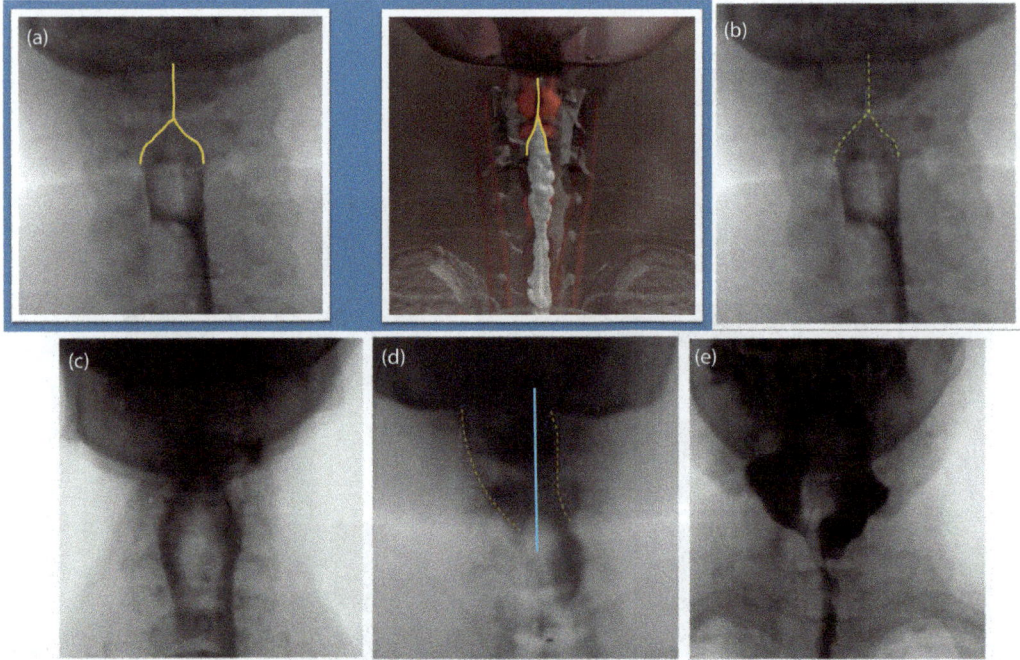

Figure 9.13 Component 13: Pharyngeal Contraction. 0 = Complete. Symmetrical shortening and complete inward compression of the pharynx. Lateral walls are relatively straight during shortening and compress against the bolus tail through the pharynx, bilaterally. 1 = Incomplete (pseudodiverticulum). Incomplete contraction represented by dynamic pouches. Typically unilateral and in the high to mid-pharynx, lateral to the valleculae. 2 = Unilateral bulging. Unilateral bulging of one pharyngeal wall extends the full length of the pharynx. May be distinguishable at rest. 3 = Bilateral bulging. Outward bulging of both pharyngeal walls.

- 0: Complete contraction with medial movement of the pharyngeal walls.
- 1: Incomplete contraction with visible pseudodiverticulae.
- 2: Unilateral bulging of the pharyngeal wall.
- 3: Bilateral bulging with significantly reduced contraction.

9.6.14 Pharyngoesophageal Segment Opening

The component evaluates the distention and duration of opening at the pharyngoesophageal segment, also known as the upper esophageal sphincter (UES), during bolus passage and maximum distention of PES through closure. Adequate PES opening is critical for bolus clearance into the esophagus. Impaired opening can cause residue in the pyriform sinuses and backflow into the pharynx, increasing aspiration risk (Figure 9.14a–e).

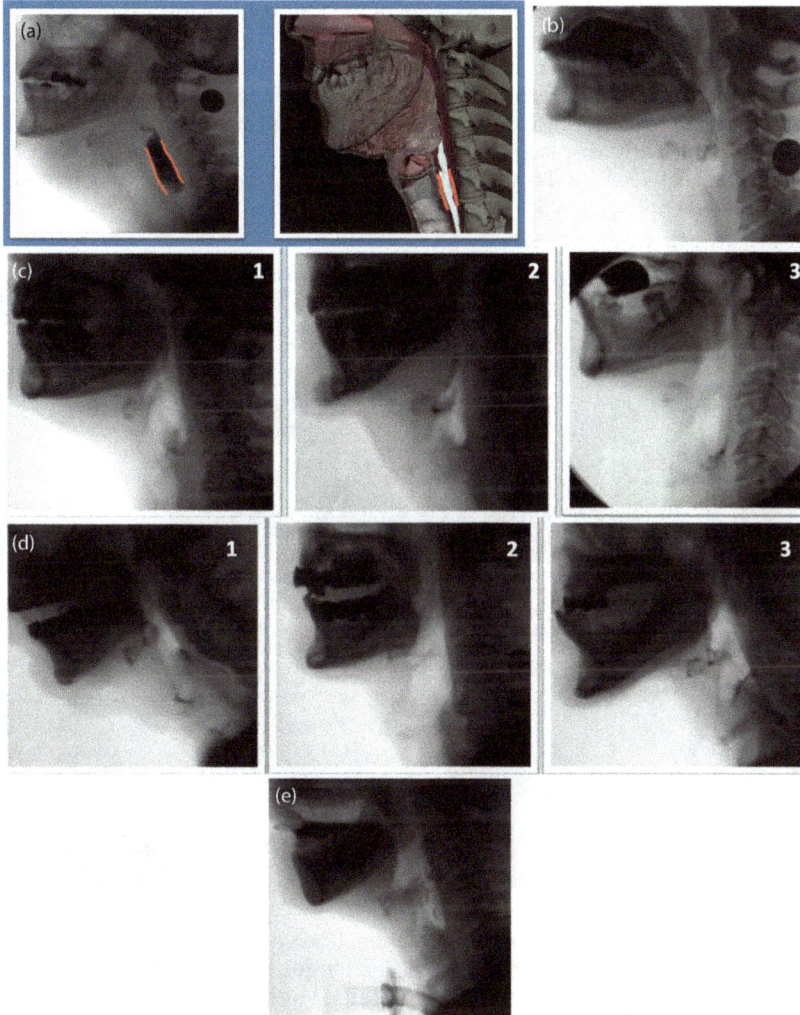

Figure 9.14 Component 14: Pharyngoesophageal Segment Opening. 0 = Complete distension, complete duration, no obstruction of flow. Straight edges throughout the segment with no appreciable narrowing from the pharynx to the proximal esophagus. PES remains distended long enough for the entire bolus to pass through the esophageal inlet. **1 = Partial distension, partial duration, partial obstruction of flow.** A score of (1) can be represented in several ways: (1) Narrowing of the PES at the esophageal inlet while maintaining opening long enough for most of the bolus to pass. (2) Adequate distension of the PES but with early collapse allowing most of the bolus to pass. (3) Both narrowing and early collapse of the PES resulting in partial obstruction. **2 = Minimal distension, minimal duration, marked obstruction to flow.** A score of (2) can appear as follows: (1) Significant narrowing of the PES resulting in resistance to bolus passage. (2) Rapid collapse of the PES allowing only a minimal portion of the bolus to pass. (3) Both significant narrowing and rapid collapse of the PES resulting in marked obstruction. **3 = No distension with total obstruction to flow.** The PES does not open, and there is no bolus clearance. Generally results in the need for the patient to expectorate. Escape into the laryngeal vestibule or nasal cavity is common.

- 0: Complete distention and appropriate duration.
- 1: Partial distention and/or shortened duration.
- 2: Minimal distention with marked obstruction.
- 3: No opening of the PES.

9.6.15 Tongue Base Retraction

This component evaluates the posterior movement of the tongue base toward the posterior pharyngeal wall during the pharyngeal phase of swallowing.

Adequate tongue base retraction is necessary to generate pharyngeal pressure and ensure efficient bolus propulsion. Inadequate retraction leads to vallecular residue and incomplete bolus clearance. Here we study the posterior retraction of the tongue resulting in approximation of the tongue base (TB) with the anteriorly displacing pharyngeal wall (PW) and especially the presence and degree of bolus or air between the TB and PW, during maximal retraction of the tongue and maximum posterior movement (Figure 9.15a–f).

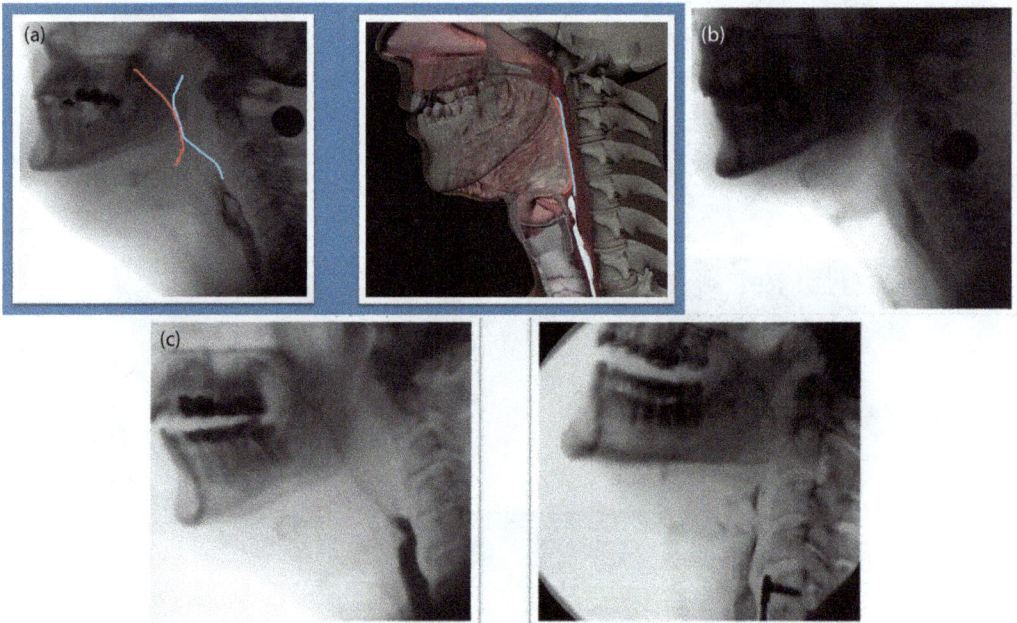

Figure 9.15 Component 15: Tongue Base Retraction. 0 = No contrast between TB and PW in the lateral viewing plane; it resembles a "merging" of the tongue base and pharyngeal wall. 1 = Trace column of contrast or air between TB and PW. Represented by only a trace column of contrast or air between the TB and PW. 2 = Narrow column of contrast or air between TB and PW. Resembles an amount of air or contrast similar to "collection" (Components 5 and 16). 3 = Wide column of air or contrast between TB and PW. 4 = No visible posterior motion of TB. Despite initiating a swallow, the patient below demonstrates no appreciable posterior motion of the TB.

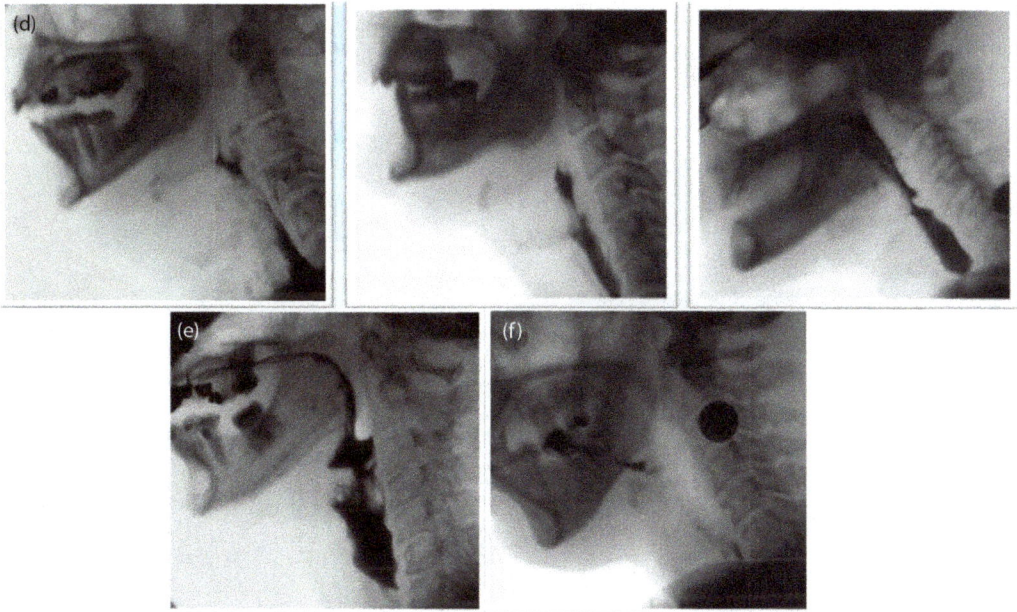

Figure 9.15 Continued.

- 0: Complete contact between tongue base and posterior pharyngeal wall.
- 1: Trace column of contrast or air between structures.
- 2: Narrow column of contrast or air.
- 3: Wide column of contrast or air.
- 4: No visible posterior movement of the tongue base.

9.6.16 Pharyngeal Residue

Here we study contrast material remaining in the pharynx after completion of the first swallow, or following the last swallow of the sequential swallowing task (Figure 9.16a–f).

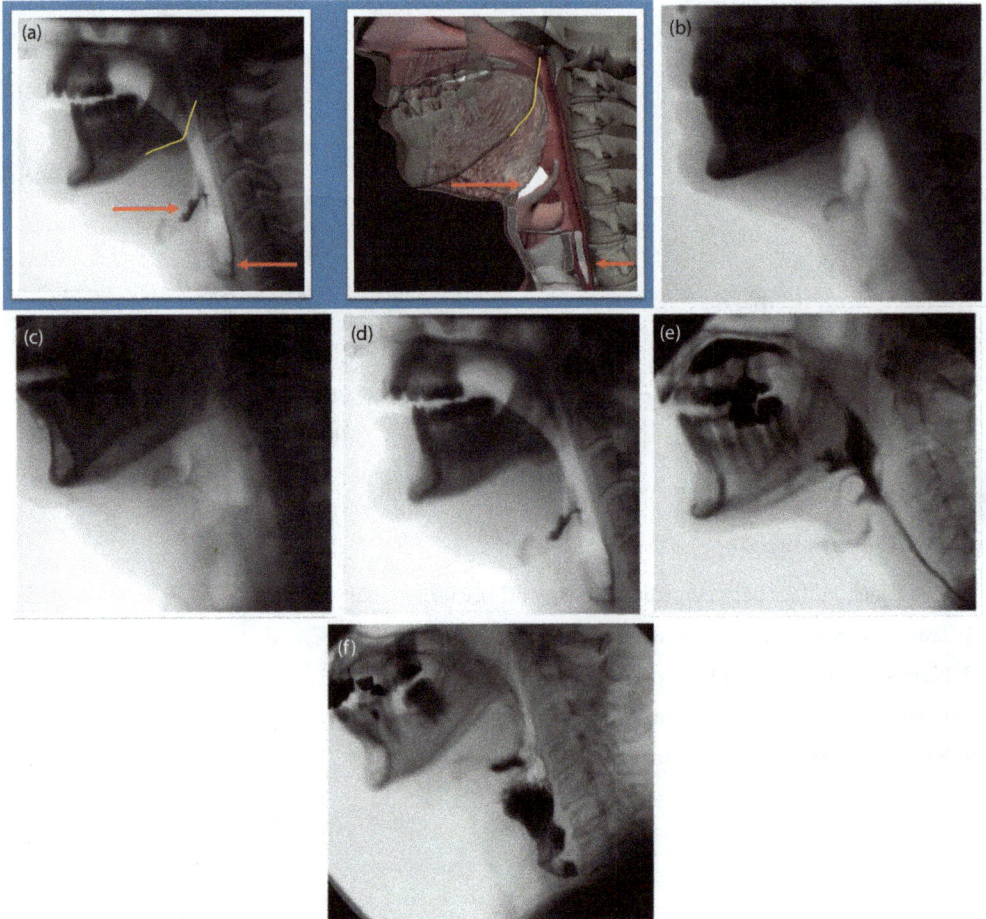

Figure 9.16 Component 16: Pharyngeal Residue. 0 = Complete pharyngeal clearance. 1 = Trace residue within or on pharyngeal structures. Trace, or lining, of residue within or on any of the pharyngeal structures. 2 = Residue collection within or on pharyngeal structures, an amount sufficient to extract or "scoop" from the pharynx. 3 = Majority of contrast within or on pharyngeal structures; > half of the bolus remains in the pharynx, relative to the bolus size. 4 = Minimal to no pharyngeal clearance.

- 0: Complete clearance.
- 1: Trace retention.
- 2: Collection of residue within or on pharyngeal structures.
- 3: Majority of contrast within or on pharyngeal structures.
- 4: Minimal to no pharyngeal clearance.

9.6.17 Esophageal Clearance

This component observes the bolus as it moves through the esophagus while the patient is in an upright seated position. Impaired esophageal motility or obstruction may result in bolus retention or retrograde flow. Identification is critical for appropriate referral (Figure 9.17a–f).

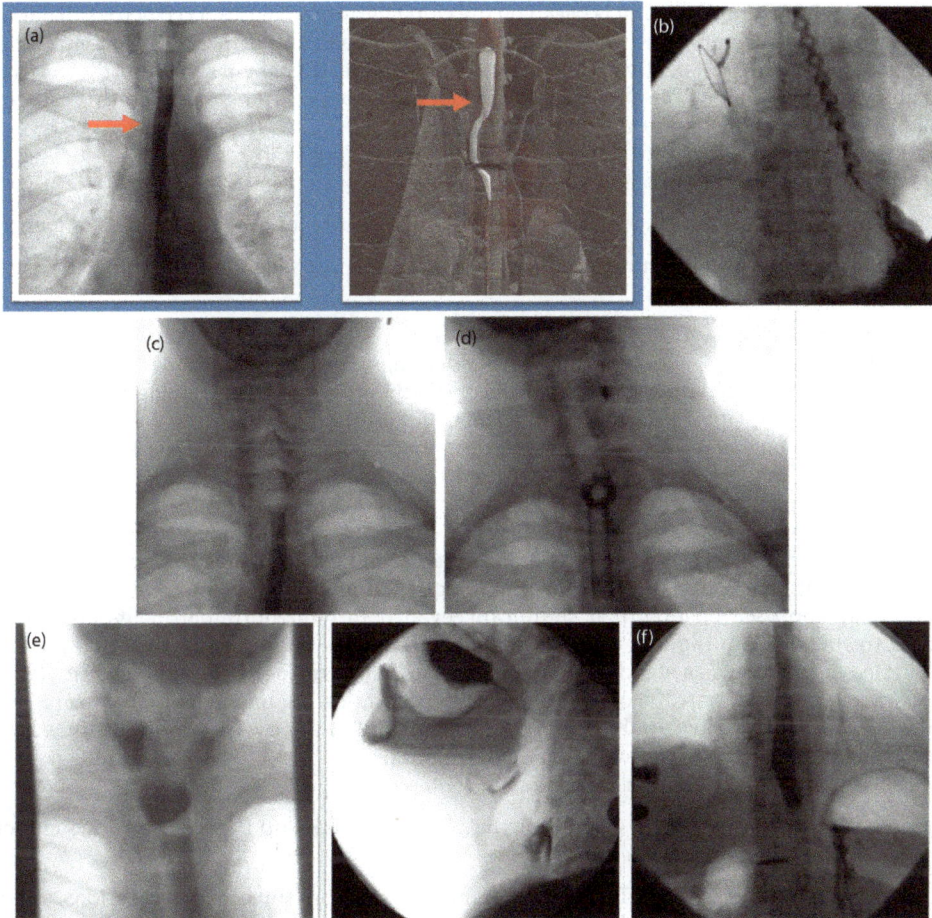

Figure 9.17 Component 17: Esophageal Clearance. 0 = Complete clearance, esophageal coating, after a primary or secondary wave of contraction. There may be esophageal coating resembling a trace outline of the lining of the esophagus. 1 = Esophageal retention. Esophageal retention after a primary or secondary wave of contraction. May resemble a "collection" of contrast material anywhere along the full length of the esophagus. 2 = Esophageal retention with retrograde flow below the PES. 3 = Esophageal retention with retrograde flow through the PES. 4 = Minimal to no esophageal clearance.

- 0: Complete clearance.
- 1: Residue remaining.
- 2: Retrograde flow below PES.
- 3: Retrograde flow through PES.
- 4: Minimal to no esophageal clearance.

9.7 SCORING AND INTERPRETATION

The scoring system of the MBSImP is one of its most critical features, offering a structured, objective framework to interpret physiological swallowing performance. Each of the 17 components is rated on an ordinal scale where a score of "0" reflects normal function. Higher scores indicate increasing severity of impairment, with each level clearly defined by observable criteria.

Importantly, the MBSImP scoring is based on the worst performance observed across all administered boluses for each component. This approach ensures that all clinically significant impairments are captured, even if inconsistently demonstrated. For example, if a patient shows normal lip closure for most boluses but demonstrates significant anterior bolus loss on a single trial, the higher score is retained, alerting the clinician to a potential vulnerability in functional performance.

Each score contributes to the formation of a comprehensive physiological profile. Clinicians summarize this information into two main outcomes:

- The **Component Score Sheet**, which records the ordinal score for each individual component.

- The **Impairment Profile Summary**, which identifies the most severely impaired score for each component across bolus trials.

From these, clinicians may derive a **Profile Total Score**, a cumulative measure that can be useful in tracking patient progress over time or conducting research. The Profile Total Score (PTS) is an optional but valuable metric derived from the MBSImP that offers a single numerical value representing the cumulative severity of impairment across the 17 swallowing components. While individual component scores provide detailed, component-specific insights, the PTS offers a consolidated measure that can be especially useful for tracking global progress over time, facilitating research, and comparing patient populations.

To calculate the PTS, clinicians simply sum the highest scores obtained for each component throughout the videofluoroscopic study. Because the PTS reflects the most impaired performance per component, it represents a worst-case physiological profile rather than an average or typical swallow. This approach ensures that significant, even if infrequent, impairments are acknowledged in treatment planning and clinical documentation. It is important to note that the PTS is not designed to function as a standalone diagnostic label or to replace clinical judgment. Rather, it serves as an aggregated snapshot of overall physiologic swallowing impairment. For example, two patients may have identical PTS values but very different patterns of dysfunction and clinical needs, underscoring the necessity of individualized interpretation.

The PTS is particularly useful in the following contexts:

- *Tracking functional improvement*: Comparing baseline and follow-up PTS values allows clinicians to quantify therapeutic outcomes objectively.

- *Research and clinical trials*: The PTS facilitates comparison across subjects, interventions, and time points in a statistically measurable format.

- *Communication across teams*: The numerical value can complement detailed narrative findings and visual images, aiding in interdisciplinary care planning.

Ultimately, the PTS enhances the MBSImP by providing an efficient way to summarize complex physiological data and contribute to evidence-based practice and outcome measurement in dysphagia management.

9.8 THE PENETRATION-ASPIRATION SCALE

In addition to the MBSImP scoring system, many clinicians also incorporate the Penetration-Aspiration Scale (PAS) during videofluoroscopic swallow studies to evaluate the safety of airway protection. Developed by Rosenbek et al. in 1996, the PAS is an 8-point ordinal scale designed to categorize the depth and patient response to penetration or aspiration events during swallowing.

The PAS provides valuable information that complements the MBSImP by specifically addressing the relationship between the bolus and the airway. The scale ranges from:

- **1**: Material does not enter the airway (normal).

- **2–5**: Material enters the airway (penetration), but does not pass below the vocal folds or is expelled.

- **6–8**: Material enters the airway (aspiration), passes below the vocal folds, and is either expelled or remains, with or without a patient response.

Unlike the MBSImP, which focuses on the physiological processes underlying swallowing impairment, the PAS centers specifically on the outcome of bolus-airway interaction. The two systems are often used together: the MBSImP identifies why aspiration may be occurring (e.g., delayed pharyngeal swallow, reduced laryngeal elevation), while the PAS quantifies how severe the aspiration event is.

Together, the MBSImP and PAS provide a robust, complementary diagnostic framework for dysphagia evaluation. The MBSImP guides therapy based on physiological targets, while the PAS highlights the urgency and nature of airway compromise, often informing recommendations regarding diet texture, compensatory strategies, and medical referrals.

The PAS is calculated by observing and scoring the most severe penetration or aspiration event that occurs during the VFSS. The scoring is performed by a trained clinician, based on real-time or frame-by-frame fluoroscopic analysis. Each swallow trial is individually evaluated for bolus interaction with the airway.

The rater determines the PAS score using the following criteria:

- *Depth of entry*: Whether the bolus enters the airway above (penetration) or below (aspiration) the level of the vocal folds.

- *Response to entry*: Whether the patient makes an effort to eject the material from the airway (i.e., cough or throat clear) and whether that effort is successful.

The PAS does not consider the cause of the event, only the outcome. It is a descriptive tool, not a diagnostic one, and must be used in conjunction with clinical interpretation and physiological assessment, such as the MBSImP, for example.

Only the worst PAS score observed during the study is typically recorded for clinical documentation. However, multiple scores may be noted if specific bolus consistencies produce varying airway responses. For example, a patient may score a 2 with nectar-thick liquid but a 7 with thin liquid, indicating a higher aspiration risk for less viscous consistencies.

Proper calculation and interpretation of the PAS require training and familiarity with laryngeal anatomy and VFSS imaging. The PAS is widely validated and has demonstrated strong inter-rater reliability when used by experienced clinicians. Its simplicity and clarity make it a useful adjunct to the more detailed physiological data provided by the MBSImP.

PAS SCORE DESCRIPTIONS (1–8)

Score 1: Material does not enter the airway.

- Normal swallow with complete airway protection.

Score 2: Material enters the airway, remains above the vocal folds, and is ejected from the airway.

- Mild penetration with effective protective response.

Score 3: Material enters the airway, remains above the vocal folds, and is not ejected.

- Penetration with no response; material stays in the supraglottic space.

Score 4: Material contacts the vocal folds and is ejected.

- Transient glottic invasion, but cleared by a reflexive response.

Score 5: Material contacts the vocal folds and is not ejected.

- Deep penetration without effective response.

Score 6: Material passes below the vocal folds and is ejected into the larynx or pharynx.

- Aspiration with a successful cough or clearing response.

Score 7: Material passes below the vocal folds and is not ejected from the trachea despite effort.

- Aspiration with an ineffective cough or clearance.

Score 8: Material passes below the vocal folds with no effort to eject.

- Silent aspiration; no cough or observable reaction to material in the airway.

While the PAS and the MBSImP are both essential tools in swallowing assessment, they serve different yet complementary purposes. The MBSImP evaluates the physiological mechanisms that contribute to swallowing, while the PAS quantifies the outcome in terms of airway invasion. Table 9.1 provides a conceptual comparison of their characteristics.

9.9 ESOPHAGEAL ANALYSIS DURING MBS

While the MBSImP extends to the esophagus, it is not meant to evaluate esophageal morphology and its motility patterns. In our institution (FBF Hospital, Benevento, Italy), we approach the esophageal analysis by considering the esophagus not as a whole, but a structure made of nine different portions, including the pharynx, according to Brombart's radiologic anatomy: pharynx, upper esophageal sphincter paratracheal, aortic, interaortobronchial, bronchial cardiac, epiphrenic, hiatal, and subfrenic portions. Each of these portions is singularly scored for the presence of different items, which may configure specific motility patterns or diseases: hypotonia, spasm, dilation, stasis, profile alteration (mass/diverticulum); bird-beak sign is applied to hiatal and subfrenic portions, only in the case of achalasia. Each item is scored in severity, with the aid of a structured report, on a scale from 0 to 10 and, overall, on a scale from 0 to 50 to form the esophageal overall impression (EOI), which is meant as an esophageal equivalent of the PTS, not to be used to compare different patients but to monitor the same patient before and after therapy and surgery. This structured approach, derived from the FBF scoring system we developed years ago, makes esophageal analysis and reporting accessible and easier even for inexperienced readers.

9.10 FBF SCORING SYSTEM FOR ACHALASIA

Our scoring system, named after the institution in which it was developed, the Fatebenefratelli Hospital in Benevento, Italy, should not be considered as just a mere tool to obtain patient stratification; even though that was the main aim when first implemented in our clinical practice, its use prompted the development of the checklist we have gone through in the last few pages, and, subsequently, almost inadvertently, it helped form the basis for a new, clinically oriented structured reporting form. After a period of empiric observation, we came to the conclusion that, in order to obtain an effective radiographic profiling that reflected the new advances of pathophysiology, only five findings (or parameters) were to be focused on. Of these parameters, one, namely the bird-beak sign, is in common to all achalasia subtypes and is somewhat pathognomonic, allowing the disease to be radiographically recognized; some others might be in common to the different subtypes, albeit in varying degrees, such as dilation and endoluminal stasis. In the end, we have the two remaining findings on complete opposite sides: hypotonia, typical of atonic subtype 1 achalasia, and spasm, typical of spastic, also known as "vigorous" subtype 3 achalasia. This made the search for a finding or parameter characterizing subtype 2 rather useless or even confusing, at worst. The scoring system has been developed as a series of questions to be answered while analyzing the morphodynamical examination that leads to diagnosis confirmation and patient stratification. A variable amount of points is awarded to each question when positively responded to; at the end of the questionnaire, points are summed up and the final result will position the patient exactly in his subtype. Of course, this final result will be a great support to the manometric and endoscopic diagnosis, allowing the radiologist, for the first time, to give pathophysiologic information to the clinician and not just a mere and pointless morphological description of images. Our aim when developing this scoring system was to train the mind of the radiologist to think and critically elaborate the images, to internalize the whole morphodynamical diagnostic process. Considering many diagnoses of achalasia are still missed today, though, especially in the case of subtype 2 or 3 (because they do not necessarily reflect the "typical" achalasia findings trainees are taught to look for), a scoring system such as ours was created to serve as a guide, especially for the less expert observer and an easily

Table 9.1 Main Differences between MBSImP and PAS

Feature	MBSImP	PAS
Primary Focus	Swallowing physiology	Airway safety outcome
Number of Scores	17 components	Single score per swallow (1–8)
Scoring Basis	Worst impairment across trials	Worst airway event per trial
Clinical Use	Therapy targeting physiology	Risk stratification and dietary decisions
Quantifies ...	Oral, pharyngeal, esophageal impairment	Penetration and aspiration severity

readable support for the clinician. Many of the findings, namely bird-beak sign, stasis, hypotonia, and dilation <4 cm are given 2 points each when present; the only exceptions being spasm, awarded –2 points, and the higher degrees of dilation being given 4, between 4 and 6 cm, and 6 points, when caliber is >6 cm.

Now, summing up all the points in each patient, all the possible combinations will lead to one of three subtypes, which are perfectly comparable to the Chicago Classification subtypes:

- *Subtype 1*: When the score is 8 or higher.

- *Subtype 2*: When the score is 6 or 8 (when hypotonia is present, score 8 should be considered subtype 1).

- *Subtype 3*: When the score is from 0 to 6 (when spasm is present, score 6 should be considered subtype 3).

As you might have noticed, this scoring system and our overall approach to achalasia is very much clinically and pathophysiologically oriented; the scoring system was developed in order to drastically separate the "extreme" subtypes, 1 and 3, obtaining the same, by consequence, for what stays in the middle, subtype 2. Apart from the patient stratification implications that could help communicate with clinicians and surgeons, we reckon the whole approach and checklist should be adopted as a modus operandi for the reporting of achalasia, a process that starts during the execution of the exam.

REFERENCES

1. Fontanella, G, Fronda, M, & Bonatti, G. A proposal for a new prognostic grading system in achalasia using dynamic barium swallow: the FBF score. *EMJ Radiology*, 2021;2(1):34–36.
2. Chen, H. W., & Du, M. Minimally invasive surgery for esophageal achalasia. *Journal of Thoracic Disease*, 2016;8(7):1834–1836.
3. Pandolfino, J. E., & Gawron, A. J. Achalasia: A systematic review. *JAMA*, 2015;313(18):1841–1852.
4. Goldblum, J. R., Whyte, R. I., Orringer, M. B., & Appelman, H. D. Achalasia: a morphologic study of 42 resected specimens. *American Journal of Surgical Pathology*, 1994;18(4):327–337.
5. de Oliveira, J. M., Birgisson, S., Doinoff, C., et al. Timed barium swallow: a simple technique for evaluating esophageal emptying in patients with achalasia. *AJR American Journal of Roentgenology*, 1997;169:473–479.
6. Vaezi, M. F., Baker, M. E., & Richter, J. E. Assessment of esophageal emptying post-pneumatic dilation: use of the timed barium esophagram. *American Journal of Gastroenterology*, 1999;94:1802–1807.
7. Vaezi, M. F., Baker, M. E., Achkar, E., et al. Timed barium oesophagram: better predictor of long-term success after pneumatic dilation in achalasia than symptom assessment. *Gut*, 2002;50:765–770.
8. Rohof, W. O., Hirsch, D. P., Kessing, B. F., et al. Efficacy of treatment for patients with achalasia depends on the distensibility of the esophagogastric junction. *Gastroenterology*, 2012;143:328–335.
9. Bredenoord, A. J., Fox, M., Kahrilas, P. J., et al. Chicago classification criteria of esophageal motility disorders defined in high resolution esophageal pressure topography. *Neurogastroenterology & Motility*, 2012;24(Suppl 1):57–65.
10. Nicodeme, F., de Ruigh, A., Xiao, Y., et al. A comparison of symptom severity and bolus retention with Chicago classification esophageal pressure topography metrics in patients with achalasia. *Clinical Gastroenterology and Hepatology*, 2013;11:131–137:quiz e15.
11. Rohof W. O., Lei, A., & Boeckxstaens, G. E. Esophageal stasis on a timed barium esophagogram predicts recurrent symptoms in patients with long-standing achalasia. *American Journal of Gastroenterology*, 2013;108:49–55.
12. Clayton, S. B., Patel, R., & Richter, J. E. Functional and anatomic esophagogastric junction outflow obstruction: manometry, timed barium esophagram findings, and treatment outcomes. *Clinical Gastroenterology and Hepatology*, 2016;14:907–911.
13. Kostic, S., Andersson, M., Hellstrom, M., et al. Timed barium esophagogram in the assessment of patients with achalasia: reproducibility and observer variation. *Diseases of the Esophagus*, 2005;18:96–103.
14. Sackett, D. L., & Haynes, R. B. The architecture of diagnostic research. *BMJ*, 2002;324:539–541.

15. Martin-Harris, B., Brodsky, M., Michel, Y., Castell, D., Schleicher, M., Sandidge, J., Maxwell, R., & Blair, J. MBS measurement tool of swallow impairment—MBSImP: establishing a standard. *Dysphagia*, 2008;23(4):392–405.

16. Hazelwood, R. J., Armeson, K. E., Hill, E. G., Bonilha, H. S., & Martin-Harris, B. Identification of swallowing tasks from MBSS that optimize the detection of physiologic impairment. *Journal of Speech, Language, and Hearing Research*, 2017;60:1855–1863.

17. Martin-Harris, B., Humphries, K., & Garand, K. The Modified Barium Swallow Impairment Profile (MBSImP™)—Innovation, dissemination and implementation. *Perspectives of the ASHA Special Interest Groups*, 2017;2:129. doi:10.1044/persp2.SIG13.129.

18. Clain, A. E., Alkhuwaiter, M., Davidson, K., & Martin-Harris, B. Structural validity, internal consistency, and rater reliability of the Modified Barium Swallow Impairment Profile: breaking ground on a 52,726-patient, clinical data set. *Journal of Speech, Language, and Hearing Research*, 2022;65(5):1659–1670.

19. Alkhuwaiter, M., Lee, J., & Martin-Harris, B. Diagnostic validity of clinical observations for detecting physiologic swallowing impairment. *Dysphagia*, 2024;40(4):775–785. doi: 10.1007/s00455-024-10775-2.

20. Milford, E. M., Wang, B., Smith, K., Choi, D., Martin-Harris, B., & Garand (Focht), K. L. Aging and sex effects on mastication performance in healthy, non-dysphagic community-dwelling adults. *American Journal of Speech-Language Pathology*, 2020;29(2):705–713.

21. Bhutada, A. M., Dey, R., Martin-Harris, B., & Garand, K. L. Factors influencing initiation of pharyngeal swallow in healthy adults. *American Journal of Speech-Language Pathology*, 2020;29(4):1956–1964. doi:10.1044/2020_AJSLP-20-00027.

22. Pearson, W. G., Taylor, K., Blair, J., & Martin-Harris, B. Computational analysis of swallowing mechanics underlying epiglottic inversion. *Laryngoscope*, 2016;126(8):1854–1858. doi:10.1002/lary.25788.

23. Gullung, J., Hill, E. G., Castell, D. O., & Martin-Harris, B. Oropharyngeal and esophageal swallowing impairment: association and predictive value of Modified Barium Swallow Impairment Profile and combined multichannel intraluminal impedence-esophageal manometry. *Annals of Otology, Rhinology, and Laryngology*, 2012;121(11):738–745.

24. Garand (Focht), K. L., Culp, L. S., Wang, B., Davidson (Humphries), K., & Martin-Harris, B. Aging effects on esophageal transit time in the upright position during videofluoroscopy. *Annals of Otology, Rhinology & Laryngology*, 2020;129(6):618–624.

25. Garand, K. L., Beall, J., Hill, E. G., Davidson, K., Blair, J., Pearson Jr, W., & Martin-Harris, B. Effects of presbyphagia on oropharyngeal swallowing observed during modified barium swallow studies. *Journal of Nutrition, Health & Aging*, 2022;26(11):973–980.

26. Ambrocio, K. R., Miles, A., Bhutada, A. M., Choi, D., & Garand, K. L. Defining normal sequential swallowing biomechanics. *Dysphagia*, 2023;38(6):1497–1510.

27. Garand, K. L., Armeson, K., Hill, E. G., Blair, J., Pearson, W., & Martin-Harris, B. Quantifying oropharyngeal swallowing impairment in response to bolus viscosity. *American Journal of Speech-Language Pathology*, 2024;33(1):460–467.

28. Garand, K. L., Armeson, K., Hill, E. G., Martin-Harris, B. Identification of phenotypic patterns of dysphagia: a proof of concept study. *American Journal of Speech Language Pathology*, 2018;27(3):988–995.

29. Clain, A. E., Samia, N., Davidson, K., & Martin-Harris, B. Characterizing physiologic swallowing impairment profiles: a large-scale exploratory study of head and neck cancer, stroke, chronic obstructive pulmonary disease, dementia, and Parkinson's disease. *Journal of Speech, Language, and Hearing Research*, 2024;67(12):4689–4713. doi: 10.1044/2024_JSLHR-24-00091.

30. Bealll, J., Hill, E. G., Armeson, K., Garand (Focht), K. L., Davidson (Humphries), K., & Martin-Harris, B. Characterizing swallowing impairment severity: a latent class analysis of Modified Barium Swallow Impairment Profile scores. *American Journal of Speech-Language Pathology*, 2020;29(2S):1001–1011.

31. Beall, J., Li, H., Martin-Harris, B., Neelon, B., Elm, J., Graboyes, E., & Hill, E. Bayesian hierarchical profile regression for binary covariates. *Statistics in Medicine*, 2024;43(18):3432–3446

32. Bonilha, H. S., Blair, J., Carnes, B. N., Huda, W., Humphries, K., McGrattan, K., Michel, Y., & Martin-Harris, B. Preliminary investigation of the effect of pulse rate on judgments of swallowing impairment and treatment recommendations. *Dysphagia*, 2013;28(4):528–538

33. Bonilha, H. S., Humphries, K., Blair, J., Hill, E.G., McGrattan, K., Carnes, B. N., Huda, W., & Martin-Harris, B. Radiation exposure time during MBSS: influence of swallowing impairment severity, medical diagnosis, clinician experience, and standardized protocol use. *Dysphagia*, 2013;28(1):77–85.
34. Bonilha, H. S., Wilmskoetter, J., Tipnis, S., Horn, J., Martin-Harris, B., & Huda, W. Relationships between radiation exposure dose, time, and projection in videofluoroscopic swallowing studies. *American Journal of Speech-Language Pathology*, 2019;28(3):1053–1059.
35. Bonilha, H. S., Huda, W., Wilmskoetter, J., Martin-Harris, B., & Tipnis, S. V. Radiation risks to adult patients undergoing modified barium swallow studies. *Dysphagia*, 2019;34(6):922–929.
36. Wilmskoetter, J., Martin-Harris, B., Pearson, W. G., Bonilha, L., Elm, J. J., Horn, J., & Bonilha, H. S. Differences in swallow physiology in patients with left and right hemispheric strokes. *Physiology and Behavior*, 2018;194:144–152.
37. Wilmskoetter, J., Bonilha, L., Martin-Harris, B., Elm, J., Horn, J., & Bonilha, H. Mapping acute lesion locations to physiological swallow impairments after stroke. *NeuroImage: Clinical*, 2019;22:101685.
38. Wilmskoetter, J., Bonilha, L., Martin-Harris, B., Elm, J., Horn, J., & Bonilha, H. Factors influencing oral intake improvement and feeding tube dependency in patients with post-stroke dysphagia. *Journal of Stroke and Cerebrovascular Disease*, 2019;28(6):1421–1430.
39. Martin-Harris, B., Canon, C. L., Bonilha, H. S., Murray, J., Davidson, K., & Lefton-Greif, M. A. Best practices in modified barium swallow studies. *American Journal of Speech-Language Pathology*, 2020;29(2S):1078–1093.
40. Martin-Harris, B., Bonilha, H. S., Brodsky, M. B., Francis, D. O., Fynes, M. M., Martino, R., ... Zarzour, J. The modified barium swallow study for oropharyngeal dysphagia: recommendations from an interdisciplinary expert panel. *Perspectives of the ASHA Special Interest Groups*, 2021;6(3):610–619.
41. Hazelwood, R. J., Armeson, K. E., Hill, E. G., Bonilha, H. S., & Martin-Harris, B. Relating physiologic swallowing impairment, functional swallowing ability, and swallow-specific quality of life. *Dysphagia*, 2022;38(4):1106–1116. doi: 10.1007/s00455-022-10532-3.
42. Garand, K. L., Schwertner, R., Chen, A., & Pearson, W. G. Computational analysis of pharyngeal swallowing mechanics in patients with motor neuron disease: a pilot investigation. *Dysphagia*, 2018;33(2):243–250.
43. Krekeler, B. N., Davidson, K., Kantarcigil, C., Pearson, W., Blair, J., & Martin-Harris, B. Determining swallowing biomechanics underlying Modified Barium Swallow Impairment Profile scoring using computational analysis of swallowing mechanics. *Journal of Speech, Language, and Hearing Research*, 2022;65(10):3798–3808. doi: 10.1044/2022_JSLHR-22-00047.

10 Pharyngeal Disorders

10.1 NEUROMUSCULAR DISORDERS

Neuromuscular disorders of the esophagus and hypopharynx have several origins. Dysphagia is the primary symptom of these illnesses, which are caused by impairment of the swallowing system. This group of disorders is typically divided into systemic diseases that affect the muscles involved in deglutition, local toxic myopathies, and lesions that disrupt the normal reflex arc controlling deglutition. While we will present specific disease-related images here, we invite the reader to go back to the extensive image collection in Chapter 9, which includes every possibility one may encounter in case of pharyngeal disorders [1].

10.1.1 Reflex-Arc Lesions

Multiple lesions disrupt the usual reflex pathway to the muscles of the orohypopharynx and esophagus. These can be categorized according to location as cerebral, intermediate, or peripheral. The subsequent complications may be either acute or persistent. Acute brain lesions typically persist longer and result in more significant incoordination than acute peripheral lesions. Peripheral lesions generally exhibit a reduced duration and result in a diminished level of impairment. The radiologic characteristics are predominantly vague and many, primarily indicating compromised functionality of the swallowing process. The symptoms of dysphagia typically serve as the initial indication of a significant impairment, necessitating further investigations. The patient's age and medical history are critically significant. Neuromuscular degenerative alterations in the aged must be distinguished from more severe disorders of the nervous system. The radiologic abnormalities are most effectively observed during fluoroscopy or cineradiography, necessitating a meticulous assessment of the oropharynx and hypopharynx functions. Because the liquid bolus passes through these locations quickly, they are often very briefly checked during an upper gastrointestinal system inquiry. Early difficulties initiating the swallowing act, segmentation, and asymmetrical passage of the bolus, patchy or irregular coating of the pharyngeal walls, nasal and/or tracheal spillage, pharyngoesophageal sphincter spasm (Figure 10.1), widening or overdistension of the hypopharynx, and failure of the epiglottis to fold over the larynx should all be carefully looked for. There may also be a delay in the bolus's propulsion due to weak or nonexistent peristalsis and an inability to swallow forcefully. Prolonged retention of barium in the valleculae (the vallecular sign, Figure 10.2) and regurgitation

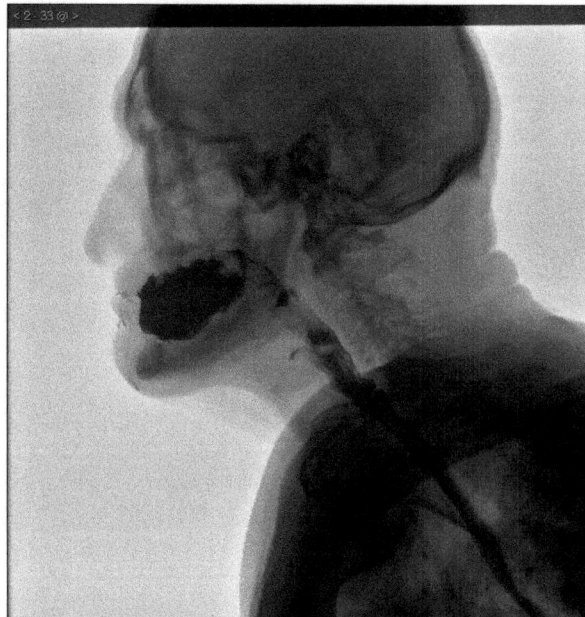

Figure 10.1 Pharyngoesophageal sphincter spasm.

DOI: 10.1201/9781003508113-10

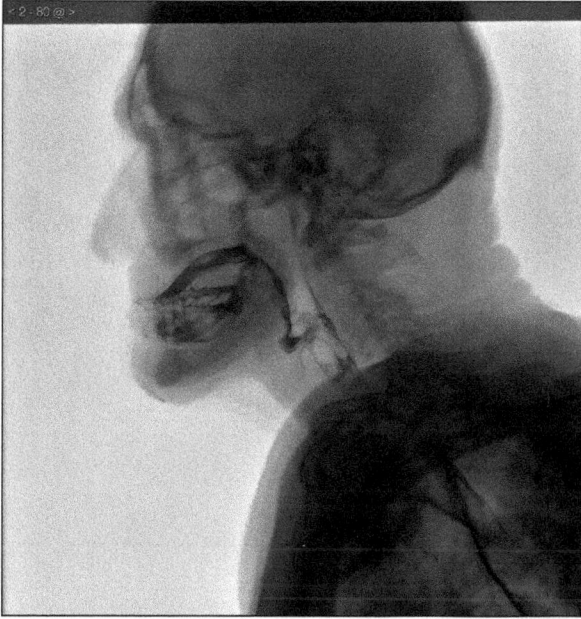

Figure 10.2 Vallecular sign, lateral projection.

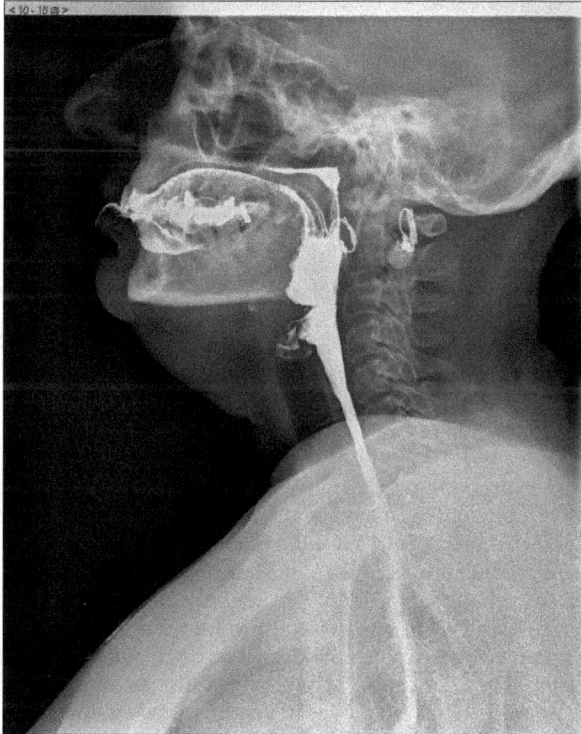

Figure 10.3 Barium in the nasopharynx.

of barium into the nasopharynx and trachea (pharyngeal incoordination) (Figures 10.3 and 10.4) typically suggest a significant organic lesion. The causal lesion may occur at many sites or even extend from one area to another, despite the fact that neuromuscular disorders affecting the swallowing mechanism have been categorized according to their locations.

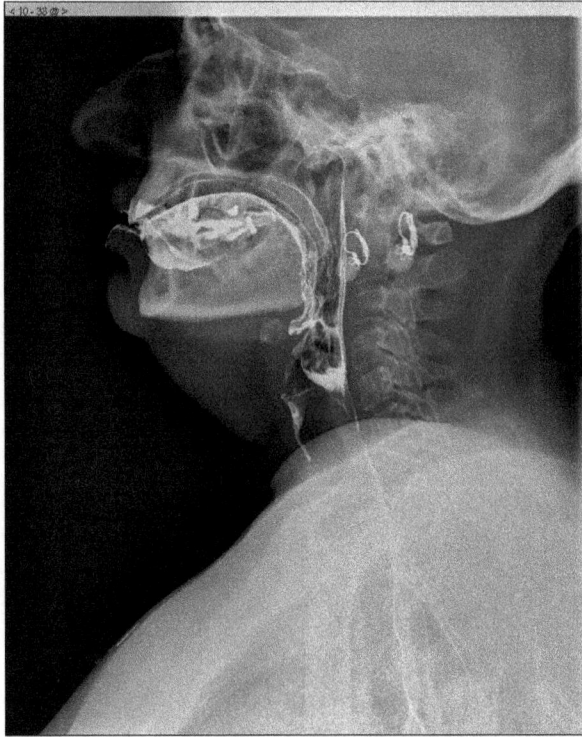

Figure 10.4 Barium aspiration.

10.1.2 Cerebral/Intermediate Lesions

The most dramatic cause of dysphagia's abrupt onset is cerebrovascular accidents. A vascular embolization, thrombosis, or hemorrhage that affects the swallowing center or breaks the reflex arc to the muscles controlling the swallowing mechanism is typically the cause of the cerebral episode. The propulsive mechanism in the oro- and hypopharynx fails in the majority of cases due to abrupt involvement of the sphincter and upper constrictors; however, the degree of paralysis varies. The barium bolus does not go much past the hypopharynx at fluoroscopy. Due to the upper sphincter's inability to open, it gathers there and is held there for a long period. When more barium is administered, the hypopharynx floods, causing nasal regurgitation and barium to stream into the trachea and larynx. This is suggestive of a severe swallowing disorder. However, the underlying brain pathologic process will determine when the patient's symptoms progress.

10.1.3 Pseudobulbar and Bulbar Palsy

Bulbar palsy is an uncommon condition that causes problems with speech, deglutition, and mastication, primarily due to atrophy of the pharyngeal and hypopharyngeal muscles. There are degenerative alterations in the motor cells of the medulla oblongata and pons. Numerous different brain lesions that impact the bulbar nuclei and cause symptoms resembling those of bulbar poliomyelitis, syringomelia, epidemic encephalitis, Parkinsonism, etc. can cause pseudobulbar palsy. A positive vallecular sign (Figures 10.4 and 10.5), barium spilling into the trachea, and atonia characteristic of paralysis of the brain center-controlled masticatory or deglutition muscles will be seen during a fluoroscopic examination. Both the inferior constrictor muscles and the sphincter zone's muscular components become paralyzed in bulbar poliomyelitis. The barium bolus flows slowly down one side of the lateral channels due to the asymmetrical paresis (Figure 10.6), which causes partial paralysis. The bulbar nuclei are affected in Parkinsonism, which results in decreased esophageal peristalsis. Additionally, muscle stiffness causes difficulty with mastication. Even before the onset of dysphagia, a particular series of alterations has been documented on fluoroscopic evaluation using barium that has been taken orally. The first sign of lingual impairment is a slowing of the swallowing time. The involvement of the pharyngeal muscles leads to dysphagia, which is characterized by a greater impairment of motility. Esophageal reflux and tertiary contractions gradually

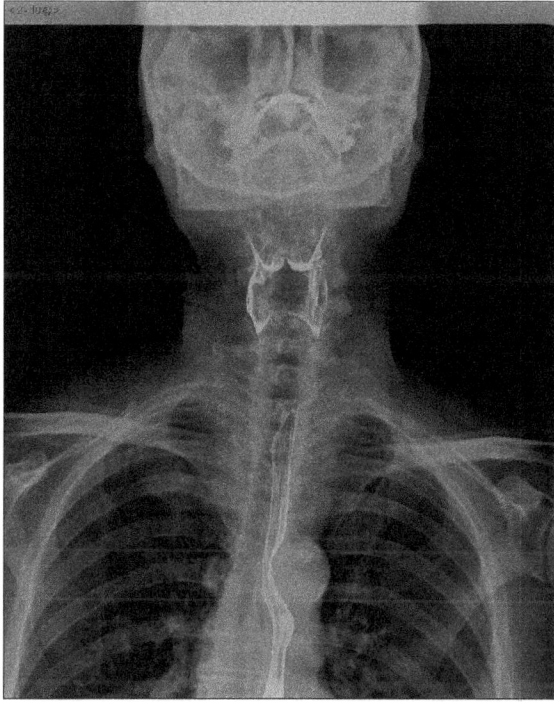

Figure 10.5 Vallecular sign, anteroposterior projection.

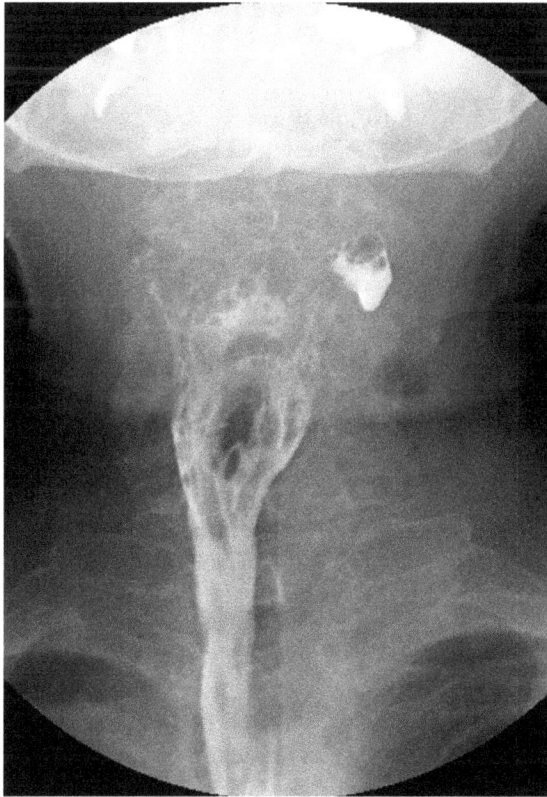

Figure 10.6 Asymmetrical paresis.

emerge, affecting the lower end of the esophagus. There is frequently associated pharyngoesophageal sphincter spasm.

10.1.4 Brain Tumors

The nerve pathways governing the masticatory and swallowing muscles may also be disrupted by brain tumors or other cerebral mass abnormalities, such as a gumma. The swallowing process can also be impacted by aneurysms, trauma, lesions of the jugular foramen, and tumors of the glossopharyngeal nerve and cerebellopontine angle. The location and size of the lesion determine the radiologic results. If the patient survives the initial brain injury, there is typically a pretty quick progression of improvement and occasionally total recovery.

10.1.5 Avellis Syndrome

An intramedullary lesion affecting the nucleus ambiguous or the vagal and spinal accessory nerves feeding the vocal cords and soft palate is known as Avellis syndrome. Additionally, Horner's syndrome is present with more extensive involvement. Numerous conditions, such as neoplasms, trauma, vascular accidents, inflammatory lesions, or even poisonous chemicals, might result in Avellis syndrome. During a fluoroscopic examination, regurgitation into the nose indicates swallowing difficulties (Figure 10.3). Stasis of barium in the valleculae is seen, and unilateral transfer of barium occurs in the hypopharynx region. Unilateral paralysis of the vocal cords is a common condition that may be detected with the use of laryngeal tomographic investigations.

10.1.6 Lateral Amytrophic Sclerosis

The anterior horn cells of the spinal cord and pyramidal tract are affected by degenerative alterations in amyotrophic lateral sclerosis, which results in decreased or nonexistent esophageal peristalsis involving both the upper and lower sphincters. Complete atonia or paralysis of the esophagus and hypopharynx may be visible during fluoroscopy. There is no peristalsis in the esophagus itself, and both sphincters relax and become patent. The esophagus seems uniform in size and inflexible, and its diameter is significantly diminished. The flow will be noticeably reduced after ingesting barium paste or liquid barium, leaving only a long, thin strand of barium that extends from the oropharynx to the stomach and lacks the typical sphincteric contraction zones. As a result, the esophagus will look like a long tube.

10.1.7 Multiple Sclerosis

The central nervous system's motor pathways undergo widespread degenerative alterations in multiple sclerosis. Radiographic results resemble those in amyotrophic lateral sclerosis if the motor circuits governing the swallowing mechanism are affected.

10.1.8 Peripheral Lesions

Numerous lesions may disrupt the reflex arc to the muscles involved in deglutition, hence disrupting the swallowing mechanism through peripheral pathways. The modifications are often unilateral, asymmetrical, and only partially implemented. Infectious or inflammatory diseases, as well as esophageal cancer, can affect the vagus and recurrent laryngeal nerves. Both sensory and motor alterations occur when local variables and toxic systemic consequences are to blame. Metabolic alterations that impact the peripheral nerves result in diabetic peripheral neuropathy. The swallowing mechanism becomes disrupted when the vagus nerve is activated. There is evidence of limited esophageal peristaltic action, which results in delayed emptying. There are also tertiary contractions. These tertiary contractions, which are common in the elderly and are brought on by degenerative changes, must indicate diabetic neuropathy in a young person. Metabolic alterations that impact the peripheral nerves result in diabetic peripheral neuropathy. The swallowing mechanism becomes disrupted when the vagus nerve is activated.

10.2 TOXIC MYOPATHIES

Numerous illnesses generate both systemic and locally active toxins that impair the masticatory muscles and result in dysphagia [2].

10.2.1 Diphtheritis

The toxic symptoms of this infectious disease take precedence over diphtheritic paralysis. Although the esophagus may also be affected, the muscles of the pharynx, soft palate, and larynx are typically affected. Both the vagus nerve and autonomic innervation are implicated. It affects both sensory

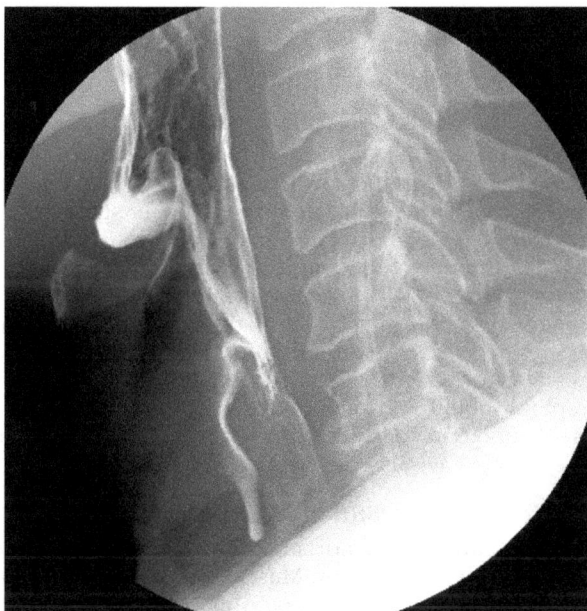

Figure 10.7 Barium aspiration.

and motor activities. The radiologic findings show slow to nonexistent peristaltic activity and partial or perhaps complete paralysis. When the patient swallows thick barium paste, this becomes more noticeable. The vallecular sign is typically present (Figure 10.5), and the transit duration is noticeably longer.

10.2.2 Botulism

Additionally, botulism can cause paralysis, especially of the pharyngeal constrictors. The effects of the botulinum toxin on the brain's swallowing centers cause the paralysis as a subsequent effect. Progressive dryness of the pharynx and eventual paralysis of the pharyngeal muscles, including the soft palate, are the subtle signs. It is tough to consume liquids because of aspiration (Figure 10.7). Pharyngeal and esophageal paralysis are observed on fluoroscopic examination, together with a positive vallecular sign and no peristalsis. Due to the toxin generated in this condition, tetanus causes clonic spasms of the masticatory muscles. The swallowing mechanism is impaired as a result of the disruption of the neural circuits that govern these muscles.

10.2.3 Rabies

The central nervous system is impacted by rabies. Respiratory and swallowing difficulties may be prevalent in the early stages. When breathing and drinking are interfered with, reflex spasm occurs. Then paralysis takes place. It is possible to mimic the symptoms of acute bulbar paralysis and even tetanus. Other clinical information and the history are useful. The pharyngoesophageal sphincter spasm and reduced function are the initial radiologic characteristics. These are followed by findings linked to total paralysis.

10.3 MUSCULAR DISORDERS

10.3.1 Myasthenia Gravis

Skeletal muscles are affected by myasthenia gravis, an endocrine or metabolic condition. Early tiredness and muscle weakness are its hallmarks. The reason could be a thymic tumor. There are no signs of muscular atrophy or sensory impairment. When the terminal nerve end plates or myoneural junction are "blocked," muscle contraction is not possible. After an initial oral phase, pharyngeal muscle weakness develops. Deglutition is hampered by slow tongue movements. The orohypopharyngeal muscles then undergo paresis, which causes dilation and stasis. It appears that the sphincters are not implicated. The larynx is unable to ascend and the epiglottis is unable to fold over when examined under a microscope. As a result, a positive valve sign appears, where the barium spills into the throat and larynx (Figure 10.4). A favorable reaction to cholinergic medications may be expected as the underlying problem involves a chemical block of the neuromuscular junction. Aspiration, penetration, and nasal regurgitation are all hallmarks of this disease (Figure 10.3) [3].

10.3.2 Muscular Dystrophy

Skeletal muscle atrophy and myotonia are hallmarks of myotonic dystrophy (also known as muscular dystrophy), an illness of unclear etiology. Chalasia, or the free regurgitation of food from the esophagus into the pharynx, is caused by atony of the upper sphincter of the esophagus. The handle portion of the typically racket-shaped image of the dilated sphincter appears larger and more tubular than usual due to atony of the sphincter in anteroposterior view of the barium-filled cervical esophageal cavity in a patient with myotonic dystrophy. It is normal for barium to spill into the trachea and cause pneumonia. Radiologic abnormalities resembling achalasia, scleroderma, or paralytic lesions involving the sphincters are produced by the reduced peristalsis, dilation, and inadequate esophageal emptying. When there is no apparent cause for a dilated esophagus (and colon), myotonic dystrophies should be taken into consideration. Along with the previously mentioned alterations, this condition may also cause an enlarged skull with small sella turcica and prominent frontal sinuses. There have also been reports of a rise in serum lysozyme.

10.3.3 Stiff Man's Syndrome

The rare condition known as stiff man's syndrome, which has no recognized etiology, is characterized by growing muscle rigidity and spasm. Muscle soreness and stiffness can start slowly or quickly, and the severity of the symptoms can vary. Almost always, the neck muscles involved in swallowing and deglutition are impacted. Despite the lack of particular signs, fluoroscopic examination shows abnormal esophageal motility.

10.4 OTHER DISEASES

10.4.1 Cushing Ulcers

Esophageal Cushing ulcers are related to central nervous system abnormalities that impact the hypothalamus and vagus nerve, particularly the tuber cinereum. Acute encephalitis, neoplasms, and traumatic and spontaneous hemorrhages are among the brain lesions that cause these symptoms [4]. The development of an esophageal ulcer is thought to be caused by hypersecretion and hypermotility. This could lead to localized ischemia. Most often, esophageal ulcers are acute and easily performed. Additionally, the duodenal bulb and stomach are frequently involved. In this entity, the distal third is typically where the esophageal ulcers are found.

10.4.2 Curling Ulcers

The esophagus, stomach, and duodenal bulb can potentially develop Curling ulcers as a result of severe skin burns. Usually acute, these ulcers may go "silent" until they burst. Radiologic signs of Cushing and Curling ulcers include spasm, altered motility, and the presence of a crater or niche.

10.5 INFLAMMATORY LESIONS

10.5.1 Acute Pharyngitis

Sometimes, severe edema and surrounding inflammatory reactions from simple acute pharyngitis can interfere with swallowing and the pharyngoesophageal sphincter's normal relaxing.

10.5.2 Acute Tonsillitis

An area of soft tissue enlargement including the base of the tongue and valleculae, along with downward displacement of the epiglottis, may be detectable with a lateral film of the neck in cases of acute tonsillitis. Such swelling needs to be differentiated from a tumor, a thyroglossal duct cyst, lingual thyroid tissue, and an abscess. The diagnosis is typically established by the clinical features upon direct throat inspection and the history of sudden onset. In addition to a cervical lateral film, a barium swallow aids in both the differential diagnosis and the assessment of the degree of inflammation.

10.5.3 Acute Adenoiditis

Swallowing issues can also be a symptom of acute adenoiditis. It is possible to see the adenoids, which are anterior and straightened posteriorly and typically emerge during the sixth month of life. The adenoids are more noticeable when there is inflammation or infection. Particularly in people who are comparatively asymptomatic, posterior irregularity of the adenoidal mass's outline indicates a malignant tumor. Acute epiglottitis is characterized by the quick onset of epiglottis swelling, which frequently results in total obstruction of the hypopharynx and airway. A lateral film of the neck can easily display these characteristics. A bulging epiglottis and air-filled hypopharynx are diagnostic signs. Airway blockage and involvement of the aryepiglottic folds or epiglottis may cause secondary hypopharyngeal airway distension, resulting in dysphagia and inspiratory distress during a normal cry. A "hoarse cry" is a sign of respiratory discomfort caused by acute conditions affecting the larynx, such as laryngitis, croup, foreign bodies, or paralysis of the vocal cords due to congenital problems. Edema interfering with the normal swallowing mechanism is the cause of dysphagia in acute epiglottitis.

10.5.4 Chronic Pharyngitis with Ulcers

An uncommon condition that is typically linked to aphthous stomatitis is chronic ulcerative pharyngitis. Swallowing may be hampered by cicatrizing alterations in the cricopharyngeus muscle. A noticeable cricopharyngeal impression is seen on radiologic examination, which appears to be connected to pharyngoesophageal sphincter spasm and an ulcerating pharyngeal wall. Visible on lateral plain films of the cervical area, it is situated in the center of the nasopharyngeal roof: a rounded, nicely shaped mass of soft tissue.

REFERENCES

1. Levine MS, Rubesin SE. Radiologic investigation of dysphagia. *AJR Am J Roentgenol.* 1990;154(6):1157–63. doi:10.2214/ajr.154.6.2110721.
2. Levine MS, Rubesin SE, Ott DJ. Update on esophageal radiology. *AJR Am J Roentgenol.* 1990;155(5):933–41. doi:10.2214/ajr.155.5.2120962.
3. Anatomy for Diagnostic Imaging. Saunders Ltd. Google Books.
4. Semenkovich J, Balfe D, Weyman P, Heiken J, Lee J. Barium pharyngography: comparison of single and double contrast. *AJR Am J Roentgenol.* 1985;144(4):715–20. doi:10.2214/ajr.144.4.715.

11 Esophageal Disorders

11.1 MOTILITY DISORDERS

Esophageal motility disorders are a wide array of diseases that are mainly due to hyperkinetic or spastic alterations, unlike those of the pharynx and the pharyngoesophageal junction, and with the due exception of the various forms of visceral hypotonia. At the same time, the border between normal function and esophageal dismotility is blurred, disputed, and often a source of scientific debate. Standing at this border but already on the pathology side are secondary and tertiary peristaltic contractions. On this matter, we follow the advice of Marcel Brombart: in his opinion, every paraphysiological event that puts stress and alters the normal physiology, forcing an enduring alteration and "adaptation" of the viscus, especially if it determines clinical consequences, is disease itself [1–5].

11.1.1 Secondary Contractions

Secondary contractions, peculiar alterations of the physiologic esophageal peristalsis, can be defined as follows: they are sharp contractions, arising from a single portion of the esophagus, generally the middle third, which expand both cranially and caudally. The ascending wave can send the esophageal content and, indeed, the barium up to the hypopharynx, where it can even generate a primary contraction. Radiographically, secondary peristalsis shows as a portion of extremely reduced caliber, often found in the middle third of the viscus with a dilated upper and lower esophagus, due to the ascending and descending peristaltic waves, the esophageal lumen somewhat resembling the shape of an hourglass (Figure 11.1). These contractions are more frequent to find than one might think, even though still quite rare to observe. In a few cases, especially when the contraction begins at the aortic portion, there might be only an ascending wave.

11.1.2 Tertiary Contractions

Tertiary contractions is a merely physiologic term to express a quite complex phenomenon that stands, at the same time, on the border with paraphysiology and that with frank disease. Once known as "rippling," this phenomenon is represented radiographically by a series of irregular, almost anarchic contractions, which manifest in such quick succession that they almost seem to be concomitant, interesting especially the lower two-thirds or three-quarters of the esophagus (Figure 11.2). The esophageal body will appear with an irregular caliber, due to the multiple, irregular contractions. They are generally borne out of a half-emptied esophagus, in the wake of a primary

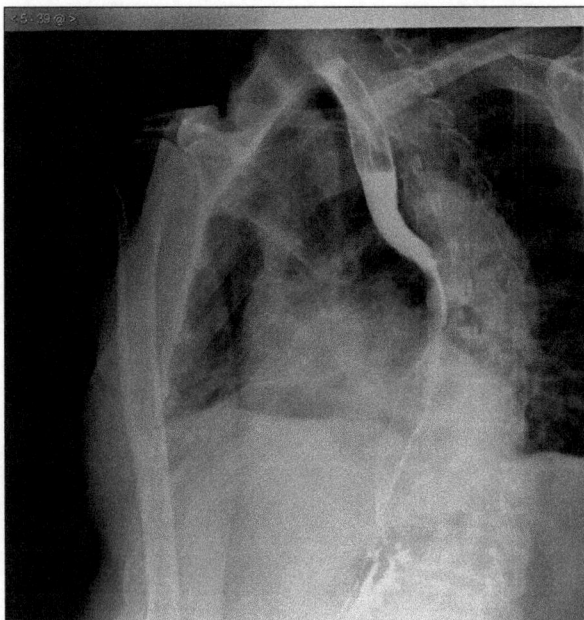

Figure 11.1 Secondary contractions.

DOI: 10.1201/9781003508113-11

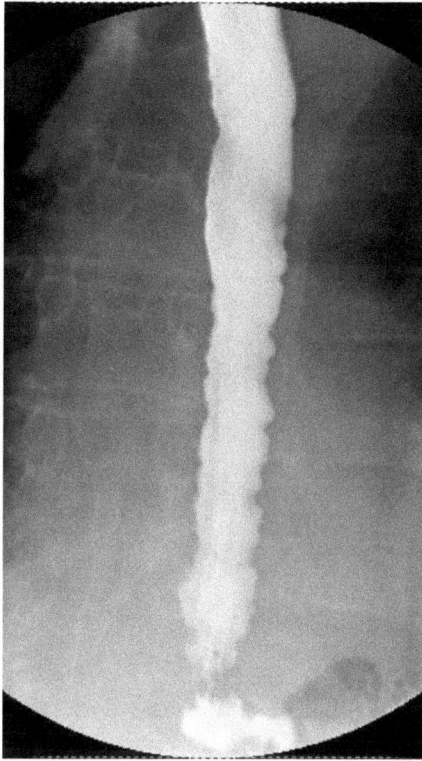

Figure 11.2 Tertiary contractions. (Image courtesy of Dr. Paul Hellerhoff, Munich.)

contraction and are, indeed, wiped out by a new primary wave. It is a very quick phenomenon that generally lasts fractions of a second and only rarely much longer. Sometimes, even though only in subjection prone to territory contraction formation, they can be elicited by making the patient swallow saliva, after a regular barium sip and when the esophagus is back in resting mode. In the vast majority of patients, they are asymptomatic and might go clinically unnoticed.

11.1.3 Achalasia

Primary achalasia is thought to be the outcome of a complicated interaction between numerous factors, according to literature. The main pathological feature of achalasia is the loss of ganglion cells both in the body of the esophagus and in patients genetically susceptible to the disease. Inflammatory and autoimmune responses, most likely triggered by viral infections, are strongly linked to the main pathological feature of achalasia: the loss of ganglion cells both in the body of the esophagus and in patients genetically susceptible to the disease. The loss of ganglion cells, especially in the lower esophageal sphincter, is significantly linked to collagen deposition and inflammation. This leads to three different potential types of disease: type I, hypotonic or classic achalasia (Figure 11.3), type II (Figure 11.4) or panpressurizing achalasia, and type III (Figure 11.5) or spastic achalasia; each of them is a specific combination of specific signs, the most important of all and common to the three types, the "bird-beak sign" (Figure 11.6) and abrupt reduction in caliber of the esophagus, which resembles a bird beak. We then find luminal dilation of different degrees, maximum in type I; spasm only found in type III; luminal stasis and pooling of barium. Advanced stages of the disease lead to a "sigmoid" esophagus (Figure 11.7) and epiphrenic diverticula formation.

11.1.4 Diffuse Esophageal Spasm

Diffuse spasm represents a neuromuscular disturbance chiefly involving the lower third of the esophagus. The disorder is primarily diagnosed in a radiologic examination. During the associated esophageal contractions, substernal discomfort simulating cardiac pain may be experienced.

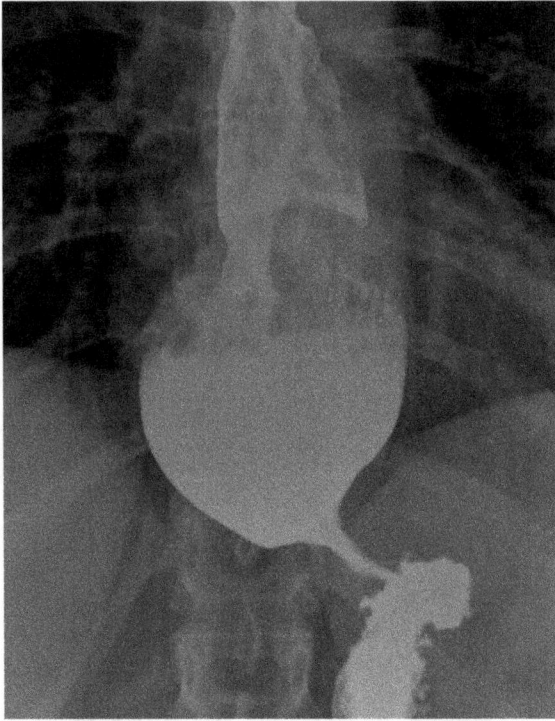

Figure 11.3 Type I achalasia.

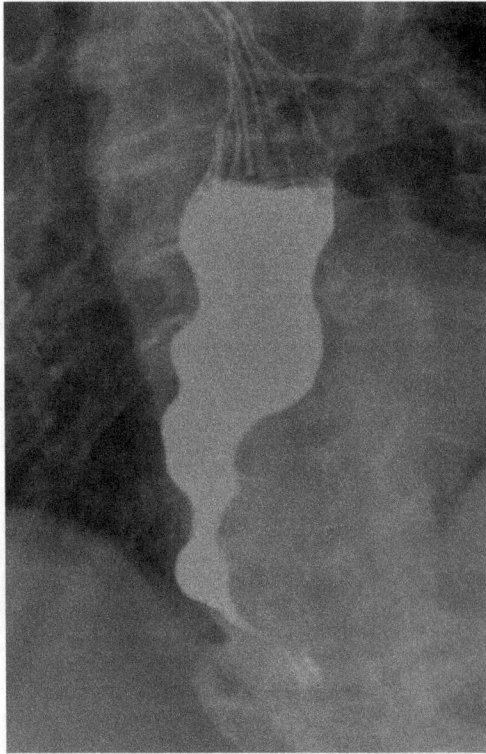

Figure 11.4 Type II achalasia.

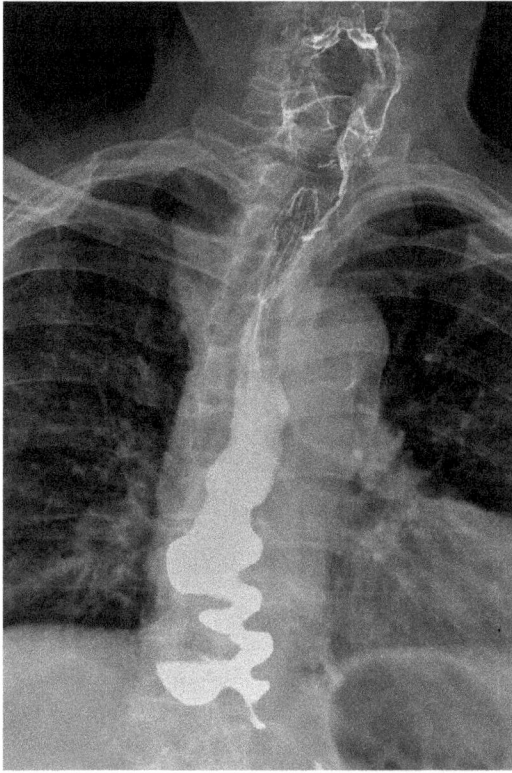

Figure 11.5 Type III achalasia.

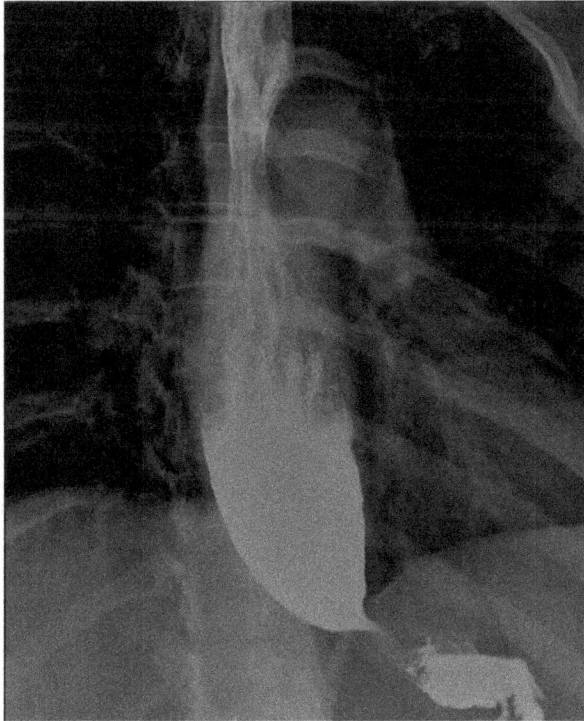

Figure 11.6 Bird-beak sign.

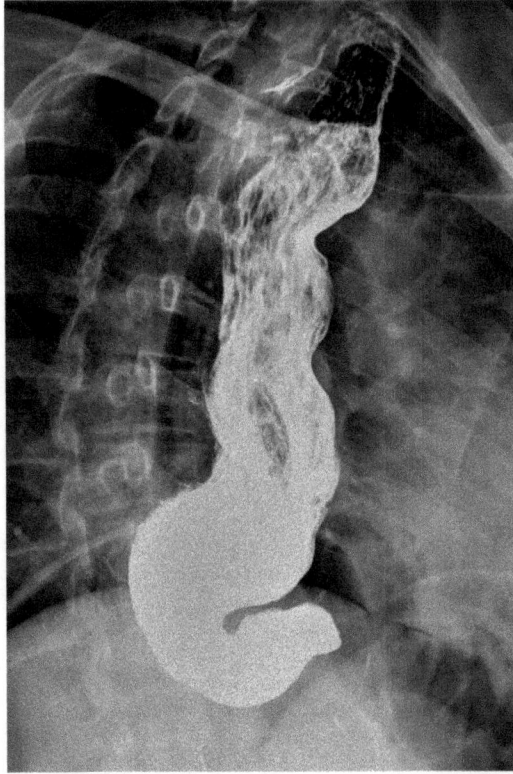

Figure 11.7 Sigmoid esophagus in late-stage achalasia.

Diffuse spasm of the esophagus simulates "curling" or the corkscrew esophagus (Figure 11.8) and is chiefly ascribed to degenerative changes in the esophageal wall. Manometric studies are helpful in confirming the diagnosis of esophageal spasm. During manometry, simultaneous, repetitive contractions of high amplitude involving the distal two-thirds of the esophagus (smooth muscle) are observed. These esophageal contractions are not responsive to the mecholyl test. A normal resting pressure is present in both the upper and lower sphincters, although pressure may be increased slightly in the lower sphincter. On radiologic examination of individuals with diffuse esophageal spasm, the primary peristaltic wave is suddenly replaced by segmental uncoordinated contractions involving the lower third of the esophagus. These abnormal waves are obliterated after ingestion of a subsequent bolus with the reappearance of normal peristaltic waves. A more severe or persistent form of diffuse spasm producing a pseudodiverticular type of contractions is called segmental spasm, being responsible frequently for substernal pain. In this disorder, the esophagus is not dilated, nor is obstruction observed. However, hypertrophy of the esophageal musculature eventually develops.

11.1.5 Elevator Esophagus

"Elevator esophagus" is a term that refers to a distinct motor dysfunction of the lower esophagus in elderly patients, associated with a serious local or distant organic disease, usually a malignancy. Fluoroscopic examination, in the upright position immediately following the ingestion of a barium mixture and especially after the first few swallows, reveals a frenzied and distinctly abnormal up and down motion of the fluid level of barium within the lower esophagus. The appearance resembles an erratic elevator. This fluoroscopic pattern disappears when the patient is examined in the prone or supine position. The cause of the disorder is thought to be secondary to an impaired neuromuscular mechanism with disturbed peristalsis of local or reflex origin. It is reminiscent of diffuse esophageal spasm.

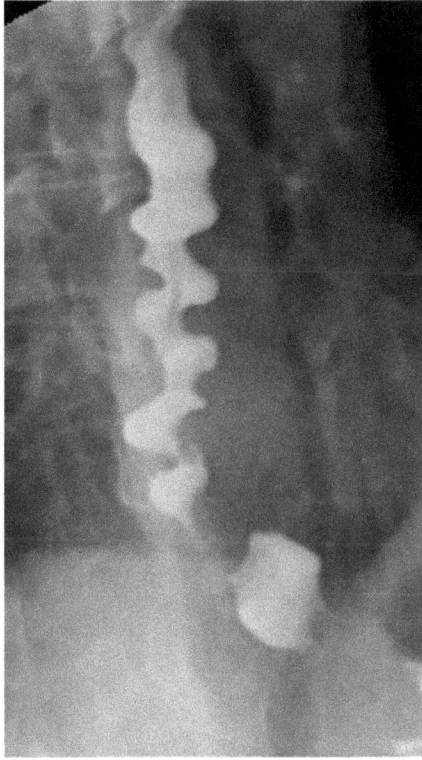

Figure 11.8 Corkscrew esophagus.

11.2 COLLAGEN DISORDERS

11.2.1 Scleroderma

The esophagus is affected by several collagen illnesses, including scleroderma. This seemingly autoimmune condition typically affects people between the ages of 30 and 50 and is more common in women than in men. Before any skin lesions show up, the esophagus may be affected by a gradual systemic form. The most prevalent kind is linked to skin lesions of the atrophic and acrosclerosis types. The esophagus exhibits fibrinoid degenerative alterations of the collagen fibers, which are the fundamental pathologic characteristics of scleroderma. Atrophy of the muscularis and sclerosis of the submucosal layer are the results of this process, which starts in the submucosal layer and subsequently spreads to the muscularis. Eventually, fibrous connective tissue takes the place of both layers. The effect is interference with the intrinsic innervation [6–10]. Atonia is also caused by the muscularis's involvement, which alters the esophageal wall's contractility. Subcutaneous edema, followed by induration and finally atrophy, are the hallmarks of the skin alterations that frequently occur before esophageal motor abnormalities. The clinical manifestation of Raynaud's disease may accompany the involvement of the skin on the face and fingers. The main cause of these alterations is vasospasm of the fingers' peripheral vessels, which leads to decreased blood flow, cutaneous sclerosis, and atrophy of the ungual tufts of the phalanges. Although this finding is not exclusive to dermatomyositis (see section on dermatomyosis), subcutaneous calcium deposits are frequently found. The esophagus is not the only organ impacted by systemic sclerosis. Collagen anomalies can occur in the heart, lungs, colon, and small intestine. The radiologic examination is crucial because esophageal motor dysfunction can sometimes occur before any other observable pathology manifests. The underlying pathologic alterations are reflected in the radiologic findings. Sclerotic alterations accompany submucosal edema as the initial mucosal abnormality in the esophagus. This impairs the esophageal motility, resulting in reduced peristalsis at first, followed by the eventual absence of normal contractility. The mucosal pattern indicates smooth atrophy as the muscularis degenerates and the mucosa thickens (Figure 11.9). Incompetence of the lower esophageal sphincter occurs. In the prone horizontal or supine posture, the bottom portion of the esophagus holds barium

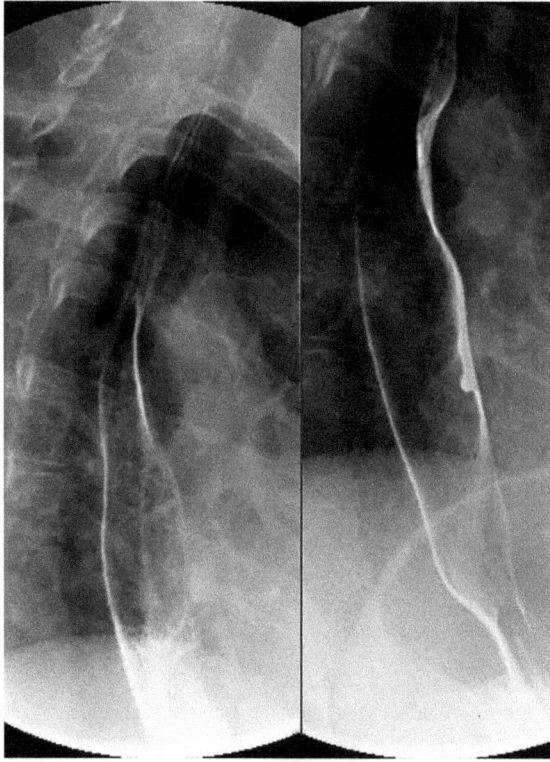

Figure 11.9 Scleroderma.

for hours, resembling a stiff tube. Because of the effects of gravity, the esophagus empties easily when standing up straight; this characteristic may be utilized to distinguish achalasia from scleroderma. Gastric regurgitation into the esophagus occurs as a result of the lower esophageal sphincter's inability to contract. Additionally, simple films show that the dilated esophagus is quickly filled with air, especially when it is horizontal. Complications are frequent due to unrestricted gastric reflux into the esophagus. At various stages, acute and then chronic esophagitis with stenosis and ulceration are frequently seen. Alongside cicatrizing alterations that cause the stomach to tuck upward are pseudodiverticula and esophageal hiatal hernias, which are caused by the esophagus shortening. When a barium enema test reveals exaggerated haustral pouches (pseudosacculations), the colon in scleroderma may become noticeably enlarged. A malabsorption or "sprue" pattern that is not unique to scleroderma (and also seen in dermatomyositis and other collagen disorders) may also manifest in the small intestine. The chest shows other notable radiologic alterations. A reticulonodular pattern, especially in the base, is a symptom of disseminated interstitial fibrosis in the lungs. Enlargement of the heart is not unusual.

11.2.2 Acrosclerosis

One type of scleroderma linked to Raynaud's disease is acrosclerosis. Although esophageal alterations occur later, they share characteristics with the radiologic signs of classical scleroderma. The concomitant vasomotor disorder involving the hands in acrosclerosis distinguishes it from scleroderma.

11.2.3 Dermatomyositis

Unlike scleroderma, dermatomyositis (polymyositis) is a collagen disease that mostly affects the upper part of the esophagus. The muscles of deglutition and the muscularis of the upper end of the esophagus acquire edema and fibrotic degenerative alterations. Due to muscle weakness and reduced esophageal motility, particularly in the upper section of the esophagus, radiologic findings on fluoroscopy show delayed transit of the barium bolus. Scleroderma rarely causes nasal regurgitation, although dermatomyositis frequently does. Scleroderma can also cause involvement of the lower end of the esophagus with sacculations or pseudodiverticula. Unlike scleroderma, there are rarely strictures or ulcerations, and the lower esophageal sphincter is not affected. Atony, distension of the middle third, segmental contractions, weak peristaltic activity, delayed transit time, and atrophic mucosa are further radiologic characteristics observed in the esophagus. Additionally, there may be impaired function of the lower and upper esophageal sphincters. There might be further gastrointestinal abnormalities, especially in the small intestine, where a "sprue" pattern could be seen. Dermatomyositis has also been found to involve the tricopharyngeal muscles. On radiologic examination, stenotic alterations of the cricopharyngeus muscle and contraction of the sphincter segment beneath the distinguishable pharyngoesophageal junction can be seen. Histologic analyses of biopsy samples taken from the cricopharyngeus muscle reveal the distinctive pathologic alterations that are exclusive to this condition. A myotomy can alleviate the accompanying symptoms. The soft tissues of the extremities and periarticular regions, especially the fingers, frequently have subcutaneous calcifications. In the later phases, digit contractures are not unusual. While less frequent than scleroderma, disseminated interstitial pulmonary fibrosis does occur.

11.2.4 Lupus Erythematous

Changes in disseminated lupus erythematosus resemble those in dermatomyositis. There may be oropharyngeal muscle weakness, which can lead to dysphagia and possibly total paralysis. A delay in esophageal emptying is frequently caused by a loss of contractile power and muscle tone of the esophagus with reduced motility, which leads to irregular or absent peristalsis.

11.2.5 Rheumatoid Arthritis

In its more severe forms, rheumatoid arthritis can also impact the esophagus, leading to a significant reduction in esophageal motility.

11.3 BENIGN STRICTURES

The main cause of restrictions is esophagitis of some kind. They can be seen anywhere in the esophagus and can range in shape from cord-like constriction to thin annular rings. Both local and systemic illness processes can cause restrictions [11–15]. Determining the cause is aided by the stricture's location, appearance, and correlation with a hiatal hernia. Corrosive agent ingestion, reflux esophagitis, esophageal ulcers, trauma (particularly from foreign bodies), hiatal hernias, ectopic and heterotopic gastric epithelialized esophagus, and congenital conditions are examples of local causes. Localized regions of muscle hypertrophy, acquired or congenital webs and rings, physiologic zones of spasm, and malignant strictures must all be distinguished from benign strictures. One crucial initial finding is the stricture's placement. The following step is to assess the obstruction's length, form, nature, and degree. A small annular stricture at or below the level of the upper sphincter may result from the presence of significant cervical spinal osteophytes. To rule out a neoplastic process, a localized area of stenosis in the aortic arch region needs to be closely examined. A benign lesion is more likely when the stricture is funneled smoothly and centrally. A neoplasm is favored by eccentric, uneven funneling above the stricture. While some distensibility of the affected segment with normal or hyperactive peristalsis supports a benign condition, rigidity of the stenotic segment with a localized aperistaltic area also promotes a malignant process. The assessment of strictures resulting from surrounding mediastinal illness presents significant complications at the mid-esophageal level. Evaluation of aberrant angulation, thickness of the esophageal wall and diverticula, fixing of any stenotic segment, and expansion of mediastinal lymph nodes is required. A healed Barrett's ulcer may result in a short, stenotic, smooth section that is somewhat below the bronchial bifurcation. The esophagus above and below this segment seems to be moving normally in this instance. The majority of esophageal strictures occur in the lower third and are typically linked to a hiatal hernia (Figure 11.10). It is important to ascertain if the sphincter stricture caused the hernia or if it came about first. Reflux esophagitis is typically the result of a large hernia that is accompanied by a stricture. Heterotopic gastric epithelium may be the secondary cause of a long, stenotic, funneled segment above a hiatal hernia. Only the sphincter zone may be affected by a stricture. Healed, traumatic perforations can also cause strictures. Chronic strictures, which result from the consumption of caustic substances, are typically long and cause stiffness and a residual beading of the stenotic segment. Because the mucosal surface of a benign stricture is destroyed after prolonged bouginage, it may resemble a malignant lesion. Malignant transformation may eventually occur in a benign stricture, and the change may be gradual enough and diagnostically modest to go

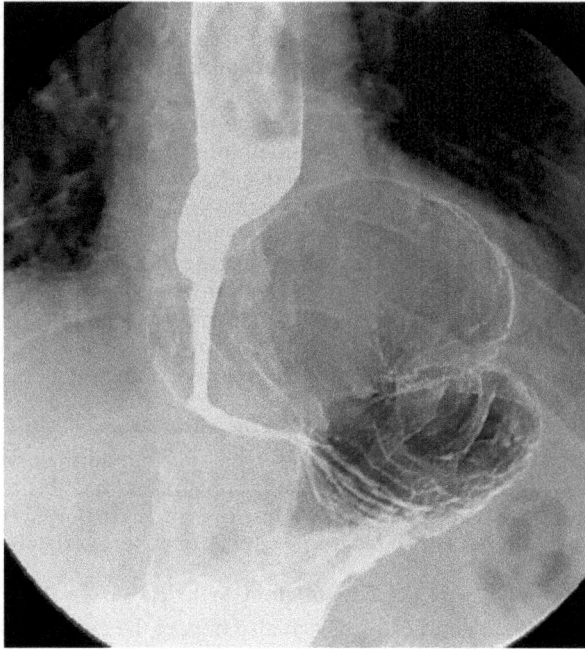

Figure 11.10   Hiatal hernia.

unnoticed. Uncertain lesions should be biopsied, and routine radiologic exams are crucial. Benign strictures exhibit some degree of movement and are somewhat more malleable than malignant lesions. Benign strictures are impacted by heart pulsations and frequently shift positions during inspiration and expiration. The wall of a malignant lesion is hard or immovable; a passing bolus can drive the lumen open, but only slightly. Because it is not as easily impacted by respiratory activity or heart pulsations, the bolus stays above the stenotic location for a longer amount of time. It is necessary to distinguish small annular strictures from localized regions of muscle hypertrophy, rings, and webs.

11.3.1 Webs

Thin membranes called webs partially or totally enclose the esophageal lumen. They can be acquired through both local and systemic sources, or they can be congenital. It is important to distinguish webs from irregular notchings that are primarily seen near the pharyngoesophageal junction. Additionally, cervical webs may develop as a result of lye strictures. Dysphagia may also result from idiopathic web-like lesions in the upper sphincter zone (Figures 11.11–11.15). There has been significant debate regarding the clinical importance of cervical and hypopharyngeal webs. In this area, asymptomatic webs are not unusual and would not have any clinical significance unless they generate the dysphagia-causing ingredient. Webs are most easily detected on radiologic examination in an esophageal or hypopharyngeal distention. It is advisable to observe the maximal narrowing caused by the web (as well as rings and strictures) right before an advancing peristaltic wave strips. Webs are typically asymmetrical and manifest as thin notchings or incisura at the barium column's edge.

11.3.2 Rings

Ring-like strictures can be acquired or congenital, and they are often wider and stiffer than webs. They can also be asymmetrical. It is common for one or more rings to be visible in the lower end of the esophagus. It is important to distinguish these from the inconstant notches that delineate the phrenoesophageal membrane's upper and lower attachments. These notches are commonly linked to hernias and hiatal insufficiency. These notches are tiny, irregular, triangular, incisure-like lesions that can be unilateral or bilateral on radiologic examination. A real ring typically covers the entire esophagus and is broader.

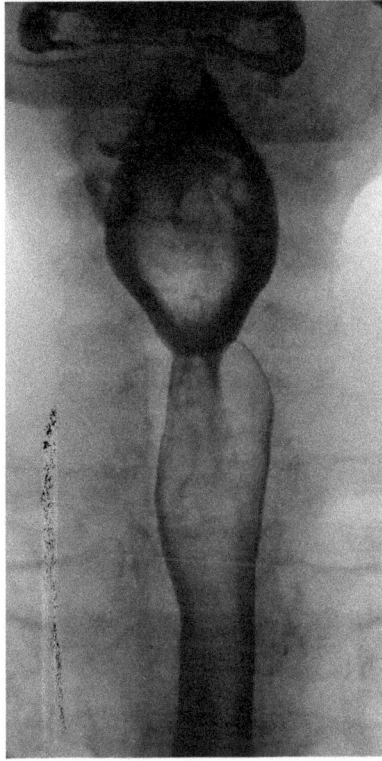

Figure 11.11 Esophageal webs. (Image courtesy of Dr. Paul Hellerhoff, Munich.)

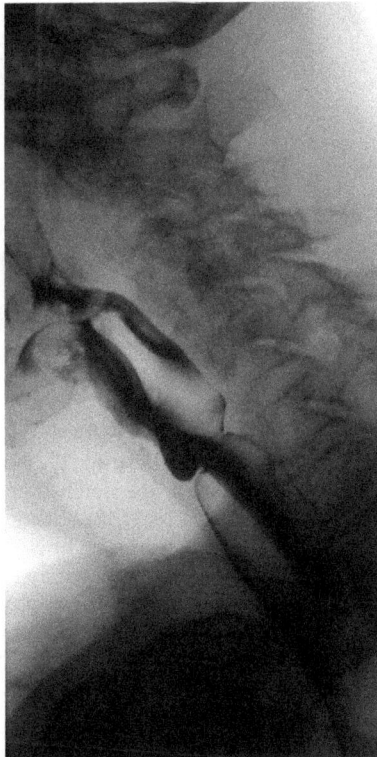

Figure 11.12 Esophageal webs. (Image courtesy of Dr. Paul Hellerhoff, Munich.)

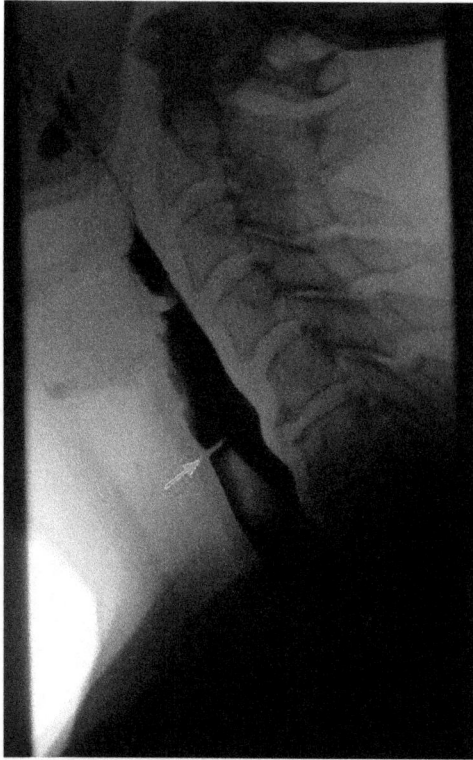

Figure 11.13 Esophageal webs. (Image courtesy of Dr. Paul Hellerhoff, Munich.)

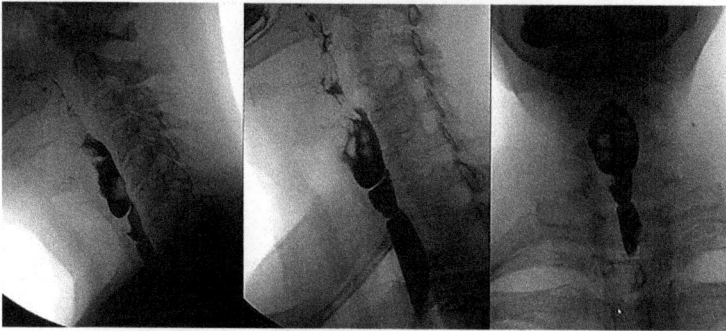

Figure 11.14 Esophageal webs. (Image courtesy of Dr. Paul Hellerhoff, Munich.)

11.3.3 Schatski's Ring

A sliding esophageal hiatal hernia is linked to Schatski's ring, which is situated at the gastroesophageal junction. When the esophagus is fully dilated, the notches appear square, thin, smooth, and symmetrical on radiologic examination (Figures 11.16–11.18). Although there is no blockage, the size of the esophageal lumen at the ring site varies depending on how much of the ring is visible. Males are more likely than females to have the Schatski ring, which may be the cause of sporadic episodes of dysphagia in both sexes. Since the ring is more common in people with reflux esophagitis brought on by a persistent duodenal ulcer, it is most likely related to the outcomes of localized acid pepsin regurgitation. At the gastroesophageal junction, the Schatski ring needs to be distinguished from rings created by strictures resulting from healed marginal ulcers. Typically, this kind of ring is stiffer and asymmetrical.

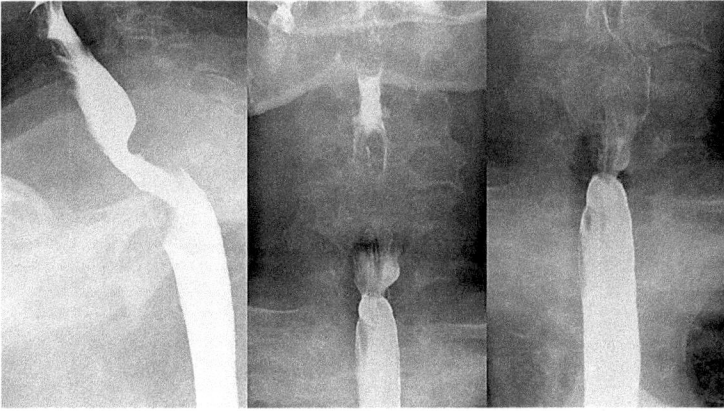

Figure 11.15 Esophageal webs. (Images courtesy of Dr. Paul Hellerhoff, Munich.)

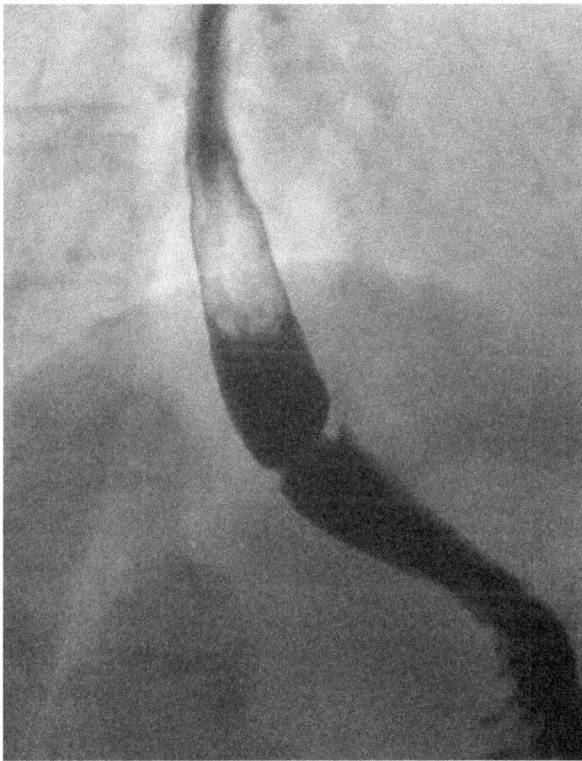

Figure 11.16 Schatski's ring. (Image courtesy of Dr. Paul Hellerhoff, Munich.)

11.3.4 Double Ring

A double ring has been seen in a number of cases linked to hiatal hernias. The upper ring seems to be situated at the level of the phrenoesophageal membrane's upper attachment, whereas the lower ring is situated at the gastroesophageal junction. Apart from a mucosal fold, a localized band of muscle hypertrophy may also be the source of these rings, particularly at the level of the membrane's top attachment.

11.3.5 Cricopharyngeal Bar

The cricopharyngeal (CP) muscle is the primary constituent of the upper esophageal sphincter (UES) [16–20]. The presence of a conspicuous bar on lateral radiographs of barium swallows,

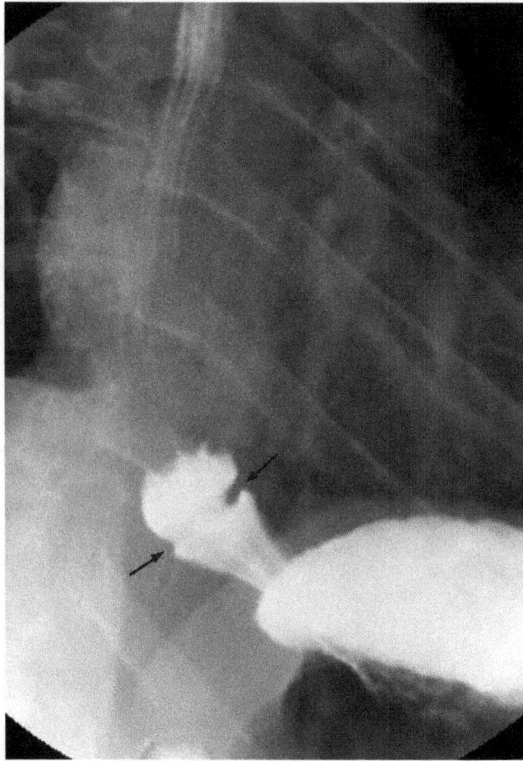

Figure 11.17 Schatski's ring. (Image courtesy of Dr. Paul Hellerhoff, Munich.)

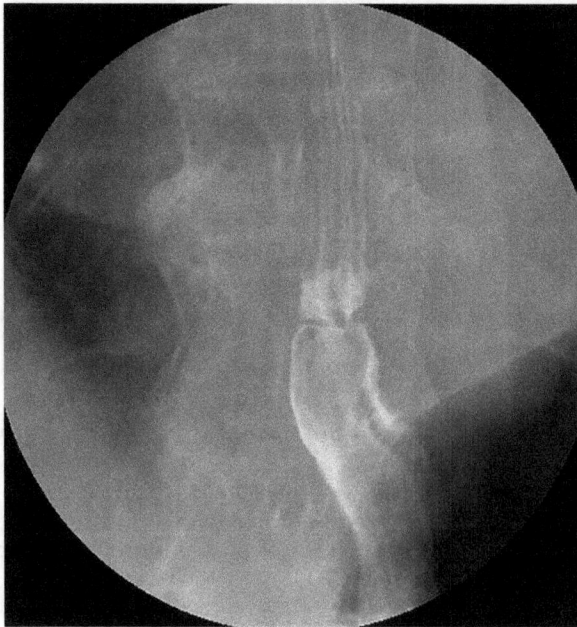

Figure 11.18 Schatski's ring.

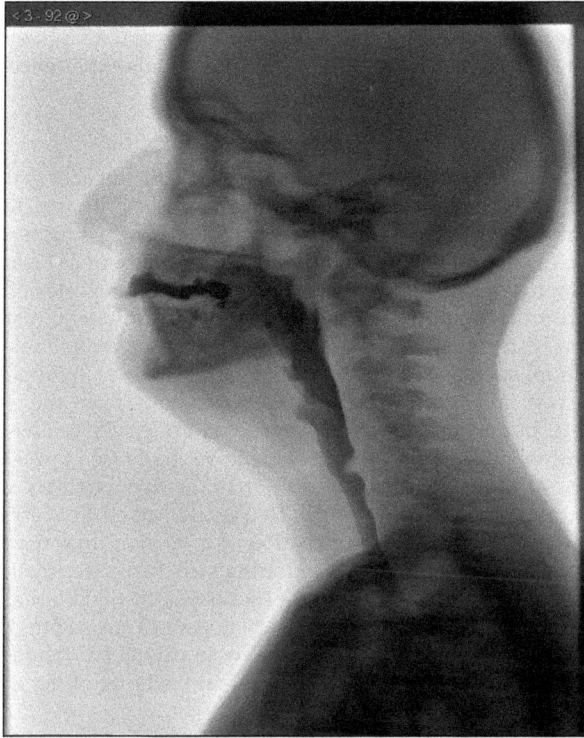

Figure 11.19 Cricopharyngeal bar.

observed in certain patients, can be identified with the CP muscle (Figure 11.19). This disease is commonly believed to be caused by a spasm or inability of the CP muscle to relax, leading to the term "cricopharyngeal achalasia," or cricopharyngeal bar, which suggests that the presence of isolated such radiologic findings is a result of defective relaxation of the upper esophageal sphincter. This could be idiopathic or due to neurologic (cerebrovascular accidents), muscular diseases (myasthenia gravis, dermatomyositis) or to occult gastroesophageal reflux disease (GERD). About half of patients with CP bars exhibit symptoms related to GERD; a fraction of these will progress toward developing a Zenker's diverticulum. Other causes could be related to muscle fibrosis. From a clinical point of view, many patients could be asymptomatic; when they are not, the main complaint is, of course, dysphagia. Voice disorders, hoarseness, bolus penetration or aspiration, with consequent pneumonia and chronic interstitial disease, as seen in our experience, are other rarer potential consequences. When either CP bar or GERD is suspected, even though CP bar is rarely a clinical suspicion and often an incidental finding, extreme attention has to be paid to these patients' pharyngoesophageal junction. Many studies have been conducted on patients with CP bars, using UES manometry, in order to assess the presence of impaired sphincter relaxation. Based on recent empirical investigations, it is postulated that the process of proper deglutitive UES opening and transsphincteric flow can be attributed to four distinct components. Initially, in the process of swallowing, the UES musculature, namely the CP muscle, experiences a temporary loss of its muscular tension lasting around 0.5 seconds. Secondly, the relaxed sphincter exhibits compliance and is easily extensible. Furthermore, the relaxation and opening of the sphincter is initiated by the application of forward traction on the larynx, which is caused by an upward and forward movement of the hyoid bone and the contraction of the thyrohyoid muscles. Last, the pressure exerted by an incoming bolus causes more distension of the sphincter compared to traction alone. The pressure exerted on the bolus is influenced by the pressure forces present within the closed pharyngeal contraction segment, which is responsible for propelling the bolus. In normal subjects, there is a notable and substantial ten-fold rise in the average transsphincteric flow rate when the volume of the ingested bolus increases from 2 to 30 mL. The primary adaptation accountable for the observed rise in flow rate is a significant increase in the dimensions and cross-sectional area of the UES, which is reliant on the volume. Meanwhile, the length of sphincter opening and the velocity of pharyngeal peristalsis exhibit minor or no alteration. Individuals with CP bars show significant anomalies, including reduced sphincter dimensions and cross-sectional areas that fail to exhibit the typical adaptive response to increased bolus volume during swallowing. Additionally, these individuals experience poor passive compliance of the UES [21–26].

11.4 DIVERTICULA

Sometimes seen in the esophagus and hypopharynx, diverticula are aberrant outpocketings of the gastrointestinal tract [27–30]. The layers of the wall in which they are situated are all present in a true diverticulum. A false diverticulum is primarily made up of the mucosal layer that protrudes via a muscle wall rupture or hole. False diverticula have a variety of causes. Diverticula are most commonly linked to other esophageal disorders. There are two categories of diverticula: acquired and congenital. Pulsion, traction, pulsion-traction, pseudo, inconsistent, resilient, and intramural diverticula are the several categories into which acquired diverticula can be classified. They can also be categorized by location, such as cervical, thoracic, epiphrenic, or hypopharyngeal. Congenital diverticula are uncommon and typically indicate leftover buds from the upper digestive tract's embryonic development. In general, acquired diverticula are easier to identify and more prevalent. Increased intraluminal pressure is hypothesized to be the cause of pulsion diverticula, which allow the mucosal lining to protrude through a section of the hypopharynx and/or esophagus that is physically weak, injured, or distended. This is frequently linked to aberrant or disturbed neuromuscular function, which all aids in the formation of a pulsion diverticulum. Secondary to an external pull from adhesions or fixation of surrounding structures are traction diverticula. A true diverticulum is created, affecting every layer of the esophageal wall. External traction and internal pulsion work together to create pulsion-traction diverticula. On a single film, pseudodiverticula are functional outpocketings that resemble diverticula. These pseudoiverticula are actually aberrant contractions that segment the esophageal lumen. Minimal wedging of the mucosal sac within the esophageal wall results in inconsistent diverticula.

11.4.1 Diverticula in the Cervical Esophagus and Hypopharynx

The most typical location for hypopharyngeal diverticula is just posterior and slightly to the left, above the pharyngoesophageal sphincter, between the oblique fibers and the "pars fundiformis" of the cricopharyngeus muscle. Zenker's diverticula is the common name for these (Figure 11.20). On rare occasions, there could be two Zenker's diverticula or a lobulated Zenker's diverticulum. The Killian–Jamieson area, a laterally positioned aperture that divides the proximal longitudinal fibers of the esophagus connected to the lower pole of the cricoid lamina from the cricopharyngeus muscle, is a less common location for diverticulum formation. This region is where the recurrent laryngeal nerve and its corresponding arteries enter the larynx. These laterally situated diverticula are situated above the sphincter zone, on either the left or right side of the pharyngoesophageal junction (Figures 11.21–11.24). Any weak or structurally flawed midline location can also have posterior midline diverticula. The pulsion type accounts for the majority of hypopharyngeal diverticula. They are particularly common in middle-aged or elderly people who have some degree of muscle atrophy or neurogenic incoordination. Since these diverticula are situated above the pharyngoesophageal sphincter, when sphincteric dysfunction results in delayed opening or increased pressure, the sphincter itself most likely causes the elevated hypopharyngeal pressure in this region. In rare cases, adhesions from trauma, fibrositis, persistent inflammatory alterations, or an infiltrating

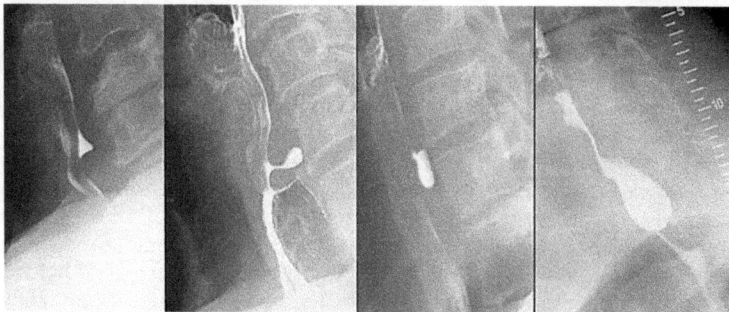

Figure 11.20   Zenker's diverticulum. (Images courtesy of Dr. Paul Hellerhoff, Munich.)

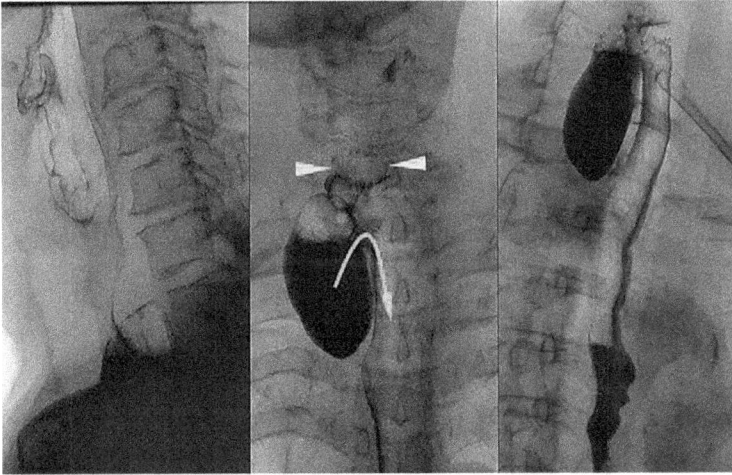

Figure 11.21 Killian–Jamieson diverticulum. (Images courtesy of Dr. Paul Hellerhoff, Munich.)

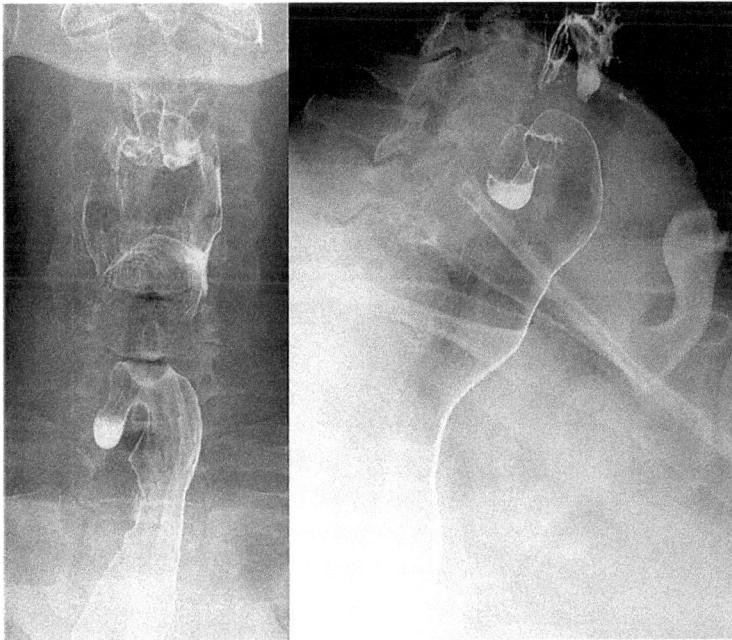

Figure 11.22 Killian–Jamieson diverticulum. (Images courtesy of Dr. Paul Hellerhoff, Munich.)

cancer may cause traction diverticula in the hypopharyngeal region. Men are more likely than women to have Zenker's diverticula, perhaps due to the additional pressure from a larger larynx. Brombart has provided a thorough description of their development and appearance at different stages (Figure 11.20). Very tiny Zenker's diverticula are frequently seen when the pharyngoesophageal area's dynamic changes are carefully examined using cine and fluoroscopy. Above the level of the contracted sphincter, at the pharyngoesophageal junction, barium stasis is common and should not be confused with a diverticulum. Due to the sluggish action of the sphincter and the relative reduction of muscular tone of the hypopharyngeal muscles, this stasis is more common among the elderly. These pseudodiverticula fluctuate in size and shape quickly. Nonetheless, it might also be inconsistent to demonstrate a little true diverticulum. Such a real diverticulum can be identified in its early stages as a thorn-like projection from the opacified lumen. As the mucosal pocket inverts during the actual swallowing act, this projection may vanish. However, while at rest, the

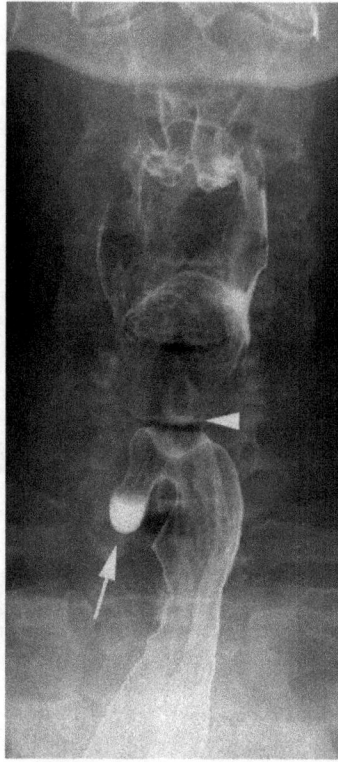

Figure 11.23 Killian–Jamieson diverticulum. (Image courtesy of Dr. Paul Hellerhoff, Munich.)

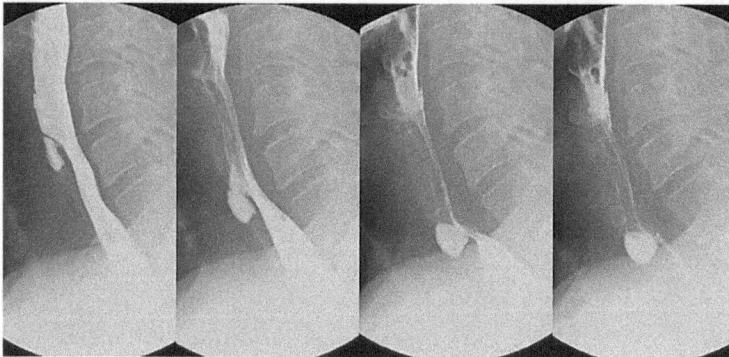

Figure 11.24 Killian– Jamieson diverticulum. (Images courtesy of Dr. Paul Hellerhoff, Munich.)

thorn-like projection resurfaces in a nearly same size, shape, and pattern. The diverticulum becomes less elastic and forms a pedicle as it gradually becomes bigger. After that, the diverticulum's sac goes through phases when it takes on an oval and pear shape before becoming pendant. Diverticula can enlarge to the point that the cervical esophagus is compressed and dislocated. The constricted sphincter zone, on the other hand, is always recognized in the resting state as a contracted segment that is a few millimeters long and lies below the pharyngoesophageal junction. A significant amount of barium is retained in the bigger diverticula due to the lack of a muscular layer that inhibits contraction and emptying. When standing up straight, a fluid level is visible. A trapped pocket of air may be visible on a plain film of the cervical area in this condition, necessitating the evaluation of abscess, pharyngocele, and laryngocele. Early detection of Zenker's diverticula can be aided by the modified Valsalva technique. It is possible to determine their level of motion, where they are, and which way they point. This technique is also useful for differentiating between diverticula of

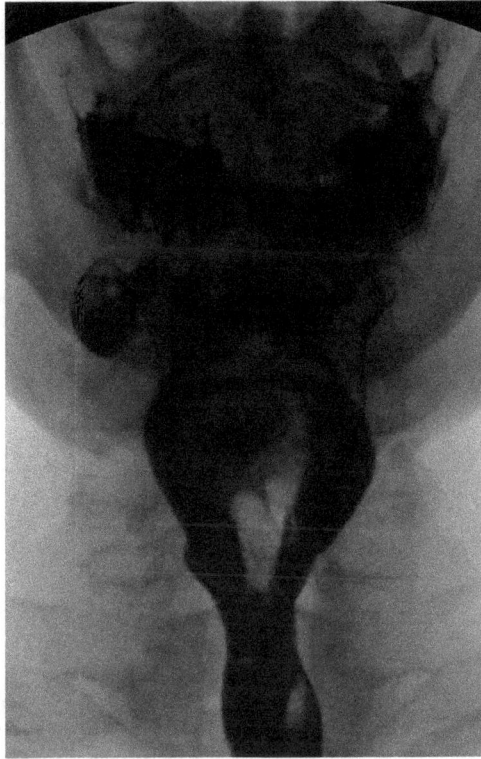

Figure 11.25   Lateral pharyngeal pouches. (Image courtesy of Dr. Paul Hellerhoff, Munich.)

the traction and pulsion types. Usually, surrounding adhesions hold traction diverticula in place. Small diverticula can be recognized in the anteroposterior view as retained barium or midline or lateral oval specks. The anteroposterior view is very useful for identifying upper lateral pharyngeal pouches or pharyngoceles, as well as lateral diverticula. There have been no reports of diverticula in the sphincter zone.

11.4.2 Lateral Pouches of the Pharynx

Lateral pharyngeal pouches may be acquired pharyngoceles or actual congenital diverticula (Figure 11.25). Congenital diverticula typically have long pedicles and are seen in the tonsillar fossa. A bulge or tear in the thyrohyoid ligament is typically the cause of acquired pharyngoceles, which can be superior or inferior to the level of the hyoid bone. The pouch reaches into the tonsillar fossa above or the pyriform fossa below. The most prevalent lateral pharyngeal pouches are found in musicians who play wind instruments or glassblowers. They can also occur in older people whose ligaments are weak or loosened. It is simple to illustrate these pharyngeal pouches—which are pulsion diverticula—using a barium swallow.

11.4.3 Laryngoceles

Laryngoceles are rare. They are either congenital or acquired, saccular or cystic dilatations of the larynx's ventricular appendix. Although laryngoceles are found inside the larynx, they can also herniate into the soft tissue of the neck through the thyrohyoid ligament, where they can be mistaken for pharyngoceles. However, because laryngoceles are found in the larynx, they are not opacified during a barium swallow. Due to the sustained intermittent increase in intraglottic pressure required to perform with these instruments, acquired laryngoceles are most common among professional horn players.

11.4.4 Diverticula of the Thoracic Esophagus

People who have chronic inflammatory illness of the apical lung segments may have pseudo, traction, or pulsion-traction diverticula of the uppermost section of the thoracic esophagus, which

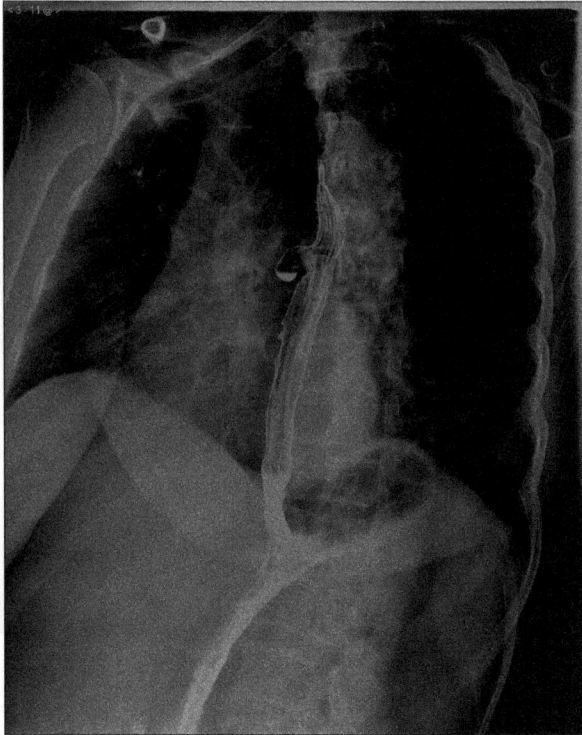

Figure 11.26 Thoracic esophagus diverticulum.

causes the esophagus to deviate and shift. Though less common, pulsion diverticula can also form in this region. Diverticula at the aortobronchial triangle are mostly of the resilient type and are not always present (Figure 11.26). This portion of the esophagus often bulges in the elderly due to air being trapped in it. The longitudinal muscles in this area of the thoracic esophagus may split apart, and an irregular protrusion through this muscular layer aperture results in a robust diverticulum or fan-like dilatation of this esophageal segment. A permanent diverticular pocket eventually develops. The carina is where esophageal diverticula most frequently occur. These areas contain diverticula of the traction type or a mix of the traction and pulsion types. The esophagus is typically impacted by persistent inflammation of the peribronchial nodes at the carina. This area frequently has calcified lymph nodes, which suggests prior inflammatory alterations primarily brought on by tuberculosis or histoplasmosis. The development of a diverticulum is rarely explained by a congenital connection of the esophagus to the tracheobronchial tree. Furthermore, hyperactive peristalsis of the upper part of the esophagus combined with spasm of the lower end of the esophagus may result in a large pressure gradient in the mid-esophagus, which facilitates the formation of diverticula. Single or several traction diverticula are easily overlooked. The right anterior wall of the middle portion of the esophagus is where they are most frequently found. The superimposition of the barium-filled esophagus may mask such a diverticulum in the anteroposterior view. Rotational and lateral views are therefore required. Cine and fluoroscopic tests are crucial. A diverticulum is easier to see when a peristaltic wave passes over its location. An esophagus at rest may not exhibit traction diverticula. Furthermore, depending on the extent of fullness and distension, diverticula may undergo form changes following repeated examination. The problem may be exacerbated by a diverticulum with a large neck that empties quickly. Located anteriorly, diverticula inferior to the tracheal bifurcation are typically tiny, irregularly walled pouches that are conical or oval in shape. It is necessary to distinguish them from ulcer niches. It is rare to see pulsion diverticula in the mid-esophageal area. They often retain barium, are tiny, have distinctly narrow necks, and move easily with the esophagus. It is also necessary to distinguish these diverticula from esophageal ulcers. Although pulsion-traction diverticula exhibit both traction and pulsion traits, they are typically locked in place by surrounding adhesions or other disease processes. Usually, there is a noticeable neck. The lower two-thirds of the esophagus are where functional or pseudodiverticula

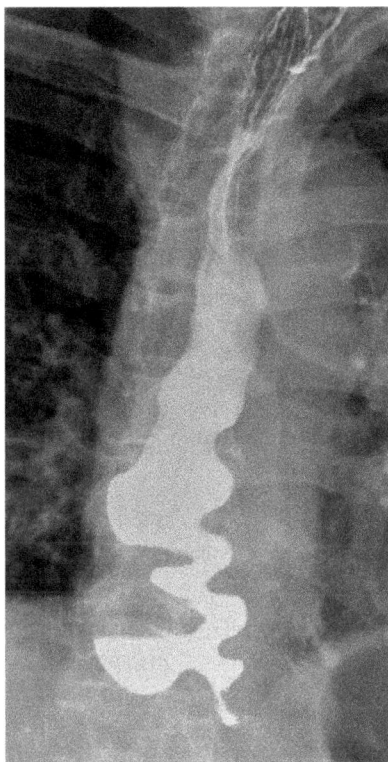

Figure 11.27 Epiphrenic diverticulum.

are most common. When the esophageal muscles contract, they are most frequently detected. They typically occur in multiples and disappear when the esophageal motility patterns relax. As bulging occurs through areas of weaker or torn muscle fibers, persistent spasm may eventually result in fixed pulsion-type diverticula at the location of pseudodiverticula, despite the fact that their shape and number tend to vary initially. In cases of disrupted innervation without accompanying muscle hypertrophies, such diverticula are seen.

11.4.5 Epiphrenic Diverticula

The lower esophageal section, right above the diaphragm, contains epiphrenic diverticula (Figure 11.27). They can be linked to achalasia, a hiatal hernia, or any other condition that causes spasms or a hypertensive lower esophageal sphincter. Primarily of the pulsion type, epiphrenic diverticula are typically seen anteriorly and to the right or left of the stomach's cardia. The size, position, and level of filling of the sacs determine their forms. As they grow, they have the potential to push the esophagus aside and give the impression of a "collar button" when they are compressed by the spine or mediastinal structures. Small epiphrenic diverticula are difficult to detect on radiologic examination, especially when the patient is upright or is ingesting a thin barium mixture. On the other hand, a little retained collection of barium is typically visible in a thick barium paste. The optimum time to observe epiphrenic diverticula is during fluoroscopy. An air fluid level at the right costophrenic angle on a plain chest film suggests the presence of an epiphrenic diverticulum. The distal end of the esophagus may have surrounding pleural adhesions, strictures, or cancer, even though epiphrenic diverticula are frequently linked to hiatal hernia and achalasia. It is necessary to distinguish an epiphrenic diverticulum from an ulcer niche, a diverticulum of the gastric cardia, a redundant esophagus with saccular dilatation as in achalasia, and the herniated section of the gastric fundus in a paraesophageal hiatal hernia. The easiest way to show saccular dilatations of the lower end of a dilated esophagus is to rotate the patient into different oblique orientations while monitoring the first barium swallow before the esophagus becomes overfilled. It is easy to identify a sliding esophageal hiatal hernia when the lower constricted sphincter zone is situated above the diaphragm. However, distinguishing a small section of stomach herniating along the left or right lateral border of the esophagus may be challenging. The diagnosis is established by the barium's flow direction and the lack of a pedicle. A precise diagnosis requires both cine and fluoroscopic tests. Usually found on the left side of the gastroesophageal junction, a diverticulum of the gastric cardia can resemble cardiac shelving. In most cases, an upright radiologic examination is necessary to make the diagnosis. Numerous esophageal diverticula problems could arise. They could bleed, perforate, or become infected. Particularly in the traction variety, a fistulous tract may form in conjunction with a nearby tumor. On rare occasions, a diverticulum may form a cancer. In rare cases, a diverticulum forms intramurally, with the sac only penetrating the deeper layers of muscle. These intramural diverticula are made up of mucosal outpocketings that do not extend through the esophagus wall's connective tissue. They could make the radiologic diagnosis more challenging. Numerous, sizable diverticula are possible. A big hiatal hernia may also contain a diverticulum.

11.5 BENIGN AND MALIGNANT ESOPHAGEAL TUMORS

Barium swallow is no longer considered a primary diagnostic tool for esophageal tumors. However, it might be possible to encounter a neoplasm as an incidental finding during an examination, so we decided to include a few basic notions about tumoral findings. A referral to CT/MRI and endoscopy is mandatory in these cases.

11.5.1 Benign Esophageal Tumors

Benign esophageal tumors are rare, accounting for less than 1% of all esophageal neoplasms. Most are submucosal and asymptomatic, often discovered incidentally.

11.5.2 Esophageal Leiomyoma

Esophageal leiomyoma is the most common benign tumor of the esophagus (60–70%). It appears as a smooth, sessile intramural mass (Figure 11.28), sharply marginated with obtuse angles against the esophageal wall. Mucosa overlying the lesion generally remains intact. It may cause extrinsic compression with gradual tapering of the barium column ("shelf effect").

11.5.3 Neurofibromas

Neurofibromas are smooth, round, or oval filling defects, well circumscribed, do not change with swallowing, and usually located in the lower third of the esophagus (Figure 11.29). They may be associated with vertebral anomalies.

11.5.4 Papillomas

Papillomas are typically seen as small, polypoid-filling defects, which may have a rough or frond-like surface, associated with HPV infection in rare cases.

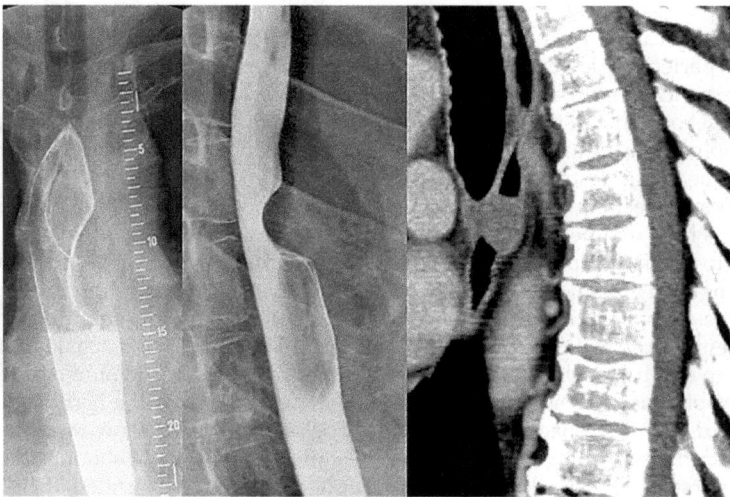

Figure 11.28 Esophageal leiomyoma.

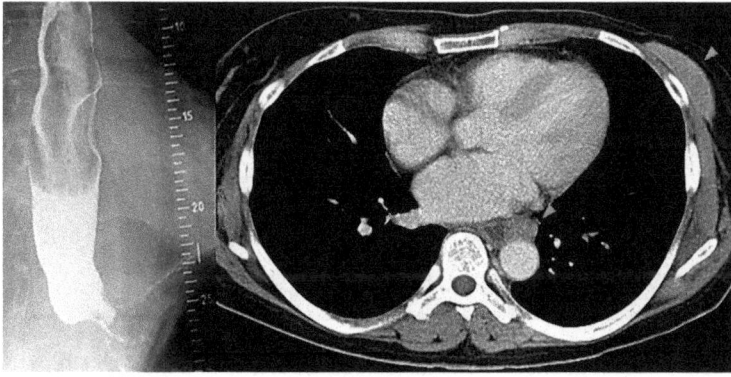

Figure 11.29 Esophageal neurofibroma. (Image courtesy of Dr. Paul Hellerhoff, Munich.)

11.5.5 Malignant Esophageal Tumors

Malignant tumors of the esophagus include squamous cell carcinoma, adenocarcinoma, and less common histologies such as small cell carcinoma, lymphoma, and metastatic disease.

11.5.6 Squamous Cell Carcinoma

The mid-esophagus being the most common site, squamous cell carcinoma appears as irregular, lobulated, or ulcerated intraluminal masses, with "shouldering" or abrupt angulation at lesion margins, determining focal narrowing with mucosal destruction (Figure 11.30). It may present as a polypoid lesion or annular constriction. Fistula formation in advanced disease is not uncommon.

11.5.7 Adenocarcinoma

Generally located in the lower third of the esophagus, adenocarcinoma is often associated with Barrett's esophagus. It appears as an irregular narrowing with mucosal nodularity, generally with ulceration and possible esophagogastric junction involvement, determining pseudoachalasia (Figure 11.31). Less commonly, it forms polypoid masses. Generally, there is a typical short segment involvement, but it can be extensive in some cases.

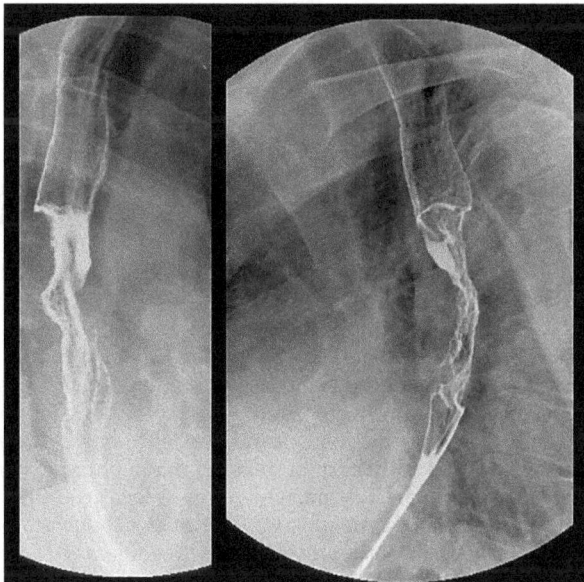

Figure 11.30 Squamous cell carcinoma. (Images courtesy of Dr. Paul Hellerhoff, Munich.)

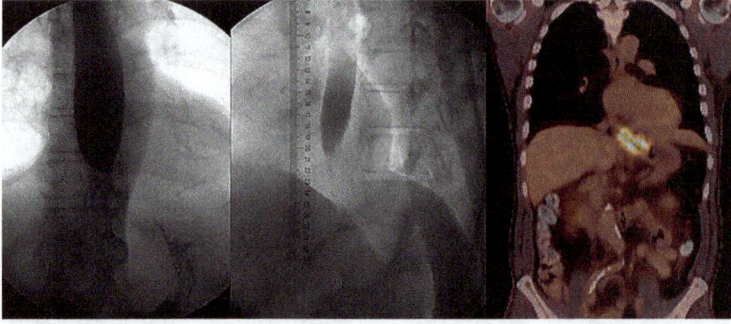

Figure 11.31 Esophageal adenocarcinoma. (Images courtesy of Dr. Paul Hellerhoff, Munich.)

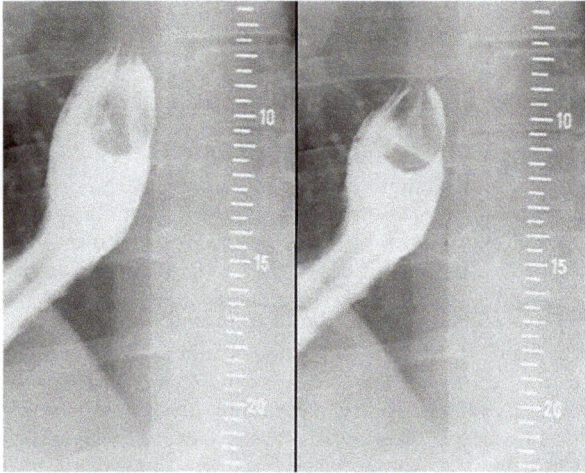

Figure 11.32 Granular cell tumor. (Images courtesy of Dr. Paul Hellerhoff, Munich.)

11.5.8 Small Cell and Other Carcinomas (Granular Cell Tumor, Melanoma)

Rapidly growing, often with submucosal spread, mall cell and other carcinomas may appear as wall thickening with minimal mucosal changes (Figures 11.32 and 11.33). They may be indistinct or subtle on barium studies.

11.6 ESOPHAGITIS

Esophageal inflammation can be caused locally or as a side effect of systemic diseases. Autopsies often reveal esophagitis, particularly in old, disabled, or chronically or critically ill individuals. Esophagitis can be either acute or chronic and can be corrosive, phlegmonous, fibrotic, catarrhal, or follicular. However, it is typically desquamative or exudative. Diffuse cellular infiltration, which may potentially be linked to superficial erosions, is a feature of exudative esophagitis. Partial separation of the esophageal lining's epithelium from the underlying esophageal wall takes place in the desquamative type. Bacterial, fungal, and parasitic agents are linked to the systemic conditions that cause esophagitis. Numerous skin conditions can cause inflammatory changes in the mucosa of the esophagus and hypopharynx. These are covered in the skin conditions section. Depending on the extent of the reparative fibrotic process that follows and the depth of the damage to the underlying tissues, acute esophagitis may either fully cure or develop into a chronic form. Acute esophagitis typically has nonspecific radiologic signs. Edema, which causes localized thickening of the mucosal folds, is the first alteration to the esophagus mucosa. The mucosal surface becomes uneven with serrated edges when superficial erosions are present. These results may regress or vanish entirely. Prolonged spasm, irregularity, and narrowing of the affected area, together with total loss of the mucosal pattern, are characteristics of progressive alterations. The cicatricial alterations are followed by a decrease in peristaltic activity. Stenosis eventually develops.

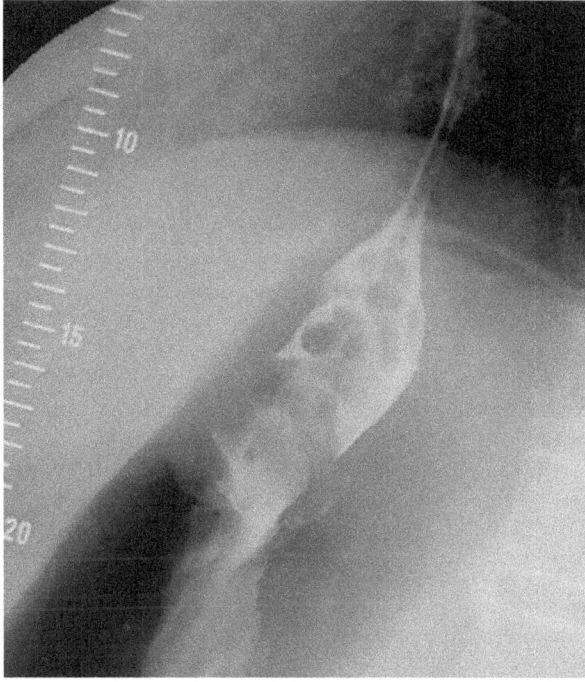

Figure 11.33 Esophageal melanoma. (Image courtesy of Dr. Paul Hellerhoff, Munich.)

11.6.1 Eosinophilic Esophagitis

Idiopathic eosinophilic esophagitis is an inflammatory condition of the esophagus marked by eosinophilia that may affect all layers of the esophageal tissue. It is predominantly observed in patients between the ages of 20 and 40. It is an uncommon disease; however, it is not rare. Patients commonly exhibit dysphagia or the sensation of food lodged in the esophagus. A particular meal or allergen typically initiates the presentation, and symptoms may endure for an extended duration thereafter. Fluoroscopy reveals a "ringed" esophagus (Figure 11.34) characterized by concentric, ring-like strictures observed during a barium swallow; these strictures may coexist with longer strictures and may be linked to esophageal spasm, dysmotility, and foreshortening.

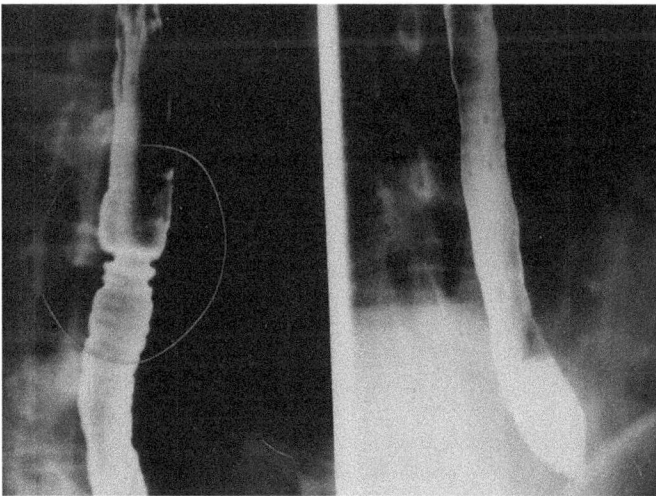

Figure 11.34 Eosinophilic esophagitis. (Images courtesy of Dr. Paul Hellerhoff, Munich.)

11.6.2 Catarrhal Acute Esophagitis

The direct extension of several inflammatory disorders, including tonsillitis, pharyngitis, laryngitis, bronchitis, and pneumonia, can result in acute catarrhal esophagitis. Irritability, hypermotility, and spasm are the main radiologic findings, which are often mild and temporary. Acute catarrhal esophagitis may also be caused by typhoid fever and exanthema, including measles and scarlet fever. Diphtheria was covered in the section on toxic myopathies. Infections from hematogenous causes linked to septicemia can also result in acute or even chronic esophagitis. There is no specificity in the radiologic findings.

11.6.3 Persisting Bacterial Esophagitis

Numerous systemic and local causes can contribute to chronic bacterial esophagitis. There are several types, including granulomatous, cystic, fibrotic, ulcerative, and follicular. Particularly in adolescents and young adults, systemic lymphoid hyperplasia is linked to chronic follicular esophagitis, which is typically caused by pharyngeal inflammation. A megaesophagus may also have this shape. After the underlying cause is removed or treated, the chronic ulcerative form of esophagitis typically goes away. Occlusion of the esophageal mucosal glands, which leads to the development of retention cysts, is a characteristic of chronic cystic esophagitis. Full recovery may result from the spontaneous bursting of these cysts. Crohn's disease can cause granulomatous esophagitis either as a primary or secondary condition.

11.6.4 Ulcerative Esophagitis

There have been reports of acute or chronic ulcerative esophagitis linked to chronic hepatitis and ulcerative colitis. A more specific association with chronic ulcerative colitis seems to be a contributing factor, even though this type of esophagitis is not uncommon in individuals who are disabled and chronically unwell, particularly those on corticosteroid treatment. According to necropsy research, esophagitis is rather common in patients with persistent ulcerative colitis. Therefore, an undetected persistent ulcerative colitis should be taken into consideration in patients with idiopathic ulcerative esophagitis. The radiologic findings are comparable to those typically observed in chronic ulcerative lesions of the esophagus, such as moniliasis. Loss of motility is seen together with an ulcerating and/or pseudopolypoid mucosal pattern. Obstruction, stenosis, and subsequent perforation may occur.

11.6.5 Renal Transplant

One gastrointestinal side effect of kidney transplantation is diffuse esophagitis. A "cobblestone" appearance of the mucosal pattern or diffuse esophageal mucosal thickening due to edema without ulcerations is observed on radiologic examination. There may also be an infection with moniliasis. Cystoisospora intestinalis pneumonia may also be linked.

11.6.6 Thrush

Infants with congenital hypogammaglobulinemia and those without lymphoid tissue in the oropharynx are frequently found to have oral thrush. A real pseudomembrane may form with expansion into the esophagus, and superficial erosions are observed. Complete esophageal blockage may occur in extreme circumstances. The radiologic abnormalities are typical of esophagitis and accompanying consequences and are often limited to the upper esophagus and hypopharynx.

11.6.7 Candidiasis

Oral thrush is typically linked to candidiasis or moniliasis, which is caused by *Candida albicans*, particularly in dehydrated infants. When the esophagus is impacted, the germinating fungus causes wide-ranging pathologic lesions and related radiologic alterations. Patients with compromised immune systems are more susceptible to moniliasis. Immunosuppressive medications, prolonged antibiotic or steroid therapy, and chemotherapeutic medicines for malignant neoplasms are significant contributing factors. However, cases of moniliasis have been documented in young individuals who do not appear to have any underlying medical conditions. The middle third of the esophagus is particularly affected, though the entire tract may be affected. As the illness worsens, the radiologic findings alter quickly. During the acute phase, the mucosal pattern takes on a "cobblestone" look after the edema-induced thickening of the mucosal folds. As the mucosal surface becomes ulcerated, the esophageal contour becomes asymmetrical, shaggy, or ragged. The lumen narrows and occasionally becomes obstructed as a result of aperistalsis and some loss of motility as the esophageal

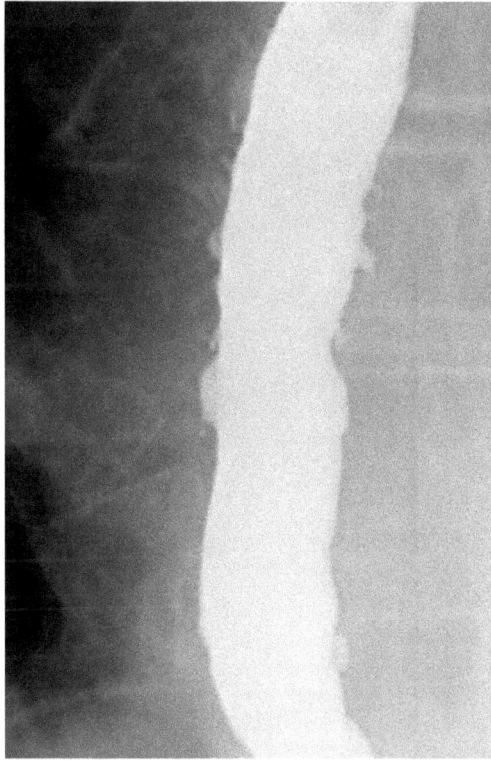

Figure 11.35 Candidiasis/moniliasis. (Image courtesy of Dr. Paul Hellerhoff, Munich.)

wall becomes more involved. The accumulation of detritus and the ongoing proliferation of monilia enhance this phase. The trend of increased involvement is followed by changes in motility. The affected segment's peristaltic movement is first seen to be slightly impaired. This is followed by increasingly slower transit, which in more advanced cases leads to total aperistalsis. Initially, the afflicted section of the esophagus is somewhat dilated, and barium coating can be observed in this area for up to an hour after a barium bolus is consumed. If left untreated, cicatricial alterations and collected debris cause the affected esophagus to constrict as the condition progresses. The mucosal pattern of the esophagus can sometimes mimic "esophageal diverticulosis" (Figure 11.35) due to dilated mucosal glands. After fungicide treatment is successful, all aberrant findings disappear.

11.6.8 Chagas Disease
The most prevalent parasite infection affecting the esophagus is Chagas disease [31–35]. It is endemic in Central and South America and is brought on by the *Trypanosoma cruzi* organism. After invading the reticuloendothelial system's host cells, the parasite finally releases into the circulatory system, where it spreads to different body regions, avoiding leishmania type T in the intestines. Cruzi is believed to release a neurotoxin that damages the myenteric plexus beneath the mucosa. A megaesophagus can be shown radiologically years later and is indistinguishable from achalasia (Figure 11.36). In the chronic stage of the disease, the early radiologic findings are linked to esophageal motor dysfunction. First, irritation and excessive contractility are observed. The esophagus gradually dilates and peristalsis gradually disappears as the sluggish process of denervation goes on. The lower esophageal sphincter fails to relax as a result. A megaesphagus eventually forms; this viscus reaches a gigantic size, exhibiting full aperistalsis and stasis of the contents of the esophagus. Similar effects may be seen in the colon. To distinguish Chagas disease from achalasia, other organs should also be implicated.

11.6.9 Schistosomiasis
A snail serves as the intermediate host for the parasitic disease schistosomiasis, which is brought on by a trematode or "blood fluke." Infected water can be consumed or bathed in to contract the sickness.

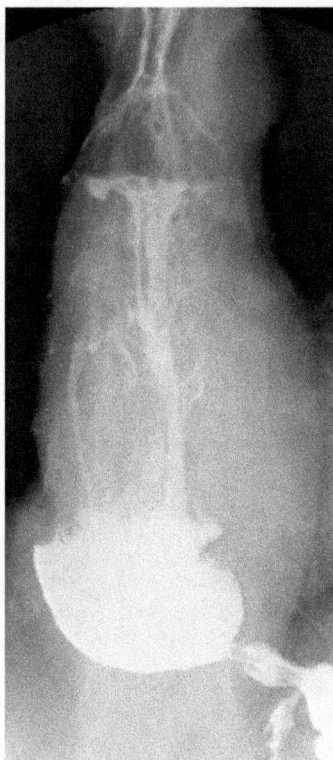

Figure 11.36 Chagas disease. (Image courtesy of Dr. Paul Hellerhoff, Munich.)

The worms' larvae develop in the intrahepatic portal veins, causing portal hypertension and chronic hepatitis, which in turn causes esophageal varices. The two most frequently found organisms that cause gastrointestinal disorders with varices are *Schistosoma mansoni* and *Schistosoma japonicum*. In various parts of the world, acquired esophageal varices in children are frequently caused by this disease. The genitourinary tract is more frequently impacted by *Schistosoma haemotobium*.

11.7 CAUSTIC AND CHEMICAL ESOPHAGITIS

11.7.1 Caustic Substances

When caustic chemicals are consumed, the esophagus experiences progressive inflammatory changes that are accompanied by radiologic abnormalities [36–43]. The main causes are accidental caustic ingestion, which occurs primarily in youngsters, and suicidal consumption in adults. Although lye is the most often consumed caustic, other potent alkali-containing substances can cause stomach, esophageal, hypopharyngeal, and oral burns. The amount and concentration of the item consumed determine the consequences.

11.7.2 Alkali Substances

Protein precipitation with deeply penetrating burns is produced by alkalis. Alkali consumption causes an instant spasm that causes vomiting of the chemical, which tends to lessen the extent of damage. Children typically develop significant mouth and subglottic burns. Prompt tracheotomy is necessary for laryngeal edema with breathing obstruction. Death, mediastinitis, and perforations could ensue.

11.7.3 Acid Agents

Acids typically only cause mild esophageal sores and superficial coagulation necrosis. Usually, the stomach is more severely affected. In regions with normal esophageal constrictions, where there is a delay in the chemical's transit, esophageal injury mostly arises (Figure 11.37). Martel has provided a thorough description of the radiologic findings using barium. In the immediate acute phase (several

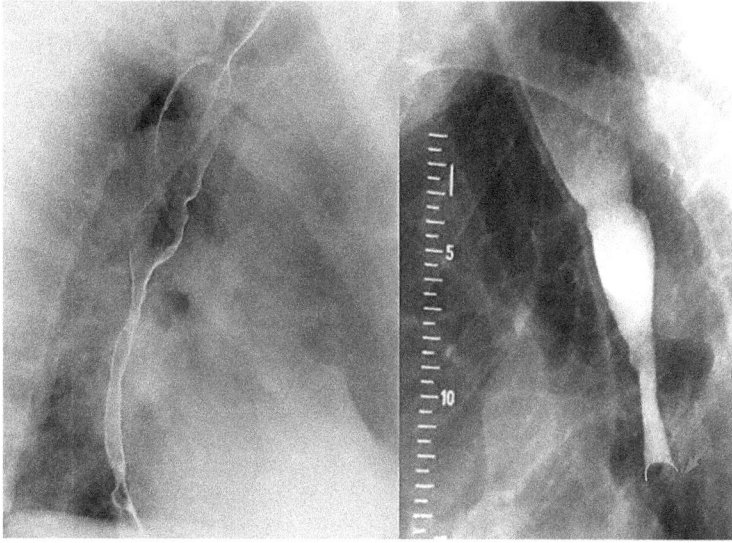

Figure 11.37 Acid-agent esophagitis. (Images courtesy of Dr. Paul Hellerhoff, Munich.)

hours after the ingestion of a caustic agent), a diffuse blurring of the esophageal mucosa occurs, secondary to edema. Slow transit of the barium column is followed by changes in the mucosal pattern, with linear streaks and plaque-like collection of barium in deep crevices or ulcers. Gaseous dilatation of the esophagus can also be observed on occasion on plain films. This dilatation is caused by the atony resulting from muscular necrosis, which occurs within 4–5 days of the acute episode. If the patient survives the acute period, the esophagus becomes denuded and a soft, granulomatous, occasionally ulcerating surface develops. The esophageal wall then shows serrated edges in the area of involvement. During this period, secondary infection may produce a diffuse, severe esophagitis, requiring several weeks to heal. A fibrotic process ensues, which continues for months. In this interval, in the absence of effective therapeutic measures, progressive narrowing of the involved area and stricture formation are observed. Eventually, complete stenosis with obstruction and an aperistaltic channel develop. The course and extent of esophageal involvement depend on the degree of damage and the response to prompt and effective therapeutic measures. With the onset of stenosis, funneling of the barium above the site of narrowing and hyperperistalsis proximal to the stricture develops. More than one stricture may exist. The residual stenosis is usually beaded in radiologic appearance.

11.7.4 Dust and Fumes

Fine chemicals are inhaled as fumes and dust by workers in several occupations. A persistent superficial esophagitis may develop, including the esophagus in addition to the lung alterations. Cellular infiltration, fibrotic alterations of the submucosa, and irregular shallow ulcerations are histological features of this type of esophagitis. The underlying pathologic alterations are reflected in the radiologic findings.

11.7.5 Alcohol and Tobacco Use

Esophagitis can also result from excessive alcohol and tobacco use. The results in chronic alcoholics are either the consequence of localized chemical irritation or the systemic development of liver cirrhosis. Periphlebitis and esophageal varices are frequently seen. Furthermore, alcohol's toxic effects may result in peripheral neuropathy of the vagus nerve. Slow peristalsis and delayed lower esophageal emptying, along with some dilation, are the outcomes of this. Usually, the lower sphincter is not used. In addition to chronic superficial esophagitis, carcinoma in situ has been documented in heavy smokers and tobacco chewers. Smokers seem to experience gastroesophageal reflux far more frequently than nonsmokers. Nicotine's relaxing effects on the lower esophageal sphincter have been linked to a decrease in the sphincter's resting pressure, which facilitates reflux and, ultimately, esophagitis. The severity of reflux and the stomach's acidity likely influence the symptoms.

11.7.6 Peptic Esophagitis

In reality, peptic esophagitis is a chemical esophagitis brought on by reflux of gastric acid. Overly acidic patients are more likely to experience symptoms. Although there are other systemic explanations for the hyperchlorhydria, a persistent duodenal ulcer is frequently linked to it. However, reflux can occur without esophagitis developing, and peptic esophagitis can exist without hyperchlorhydria. Prolonged vomiting of acid stomach contents is the most significant side effect of peptic esophagitis. The resulting esophagitis is initially acute, but a chronic variant develops after repeated or extended bouts. The esophagitis may also be caused by increased pepsin, regurgitated bile salts, and peptic fluids in addition to hydrochloric acid, especially during protracted and continuous vomiting episodes. The level of damage likely varies according to the mucosal resistance, which may be weak at first or may gradually deteriorate with frequent and lengthy infections. Only the surface epithelium is first affected, but later erosion spreads to the muscularis mucosa and submucosal surface. The first radiologic signs of peptic esophagitis include a shift in the lower esophageal mucosal pattern with ulceration, spasm, and irritability (Figure 11.38), which is followed by some degree of funneling as cicatrizing alterations take place. There are several methods to assess if gastric reflux has caused damage to the esophageal mucosa. The most prevalent symptom is most likely the burning sensation in the substernum. The patient is given acidified barium to consume in order to complete the acid barium test. When esophagitis patients ingest the acid-barium mixture, they exhibit enhanced, disorganized peristaltic action. Peristalsis does not significantly alter in people with a normal esophagus. The perfusion test is predicated on the idea that when diluted hydrochloric acid comes into contact with a healthy esophagus, no symptoms will be produced; however, in a person with esophagitis, a burning sensation beneath the chest is frequent. Studies on motility in esophagitis reveal hypermotility resembling widespread spasm. Chronic hyperacidity-induced peptic esophagitis eventually results in a long tubular stenosis without visible ulcerations. Due to the stricture's shortening of the esophagus, an upward pull is produced, which frequently leads to a sliding hiatal hernia. Peptic esophagitis was once thought to be de facto caused by the existence

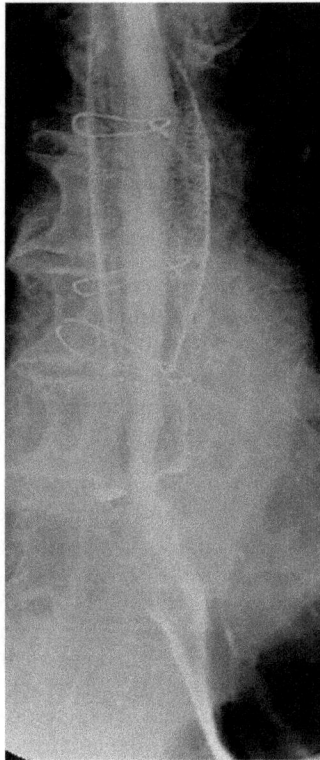

Figure 11.38 Peptic esophagitis. (Image courtesy of Dr. Paul Hellerhoff, Munich.)

of a hiatal hernia. Present-day perceptions of gastric reflux have changed due to the increased prevalence of hiatal hernias, which are now frequently seen in the elderly without any symptoms. Hyperacidity is less often a factor because the stomach's normal acid production declines with age. An inadequate lower esophageal sphincter is typically seen in patients with a preexisting hiatal hernia and related peptic esophagitis. The sphincter section is primarily impacted, and the affected region of the esophagus seems to be significantly shorter. Without abnormal epithelium, this kind of esophagitis is more likely to exhibit localized marginal ulcerations. A serrated look of the sphincter zone segment or abnormalities of the mucosal pattern are the first radiologic signs of peptic esophagitis with a hiatal hernia. A brief localized area of stenosis, with or without ulcerations, then appears. The patient's age and medical history can assist in distinguishing between peptic esophagitis and a congenitally short esophagus, which can culminate in a stricture if left untreated.

11.7.7 Heat Esophagitis

Acute edematous esophagitis can result from consuming extremely hot or cold foods because they cause thermal damage to the esophageal mucosa. Even a later consequence can be an esophageal perforation. The underlying pathologic alterations are reflected in the radiologic findings.

11.8 SKIN DISORDERS

11.8.1 Pemphigus Vulgaris

In addition to affecting the skin and mucous membranes, pemphigus vulgaris can spread to the esophagus and cause dysphagia. Skin and mucosal sores frequently worsen with time. Esophageal erosions may occur with each attack, leading to progressive stenosis and ultimately the creation of strictures. Initially, abnormal radiologic findings are typically nonexistent. Nonetheless, regions of stricturing or webs may be observed with recurrent attacks. Therefore, esophageal webs with an apparent "unknown" etiology could be caused by this disorder. The esophagus can also occasionally be affected by benign pemphigoid lesions and the uncommon bullous pemphigus variant, which can cause similar web-like strictures.

11.8.2 Herpes Simplex

Both adults and infants can have esophageal herpes simplex. In newborns with herpes simplex stomatitis, newborn herpes can spread to the esophagus, causing web-like strictures. Therefore, when this disease is present, routine radiologic examination of the esophagus is necessary. There is also an acute disseminated type that can be lethal in newborns. Herpetic esophagitis can occur in individuals who have had radiation therapy or surgery for esophageal cancer. The radiologic findings are identical to those of esophagitis moniliasis. The presence of cellular nuclear inclusion bodies characteristic of this illness in the affected esophagus mucosa histologically confirms the diagnosis.

11.8.3 Epidermolysis Bullosa

An uncommon hereditary skin condition that manifests at birth or in infancy is epidermolysis bullosa. Multiple bullous lesions form in the skin and esophageal mucosa after minor trauma. The esophageal lesions could be diffuse ulcerating, local stenotic, or both. Strictures typically form in the upper portion of the esophagus, causing pulmonary problems and stasis with food aspiration. A stricture resembling peptic esophagitis forms when the distal part of the esophagus is affected. Affected areas above the lower sphincter may exhibit symptoms resembling scleroderma or the stricture of swallowed caustics. In addition, pseudodiverticula form as a result of the inflammatory alterations. The underlying pathologic alterations are reflected in the radiologic findings. Edema and acute inflammatory alterations are the first causes of obstructive symptoms, which subsequently proceed to stenosis and stricture. These results start in childhood and could continue until adulthood. There are no particular radiologic features.

11.9 GRANULOMATOUS LESIONS

11.9.1 Tuberculosis

Esophageal tuberculosis (TB) intrinsic is uncommon. Esophageal TB can occur after esophageal trauma in a patient with active pulmonary TB who is consuming sputum contaminated with bacteria, or it can be a component of disseminated miliary TB. More frequently, a Pott's paraspinal abscess or the surrounding tuberculous mediastinal lymph nodes directly extend into the esophagus, causing secondary involvement. When there is intrinsic active disease of the esophagus, the radiologic results are indicative of nonspecific chronic esophagitis, and the pathologic changes in diffuse involvement are either ulcerative or hypoplastic in type. When a disease is localized, the mucosal pattern is effaced and the esophagus segment narrows, usually in the middle third. This causes the esophagus to dilate proximally. It is uncommon to distinguish a localized esophageal tuberculous granuloma from a tumor. External adhesions may cause the esophagus to compress, deviate, and occasionally become blocked. The esophagus may be compressed by enlarged tuberculous mediastinal lymph nodes, resulting in scalloped zones of compression and esophageal wall fixation. After the esophageal wall is directly eroded, fistulous tracts may form.

11.9.2 Syphilis

Esophageal syphilis is an uncommon condition. The pharynx, larynx, or hypopharynx may directly extend from syphilitic disease to cause it. Diffuse esophagitis and localized gumma are examples of other forms of involvement. When direct extension is the reason, the upper end of the esophagus is primarily affected. First, there are ulcerating lesions; if therapy is not received, scarring and eventually stenosis develop. A large lesion could be the first sign of a gumma. Nonspecific localized or diffuse esophagitis, gumma, or a mass lesion with irregularity and rigidity of the wall of the affected esophagus are radiologic findings that mimic a malignant tumor. After receiving appropriate antisyphilitic treatment, all of these symptoms disappear. The activity of the upper and lower esophageal sphincters may be impacted by the degenerative alterations that tabetic neuropathy causes in the posterior horn cells of the spinal cord and the posterior ganglia. In the esophagus, abnormal peristaltic waves are visible.

11.9.3 Histoplasmosis, Blastomycosis, and Actinomycosis

These entities, either as primary or secondary extensions, seldom impact the esophagus. Numerous tiny esophageal wall abscesses are among the radiologic observations; these abscesses have the potential to rupture and result in sinus tracts and fistulae. The healing phase may be followed by restrictions. There is no specificity in the radiologic results.

11.9.4 Crohn's Disease

Recent reports have shown that Crohn's disease of the esophagus is an independent lesion that is not connected to reflux esophagitis. A thickened esophageal segment that is noticeably adherent to the underlying mediastinal structures and to nearby afflicted lymph nodes is one of the pathologic signs. Similar to Crohn's disease of the small intestine, extensive submucosal fibrosis is noted, accompanied by muscularis involvement and mucosal degradation. Typically, esophageal shortening can play a role in the development of a hiatal hernia. The area of involvement's cobblestone mucosal pattern is one of the radiologic characteristics. Because of the surrounding mediastinal inflammatory changes and adenopathy, the esophageal wall's irregular shape, rigidity, and fixation may indicate a malignant lesion. It is possible to have fistulous tracts. A person with dysphagia and Crohn's disease of the small bowel (or colon) should have their esophageal involvement examined.

11.9.5 Sarcoidosis

Esophageal sarcoidosis is very uncommon. To distinguish this granulomatous illness of unknown cause from other granulomatous processes, a positive Kveim test has been employed. This test, however, seems to be less than precise, occasionally showing positive results in people with Crohn's disease or persistent adenopathy from other sources. The esophagus is seldom directly involved with sarcoidosis. Most often, swollen hilar and mediastinal nodes compress the esophagus. The wall of the affected area thickens noticeably when the esophagus is directly invaded. The extremely uncommon intrinsic type has nonspecific radiologic findings. Particularly in the early stages, only slight mucosal alterations are noticed. On the other hand, the main symptom can be a benign stricture. It is necessary to rule out Crohn's disease and other granulomatous disorders. Steroid therapy may be tried; steroids frequently result in sarcoid lesions improving or even healing, and the Roentgenologic abnormalities regress and vanish.

11.10 DEFICIENCY DISORDERS

11.10.1 Sideropenic Anemia

Iron deficiency is linked to sideropenic anemia, also known as Paterson–Brown–Kelly syndrome or Plummer–Vinson syndrome. Although it can happen to men as well, middle-aged women are

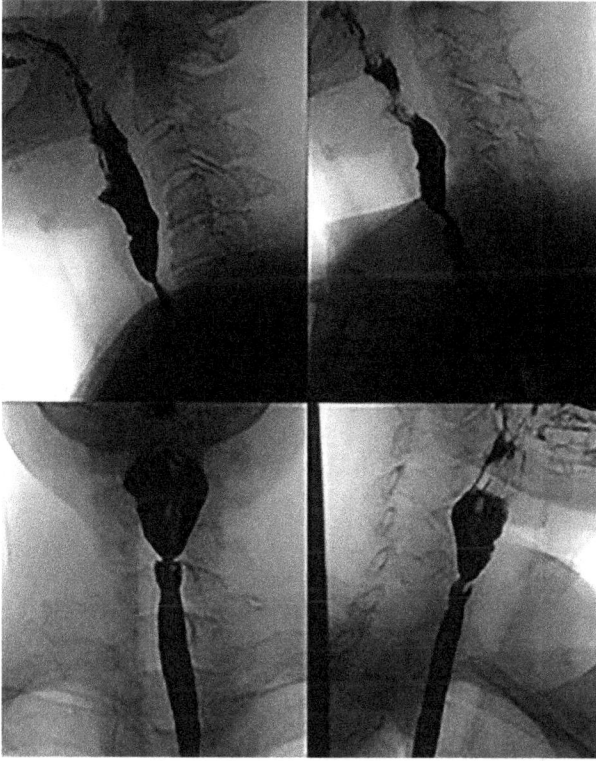

Figure 11.39 Plummer–Vinson syndrome. (Images courtesy of Dr. Paul Hellerhoff, Munich.)

more likely to have this condition. It is most common in Sweden. While some researchers think a vitamin B deficiency is the primary cause, others think hormonal imbalance is the secondary cause. In addition to tongue and mouth inflammation, there is diffuse esophagitis during the acute phase. The pharyngoesophageal sphincter is particularly affected, and the submucosal layer undergoes atrophic alterations (Figure 11.39). Later, the muscularis might also be impacted, and eventually, fibrotic changes take place, resulting in webs and mucosal atrophy, with or without obstructive symptoms. Sphincter zone narrowing may occur, accompanied by achlorhydria and hypochromic microcytic anemia. After the anemia is treated, the fibrosis and webs could still be present. This syndrome is associated with a higher incidence of hypopharyngeal cancer. The webs in this disease are primarily located anteriorly, at the pharyngoesophageal junction close to the lower pole of the cricoid lamina, and they have a distinctive appearance and placement. A complete ring may be seen occasionally, but more often than not simply a partial ring is observed. Directly beneath the web, there may also be a cuff-like constriction that corresponds to the upper sphincter zone segment. Dysphagia and blockage result from this segment's irregularity and constriction. Rarely, there may also be another web at the distal end of the upper sphincter. Particular caution is needed while demonstrating the webs in radiologic examination. Delineating the incisura characteristic of the web requires significant distension of the upper sphincter zone using barium. It is necessary to delineate views of the cervical region during swallowing in the lateral, oblique, and anteroposterior positions. Barium stasis in the hypopharynx can be seen when obstruction is present, and a positive vallecular sign is frequently linked to this condition. The differential diagnosis of esophageal webs must take into account senility, pernicious anemia, Sjögren's disease, and mucosal atrophy brought on by avitaminosis. These entities may have radiologic characteristics that are very similar to those of Plummer–Vinson syndrome.

11.10.2 Vitamin Deficiency

Esophageal motility may also be impacted by severe avitaminosis alone, leading to radiologic results that resemble achalasia.

11.11 ULCERS OF THE ESOPHAGUS

Both local and systemic factors might contribute to esophageal ulcers. Usually, there is only one ulcer, but sometimes there are several. The most frequent cause of ulcers is either acute or chronic esophagitis. It is important to distinguish between minute ulcerations and esophageal erosions. While minute ulcerations are numerous, tiny, symmetrical, superficial excavations that give the esophagus lumen a radiologically serrated appearance, erosions are typically confined, irregular patches of denuded mucosa.

11.11.1 Peptic Ulcerations

Similar to those found in the stomach and duodenal bulb, esophageal ulcers are known as "peptic" ulcerations. The degree of irritation, the extent of ulceration, the rate of change on follow-up exams, and the reaction to medical treatment all play a role in determining whether an ulcer is acute or chronic. Both benign and malignant ulcers are possible. The latter are covered in the section on cancers of the esophagus. Esophageal ulcers are diagnosed using the same radiologic criteria as other peptic ulcers. An ulcer is a mucosal surface excavation that might be superficial, deep within the muscle coat, or even perforate. The key diagnostic characteristic is the radiological display of an ulcer niche or crater using barium. The niche is a barium opacity that extends in the tangential plane of the excavation as a tiny accumulation of barium that extends past the outline of the opacified lumen. Due to the small amount of barium present, this collection has a lower density than the lumen. If the ulcer appears "en face," it is referred to as a crater. A partially coated (barium-coated) esophagus reveals the crater as a tiny, localized region of increased density. A heavily opacified esophagus may obscure or obscure the crater. A benign lesion from a malignant process can be distinguished by the ulcer's location, shape, size, contour, depth, relationship to the surrounding wall, and degree of impaired motor function at the ulcer site. Always rule out a minor esophageal diverticulum. In most cases, the subsequent outpocketing is smooth and even intermittent. Usually, there is a neck that leads to the diverticulum. Occasionally, a small ulcer that is isolated from the main lumen may develop. An ulcer's shape is more consistent throughout the inspection and is typically more irregular, holding the barium longer.

11.11.2 Barrett's Ulcer and Esophagus

In this condition, the usual squamous cells that line the esophagus are replaced by columnar epithelial cells. All other aspects of Barrett's esophagus seem normal in its uncomplicated state. In contrast to a congenitally short esophagus, where the apparent lower portion of the esophagus is actually a herniated stomach, there is no difference from any normal esophagus on radiologic examination. Under a microscope, the heterotopic columnar epithelial lining of Barrett's esophagus resembles intestinal, fundal, cardiac, or ciliated epithelium. Particularly in the proximal end of the esophagus, where squamous and columnar cells intersperse, the columnar lining may be heterogeneous in type. Furthermore, squamous epithelium may coexist with isolated islands of ectopic gastric mucosa in various parts of the esophagus, especially in the middle and upper segments. There have been no documented examples of Barrett's esophagus that affect the entire esophagus. Additionally, an inflammatory process may result in the acquisition of columnar epithelium in the lower end of the esophagus. This could result in a columnar epithelial surface that comes from the lamina propria's underlying ectopic stomach glands. The remains of defective descent during embryologic development are these glands. Elderly people who have acquired heterotopia typically have chronic esophagitis and a sliding type of hiatal hernia. Compared to normal esophageal epithelium, ectopic epithelium in the esophagus is more vulnerable to the effects of regurgitated stomach juices. As a result, ulcerations and inflammatory alterations are more common, and in particular, Barrett's esophagus is more prone to chronic ulceration than a normal esophagus. Additionally, these ulcers are typically more shallow and result in a localized, usually brief stricture, as opposed to ulcerations that develop in an esophagus lined with squamous epithelium. Deeper, more persistent, and less likely to cause cicatrization and stenosis are ulcers linked to ectopic gastric mucosa. With or without ulceration, columnar epithelial cells are also abundant in the thoracic esophagus. Thus, a stricture that may resemble a malignant tumor might also result from an inflammatory process in this region. A congenital rather than an acquired origin is suggested by a number of investigations on Barrett's esophagus, including manometric, histologic, and acid measurements. Tc 99 mm pertechnetate, which is specifically concentrated by the gastric type of mucosa present in this condition, can occasionally be used to diagnose Barrett's esophagus. Barrett's ulcers, also known as peptic ulcers of the esophagus, typically occur as a single, large ulcer in an area of ectopic gastric

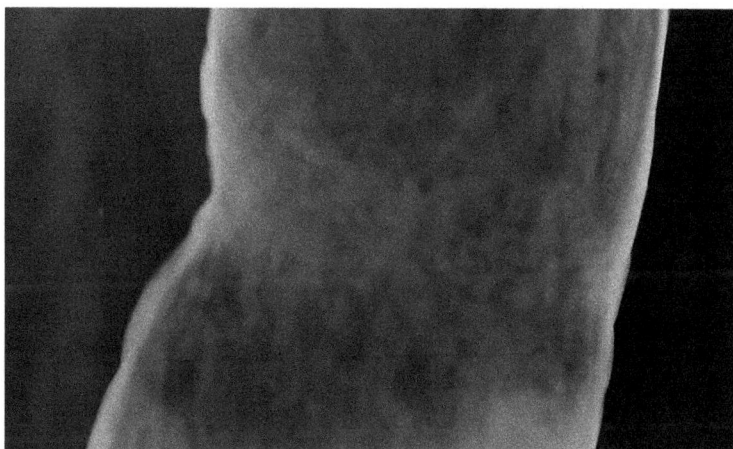

Figure 11.40 Barrett's ulcer. (Image courtesy of Dr. Paul Hellerhoff, Munich.)

epithelium in the middle third of the esophagus. The ulcer remains visible on radiologic examination as a large, deep, elongated, and strongly defined niche (Figure 11.40). Cicatrizing stenosis is typically absent, and the only noticeable functional disturbance is mild spasm or aberrant motility. There is no visible displacement or aberrant angulation of the esophagus, nor is there any fixation or bulk at the ulcer site. These ulcers eventually heal, despite the fact that they frequently defy medical intervention. Perforation is a rare consequence. It's important to distinguish a diverticulum from a Barrett's ulcer. A neoplasm must also be considered in the differential diagnosis because both ectopic and heterotopic gastric epithelium of the esophagus are predisposed to cancer.

11.11.3 Marginal Ulcers

Because of an underlying esophagitis, a marginal ulcer develops at the gastroesophageal junction. It might not be possible to identify a frequently linked hiatal hernia major. Usually severe, this kind of ulcer goes away with the right medical care. Both heterotopic gastric epithelium and such ulcers can arise. A short stenotic segment may also have a marginal ulcer at its base as a result of inflammatory alterations that impact the sphincter zone. In these cases, there is typically a hiatal hernia that either preceded or resulted from the inflammatory condition. Similar alterations are seen in younger children with a congenitally short esophagus, ulceration, and esophagitis.

11.11.4 Iatrogenic Ulcers

Iatrogenic ulcers are not uncommon after extended stomach or esophageal intubation. These ulcers are typically seem in the gastroesophageal junction (marginal). Prolonged use of corticosteroids can result in both stomach and esophageal ulcers. These ulcers are typically severe and disappear quickly with medical intervention. Any type of trauma caused by endoscopy or ingesting a foreign object can also result in iatrogenic ulcers.

11.11.5 Kissing Ulcers

"Kissing ulcers" are uncommon pressure-contact ulcers that typically occur in the postcricoid region of the hypopharynx and are common in older people with widespread cachexia. A massive, severely calcified cricoid cartilage may be the cause of the front and posterior hypopharyngeal walls' ulceration and ischemic pressure alterations. These "kissing ulcers" can also result from vascular alterations brought on by the prolonged lodgement of foreign objects, intubation, or the use of tracheotomy tubes. The extreme inflammation frequently results in marked spasm. In rare cases, such ulcers may be visible on radiologic evaluation during the administration of a barium swallow. It is frequently only after necropsy that these "kissing ulcers" are found.

11.12 OTHER CONDITIONS

11.12.1 Esophageal Atresia

The term "esophageal atresia" describes a lack of esophageal continuity brought on by an improper partition of the primordial foregut into the trachea and esophagus. It is caused by the primordial

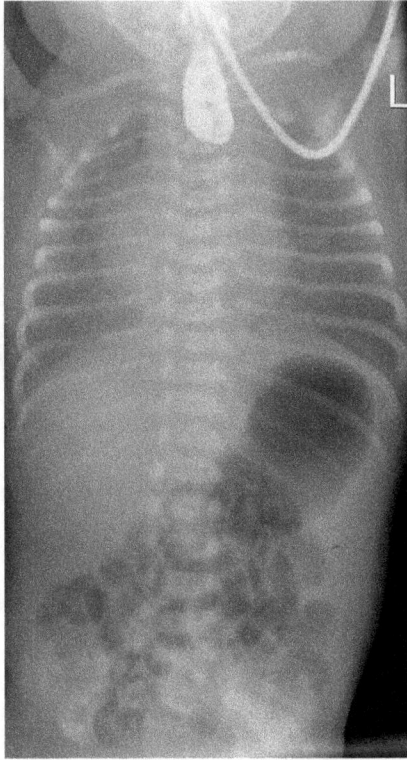

Figure 11.41 Esophageal atresia. (Image courtesy of Dr. Paul Hellerhoff, Munich.)

foregut's inability to split into the esophagus posteriorly and the trachea anteriorly. Usually, this occurs during the fourth week of pregnancy. Teratogenic effects resulting from early pregnancy use of antithyroid medications are part of general pathophysiology. This is the most prevalent esophageal congenital abnormality. It is estimated to occur in between 1300 and 4500 live births; 50–75% of esophageal atresia patients are linked to other abnormalities. Among them are an additional intestinal atresia (duodenal, jejunal, or anal), annular pancreas, pyloric stenosis, VACTERL association, CHARGE syndrome, and trisomies. Aspiration during early feeding, difficulty passing a nasogastric tube into the stomach, or difficulty swallowing milk or saliva can all raise suspicions for esophageal atresia in neonates or on prenatal ultrasounds (see below). Contrast swallow may reveal indications of a tracheoesophageal fistula or contrast that blindly ends and pools in an esophageal stump (Figure 11.41). Using fluoroscopy to show an H-type fistula is especially helpful. For an H-type fistula, a withdrawal esophagogram is conducted. Under fluoroscopy, the patient is placed prone, a horizontal beam is employed, and contrast material is administered into the distal esophagus through the nasogastric tube as the tube is gradually removed. When there is a high level of suspicion and the imaging scan is unable to identify the fistula, a combination bronchoscopy and esophagoscopy is employed. A gastrostomy is used to place a Hegar dilator into the distal esophagus and a radiopaque Replogle tube into the proximal pouch in order to measure the distance between the esophageal pouches.

11.12.2 Foreign Bodies

As the most prevalent location for food impaction or ingested foreign bodies in the gastrointestinal tract, esophageal foreign bodies are commonly seen in clinical practice. Esophageal foreign bodies are more common in children, frequently as a result of inadvertently ingesting coins (Figure 11.42), batteries (Figure 11.43), toy components, pins, needles, and various foods. Adult ingestion of foreign bodies can be unintentional or deliberate, and it typically occurs in individuals with mental illnesses, intellectual disabilities, and so on. Adult impaction is most frequently caused by meat, fish (Figure 11.44) and poultry bones, and dentures.

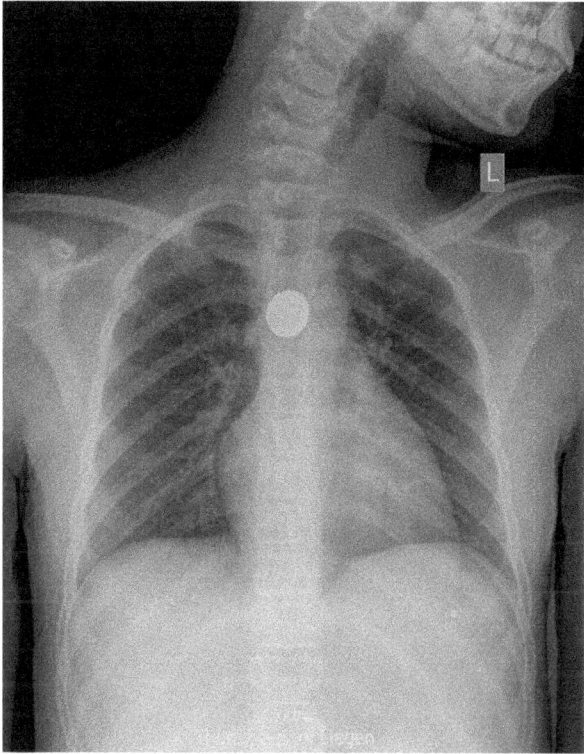

Figure 11.42 Ingested coin. (Image courtesy of Dr. Paul Hellerhoff, Munich.)

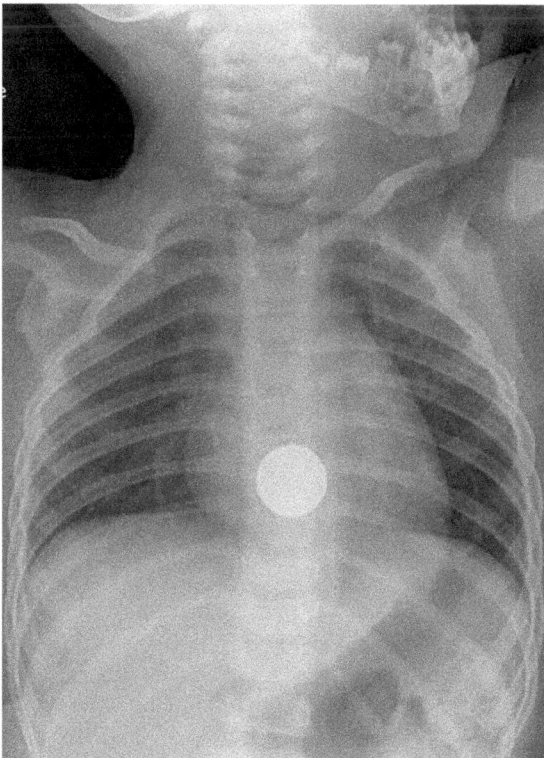

Figure 11.43 Ingested battery. (Image courtesy of Dr. Paul Hellerhoff, Munich.)

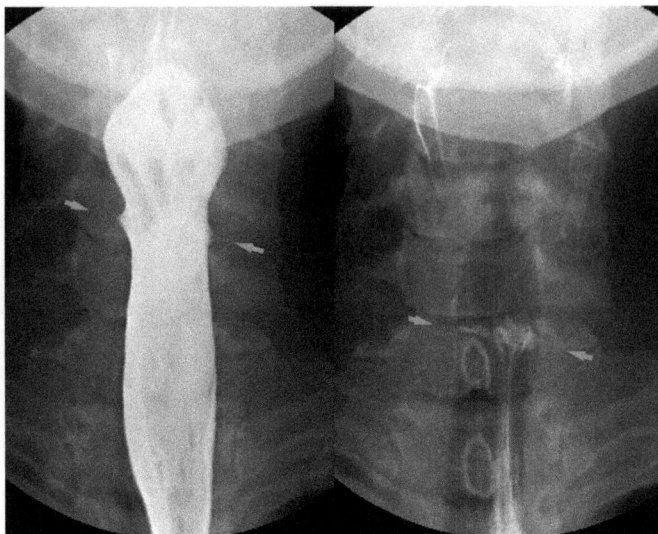

Figure 11.44 Ingested fishbone. (Images courtesy of Dr. Paul Hellerhoff, Munich.)

REFERENCES

1. Iyer R, Dubrow R. Imaging of esophageal cancer. *Cancer Imaging*. 2004;4(2):125–132. doi: 10.1102/1470-7330.2004.0022.
2. Levine MS, Rubesin SE. Diseases of the esophagus: diagnosis with esophagography. *Radiology*. 2005;237(2):414–427. doi: 10.1148/radiol.2372050199.
3. Levine MS, Rubesin SE, Laufer I. Barium esophagography: a study for all seasons. *Clin Gastroenterol Hepatol*. 2008;6(1):11–25. doi: 10.1016/j.cgh.2007.10.029.
4. Noh HM, Fishman EK, Forastiere AA, Bliss DF, Calhoun PS. CT of the esophagus: spectrum of disease with emphasis on esophageal carcinoma. *Radiographics*. 1995;15(5):1113–1134. doi: 10.1148/radiographics.15.5.7501854.
5. Zuccaro G, Jr. The use of endoscopic ultrasound in esophageal disease. *Gastroenterol Hepatol (NY)* 2007;3(3):163–164.
6. Oezcelik A, DeMeester SR. General anatomy of the esophagus. *Thorac Surg Clin*. 2011;21(2):289–297. doi: 10.1016/j.thorsurg.2011.01.003.
7. Patti MG, Gantert W, Way LW. Surgery of the esophagus. Anatomy and physiology. *Surg Clin North Am*. 1997;77(5):959–970. doi: 10.1016/S0039-6109(05)70600-9.
8. Goyal RK, Chaudhury A. Physiology of normal esophageal motility. *J Clin Gastroenterol*. 2008;42(5):610–619. doi: 10.1097/MCG.0b013e31816b444d.
9. Schraufnagel DE, Michel JC, Sheppard TJ, Saffold PC, Kondos GT. CT of the normal esophagus to define the normal air column and its extent and distribution. *AJR Am J Roentgenol*. 2008;191(3):748–752. doi: 10.2214/AJR.07.3455.
10. Moonen A, Boeckxstaens G. Current diagnosis and management of achalasia. *J Clin Gastroenterol*. 2014;48(6):484–490. doi: 10.1097/MCG.0000000000000137.
11. Farrokhi F, Vaezi MF. Idiopathic (primary) achalasia. *Orphanet J Rare Dis*. 2007;2:38. doi: 10.1186/1750-1172-2-38.
12. Ebert EC. Esophageal disease in scleroderma. *J Clin Gastroenterol*. 2006;40(9):769–775. doi: 10.1097/01.mcg.0000225549.19127.90.
13. Luedtke P, Levine MS, Rubesin SE, Weinstein DS, Laufer I. Radiologic diagnosis of benign esophageal strictures: a pattern approach. *Radiographics*. 2003;23(4):897–909. doi: 10.1148/rg.234025717.
14. Karasick S, Lev-Toaff AS. Esophageal strictures: findings on barium radiographs. *AJR Am J Roentgenol*. 1995;165(3):561–565. doi: 10.2214/ajr.165.3.7645471.
15. Benjamin SB. Esophageal foreign bodies and food impactions. *Gastroenterol Hepatol (NY)* 2008;4(8):546–548.

16. Sperry SL, Crockett SD, Miller CB, Shaheen NJ, Dellon ES. Esophageal foreign-body impactions: epidemiology, time trends, and the impact of the increasing prevalence of eosinophilic esophagitis. *Gastrointest Endosc.* 2011;74(5):985–991. doi: 10.1016/j.gie.2011.06.029.

17. Hunter TB, Taljanovic MS. Foreign bodies. *Radiographics.* 2003;23(3):731–757. doi: 10.1148/rg.233025137.

18. Fuentes S, Cano I, Benavent MI, Gomez A. Severe esophageal injuries caused by accidental button battery ingestion in children. *J Emerg Trauma Shock.* 2014;7(4):316–321. doi: 10.4103/0974-2700.142773.

19. Cianferoni A, Spergel J. Eosinophilic esophagitis: a comprehensive review. *Clin Rev Allergy Immunol.* 2016;50(2):159–174. doi: 10.1007/s12016-015-8501-z.

20. Zimmerman SL, Levine MS, Rubesin SE, et al. Idiopathic eosinophilic esophagitis in adults: the ringed esophagus. *Radiology.* 2005;236(1):159–165. doi: 10.1148/radiol.2361041100.

21. Jang KM, Lee KS, Lee SJ, et al. The spectrum of benign esophageal lesions: imaging findings. *Korean J Radiol.* 2002;3(3):199–210. doi: 10.3348/kjr.2002.3.3.199.

22. Tsai SJ, Lin CC, Chang CW, et al. Benign esophageal lesions: endoscopic and pathologic features. *World J Gastroenterol.* 2015;21(4):1091–1098. doi: 10.3748/wjg.v21.i4.1091.

23. Yang PS, Lee KS, Lee SJ, et al. Esophageal leiomyoma: radiologic findings in 12 patients. *Korean J Radiol.* 2001;2(3):132–137. doi: 10.3348/kjr.2001.2.3.132.

24. Narra SL, Tombazzi C, Datta V, Ismail MK. Granular cell tumor of the esophagus: report of five cases and review of the literature. *Am J Med Sci.* 2008;335(5):338–341. doi: 10.1097/MAJ.0b013e3181568197.

25. Sogabe M, Taniki T, Fukui Y, et al. A patient with esophageal hemangioma treated by endoscopic mucosal resection: a case report and review of the literature. *J Med Investig.* 2006;53(1–2):177–182. doi: 10.2152/jmi.53.177.

26. Lipp MJ, Broder A, Hudesman D, et al. Detection of esophageal varices using CT and MRI. *Dig Dis Sci.* 2011;56(9):2696–2700. doi: 10.1007/s10620-011-1660-8.

27. Cole TJ, Turner MA. Manifestations of gastrointestinal disease on chest radiographs. *Radiographics.* 1993;13(5):1013–1034. doi: 10.1148/radiographics.13.5.8210587.

28. Younes Z, Johnson DA. The spectrum of spontaneous and iatrogenic esophageal injury: perforations, Mallory-Weiss tears, and hematomas. *J Clin Gastroenterol.* 1999;29(4):306–317. doi: 10.1097/00004836-199912000-00003.

29. Bryant AS, Cerfolio RJ. Esophageal trauma. *Thorac Surg Clin.* 2007;17(1):63–72. doi: 10.1016/j.thorsurg.2007.02.003.

30. Young CA, Menias CO, Bhalla S, Prasad SR. CT features of esophageal emergencies. *Radiographics.* 2008;28(6):1541–1553. doi: 10.1148/rg.286085520.

31. Ballehaninna UK, Shaw JP, Brichkov I. Traction esophageal diverticulum: a rare cause of gastro-intestinal bleeding. *Springerplus.* 2012;1(1):50. doi: 10.1186/2193-1801-1-50.

32. Tao TY, Menias CO, Herman TE, McAlister WH, Balfe DM. Easier to swallow: pictorial review of structural findings of the pharynx at barium pharyngography. *Radiographics.* 2013;33(7):e189–e208. doi: 10.1148/rg.337125153.

33. Adams KM, Mahin KE. Killian-Jamieson diverticulum. *J Am Osteopath Assoc.* 2015;115(11):688. doi: 10.7556/jaoa.2015.141.

34. Conklin JH, Singh D, Katlic MR. Epiphrenic esophageal diverticula: spectrum of symptoms and consequences. *J Am Osteopath Assoc.* 2009;109(10):543–545.

35. Fasano NC, Levine MS, Rubesin SE, Redfern RO, Laufer I. Epiphrenic diverticulum: clinical and radiographic findings in 27 patients. *Dysphagia.* 2003;18(1):9–15. doi: 10.1007/s00455-002-0075-2.

36. Soreide JA, Viste A. Esophageal perforation: diagnostic work-up and clinical decision-making in the first 24 hours. *Scand J Trauma Resusc Emerg Med.* 2011;19:66. doi: 10.1186/1757-7241-19-66.

37. Teh E, Edwards J, Duffy J, Beggs D. Boerhaave's syndrome: a review of management and outcome. *Interact Cardiovasc Thorac Surg.* 2007;6(5):640–643. doi: 10.1510/icvts.2007.151936.

38. Kortas DY, Haas LS, Simpson WG, Nickl NJ, 3rd, Gates LK., Jr. Mallory-Weiss tear: predisposing factors and predictors of a complicated course. *Am J Gastroenterol.* 2001;96(10):2863–2865. doi: 10.1111/j.1572-0241.2001.04239.x.

39. Pickhardt PJ, Bhalla S, Balfe DM. Acquired gastrointestinal fistulas: classification, etiologies, and imaging evaluation. *Radiology.* 2002;224(1):9–23. doi: 10.1148/radiol.2241011185.

40. Chavez P, Messerli FH, Casso Dominguez A, et al. Atrioesophageal fistula following ablation procedures for atrial fibrillation: systematic review of case reports. *Open Heart.* 2015;2(1):e000257. doi: 10.1136/openhrt-2015-000257.

41. Jung JH, Kim JS, Kim YK. Acquired tracheoesophageal fistula through esophageal diverticulum in patient who had a prolonged tracheostomy tube - a case report. *Ann Rehabil Med*. 2011;35(3):436–440. doi: 10.5535/arm.2011.35.3.436.

42. Heckstall RL, Hollander JE. Aortoesophageal fistula: recognition and diagnosis in the emergency department. *Ann Emerg Med*. 1998;32(4):502–505. doi: 10.1016/S0196-0644(98)70182-9.

43. Kieffer E, Chiche L, Gomes D. Aortoesophageal fistula: value of in situ aortic allograft replacement. *Ann Surg*. 2003;238(2):283–290. doi: 10.1097/01.sla.0000080828.37493.e0.

12 Basics and Use of CT and MRI of the Pharynx and Esophagus

12.1 INTRODUCTION

Computed tomography (CT) and magnetic resonance imaging (MRI) have become indispensable tools in the comprehensive evaluation of diseases affecting the pharynx and esophagus [1,2]. These cross-sectional imaging modalities allow clinicians to visualize not only the luminal structures of the upper aerodigestive tract but also the surrounding soft tissues, vasculature, bones, and lymphatic drainage pathways. Their role is particularly important when conventional studies such as barium swallow or endoscopy are inconclusive, when deeper anatomical assessment is required, or when malignancy is suspected.

CT and MRI serve different yet complementary purposes. CT is widely available, fast, and particularly suited for the evaluation of acute processes, trauma, and bony structures. Its ability to detect gas, calcifications, and subtle density differences makes it ideal for identifying perforations, abscesses, or extrinsic compression. On the other hand, MRI provides unparalleled soft tissue contrast without the risks associated with ionizing radiation. This makes it a preferred modality for characterizing tumors, mapping perineural spread, assessing tissue planes, and staging cancer.

In clinical practice, these modalities are utilized across a wide spectrum of indications—from the diagnosis of squamous cell carcinoma of the oropharynx and esophagus, to the identification of benign structural anomalies, inflammatory diseases, and congenital malformations. With the increasing sophistication of imaging technology, CT and MRI are also being employed for functional evaluations, such as assessing swallowing dynamics, evaluating tumor perfusion, and guiding precision treatment planning

The purpose of this chapter is to provide an in-depth overview of how CT and MRI are used in the assessment of pharyngeal and esophageal disorders, highlighting their technical features, diagnostic strengths, clinical applications, and interpretive considerations. Understanding the capabilities and limitations of these modalities is essential for optimizing diagnostic pathways and improving outcomes for patients with complex head, neck, and upper digestive tract conditions.

12.2 CT IMAGING OF THE PHARYNX AND ESOPHAGUS

Computed tomography (CT) imaging has become a cornerstone in the evaluation of head and neck pathologies, including those involving the pharynx and esophagus [3,4]. Its rapid acquisition time, high spatial resolution, and ability to image large anatomical regions make CT particularly well-suited for both emergency and elective diagnostic imaging. Modern multi-detector CT (MDCT) scanners provide thin-slice reconstructions and the ability to generate high-quality multiplanar and 3D reformatted images, enhancing diagnostic accuracy and surgical planning.

CT imaging is especially valuable in the detection and characterization of masses within the oropharynx, hypopharynx, and upper esophagus (Figures 12.1 and 12.2). When enhanced with intravenous contrast, CT scans can delineate tumor margins, assess regional lymph node involvement, and

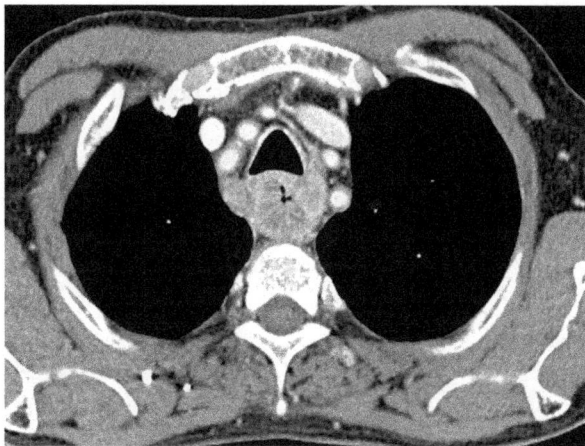

Figure 12.1 Squamous cell esophageal carcinoma.

DOI: 10.1201/9781003508113-12

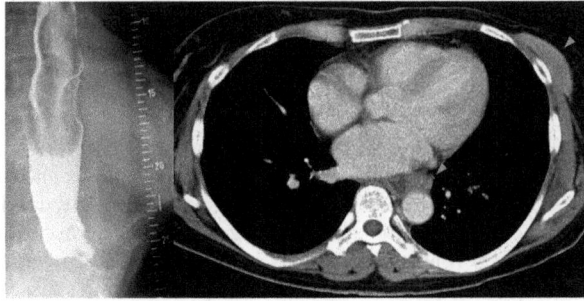

Figure 12.2 Esophageal neurofibroma.

identify vascular encasement—critical information in oncologic staging and treatment planning. In cases of suspected esophageal cancer, CT can help determine tumor extent, evaluate for tracheo-esophageal fistulas, and detect distant metastases in the chest and abdomen when included as part of a CT neck/chest/abdomen protocol.

In the acute care setting, CT is indispensable in the evaluation of deep neck space infections, abscesses, traumatic injuries, or suspected esophageal perforations (e.g., Boerhaave syndrome). The ability to detect subtle gas collections, fluid levels, and soft tissue edema allows for early diagnosis and intervention, often reducing morbidity. Moreover, the sensitivity of CT for identifying foreign bodies—particularly those that are radiopaque—makes it superior to standard X-rays in emergency scenarios.

For patients presenting with unexplained dysphagia, CT can identify extrinsic compressions of the esophagus, such as those caused by cervical osteophytes, enlarged thyroid glands, or vascular anomalies (e.g., aberrant right subclavian artery Figure 12.3, fibrovascular polyp Figure 12.4), motility disorders like achalasia (Figure 12.5). Additionally, CT plays an important role in evaluating chronic inflammatory diseases like Crohn's (Figure 12.6), congenital anomalies, postoperative anatomy, and radiation-induced changes, including fibrosis or strictures. It is useful in defining the extent of hiatal hernia (Figure 12.7).

In summary, CT imaging of the pharynx and esophagus is a highly versatile diagnostic tool that not only provides comprehensive anatomical detail but also plays a central role in a wide array of clinical settings—from oncology and infection to trauma and congenital disease.

12.3 MRI IMAGING OF THE PHARYNX AND ESOPHAGUS

Magnetic resonance imaging (MRI) is a highly valuable imaging modality for the assessment of pharyngeal and esophageal structures due to its superior soft tissue contrast and multiplanar imaging capabilities [5,6]. Unlike CT, MRI does not use ionizing radiation, which makes it ideal for repeated imaging, particularly in younger or radiation-sensitive populations, such as pediatric patients or individuals undergoing long-term cancer surveillance.

MRI provides exquisite detail of the soft tissues of the head and neck, making it the preferred modality for evaluating tumor extent in cases of oropharyngeal, hypopharyngeal, and upper esophageal cancers. It is particularly effective in identifying submucosal infiltration, perineural spread along cranial nerves, and invasion of adjacent structures such as the prevertebral fascia, carotid sheath, or skull base. This level of detail is critical for accurate tumor staging, surgical planning, and radiation therapy targeting.

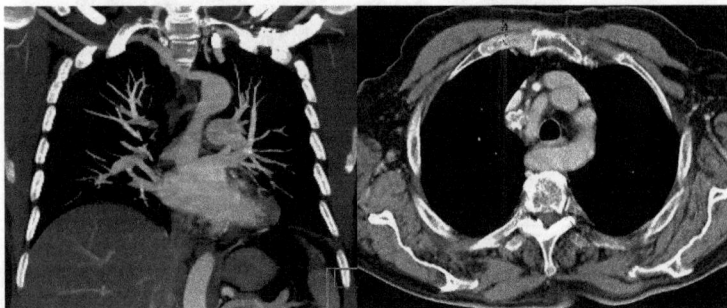

Figure 12.3 Arteria lusoria.

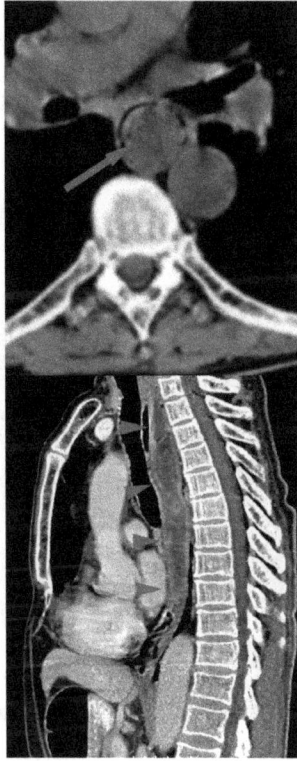

Figure 12.4 Fibrovascular polyp.

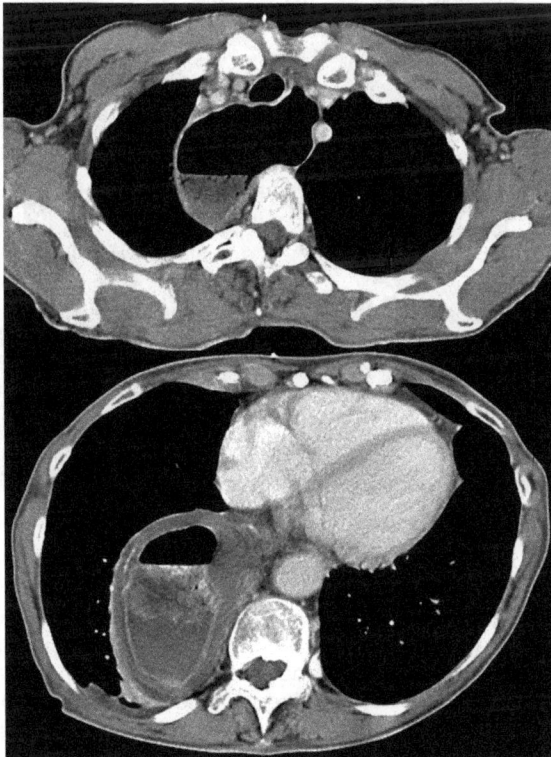

Figure 12.5 Achalasia.

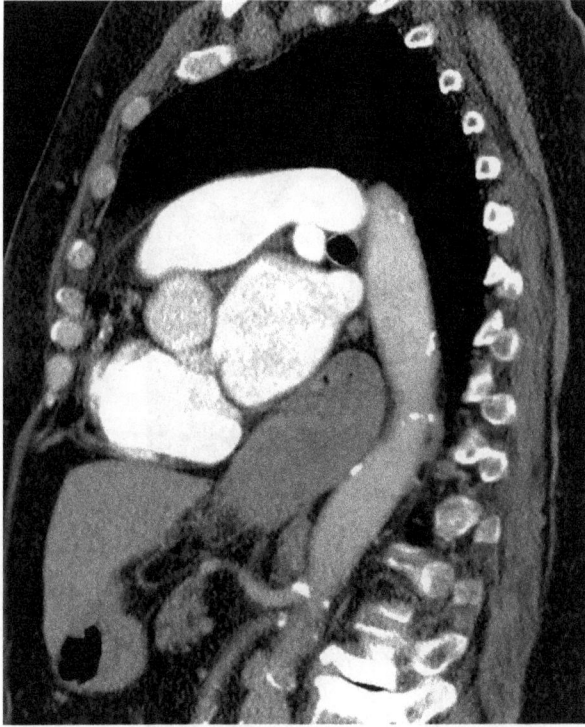

Figure 12.6 Crohn's disease.

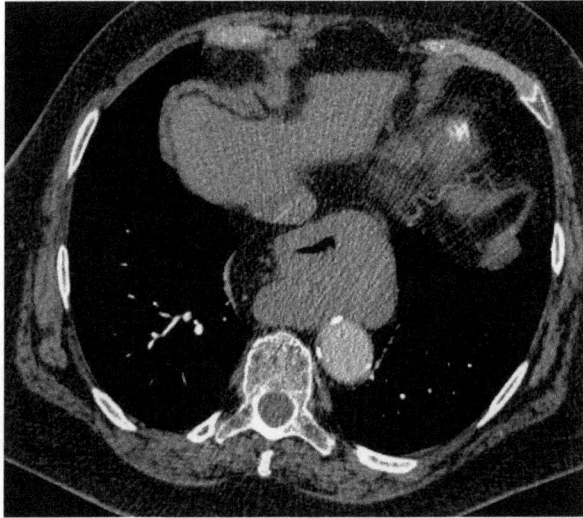

Figure 12.7 Hiatal hernia.

Standard MRI protocols typically include T1-weighted images (useful for assessing anatomy and fat planes), T2-weighted images (for highlighting fluid, edema, and cystic lesions), and post-contrast T1-weighted sequences with fat suppression. Advanced techniques such as diffusion-weighted imaging (DWI) can detect cellular density changes associated with malignancy or inflammation, while dynamic contrast-enhanced (DCE) imaging provides information about vascular anatomy and anomalies (Figure 12.8), tumor vascularity, perfusion, and treatment response.

In addition to oncologic applications, MRI is valuable in evaluating inflammatory and infectious conditions. It can differentiate between cellulitis and abscess, identify retropharyngeal edema, and

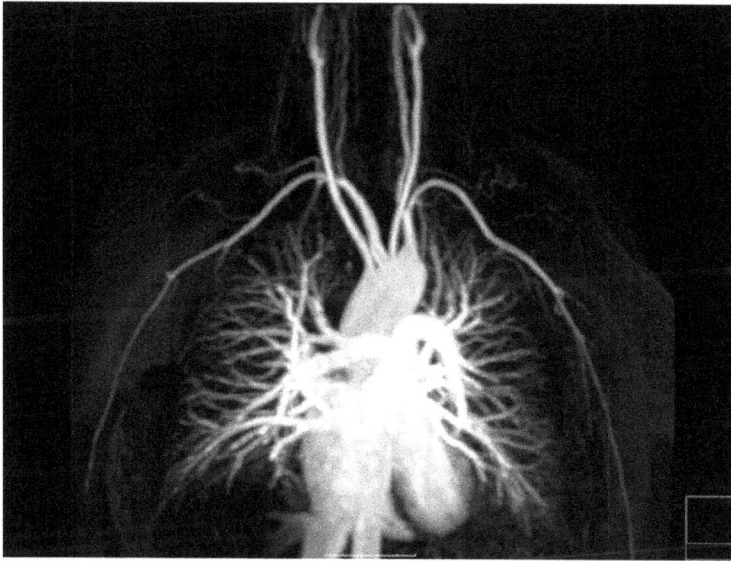

Figure 12.8 MRI reconstruction in a case of arteria lusoria.

evaluate for complications such as venous thrombosis or osteomyelitis. In trauma, MRI may be used to assess ligamentous injury, spinal cord involvement, or hematoma formation.

Although less commonly used for functional swallowing studies, emerging applications of dynamic MRI have shown promise in assessing real-time motion of pharyngeal and laryngeal structures during deglutition. These techniques, while still primarily in the research domain, may eventually complement traditional videofluoroscopic assessments, particularly in patients with complex neuromuscular disorders.

Despite its many advantages, MRI has limitations including higher cost, longer scan times, susceptibility to motion artifacts, and contraindications in patients with certain implants or claustrophobia. Nonetheless, for the detailed assessment of soft tissue pathology, MRI remains a cornerstone in modern imaging of the pharynx and upper esophagus.

12.4 COMPARATIVE ROLES OF CT AND MRI

CT and MRI serve complementary roles in the diagnostic work-up of pharyngeal and esophageal disorders, with each modality offering distinct advantages based on clinical context [7,8]. CT is generally the first-line imaging modality in acute settings due to its rapid acquisition time, wide availability, and high-resolution images of both soft tissues and bony structures. It is particularly useful in identifying structural lesions, assessing the extent of aerodigestive tract tumors, detecting calcified structures or foreign bodies, and delineating cervical lymphadenopathy.

MRI, in contrast, offers superior soft tissue contrast without the use of ionizing radiation, making it especially valuable in oncology, pediatric populations, and scenarios requiring serial imaging. It is the modality of choice when evaluating tumor infiltration into adjacent soft tissue planes, perineural spread, or post-treatment surveillance of residual or recurrent disease. MRI is also preferable for assessing pathology in areas where soft tissue resolution is paramount, such as the skull base, parapharyngeal space, or retropharyngeal area.

CT remains more sensitive in detecting bone erosion and subtle calcifications, while MRI surpasses CT in characterizing soft tissue lesions, vascular involvement, and neural structure displacement. When both modalities are used together, particularly in complex oncologic or surgical cases, they provide a comprehensive anatomical and functional map that supports precise therapeutic planning.

12.5 CLINICAL APPLICATIONS

CT and MRI are indispensable tools in the evaluation of a wide range of conditions affecting the pharynx and esophagus. In clinical practice, they are most frequently used in the context of oncologic assessment, but their applications extend well beyond cancer staging. Specific examples include [9,10]:

- *Head and neck cancer*: Both CT and MRI are used to stage tumors of the oropharynx, hypopharynx, larynx, and upper esophagus. MRI is superior in assessing soft tissue invasion, while CT is valuable for evaluating bony involvement.

- *Dysphagia with suspected mass*: When videofluoroscopic swallow study (VFSS) or endoscopy raises suspicion for extrinsic compression or a mass lesion, cross-sectional imaging is indicated to identify the source and extent of pathology.

- *Post-treatment surveillance*: In patients treated with chemoradiation or surgery for head and neck cancers, MRI is particularly useful in distinguishing post-treatment changes from residual or recurrent disease.

- *Esophageal pathologies*: While endoscopy remains the primary modality for mucosal lesions, CT and MRI are used to evaluate extraluminal masses, esophageal perforation, or mediastinal extension.

- *Infectious and inflammatory conditions*: CT with contrast is essential in diagnosing deep neck space infections, retropharyngeal abscesses, and phlegmon. MRI is used in cases where abscesses involve neurovascular structures or the spinal canal.

- *Congenital or structural abnormalities*: MRI provides excellent visualization of congenital anomalies such as laryngeal clefts, cricoid stenosis, or vascular rings that may impinge on the esophagus.

12.6 TECHNICAL CONSIDERATIONS AND PROTOCOLS

Optimizing image acquisition protocols is critical to the diagnostic value of both CT and MRI. For CT imaging of the pharynx and esophagus, the use of intravenous contrast enhances tissue differentiation and allows for better evaluation of vascular structures, mucosal thickening, and lymphadenopathy. Multiplanar reconstructions (MPRs) and three-dimensional rendering can assist in surgical planning and treatment navigation.

In MRI, the choice of sequences is tailored to the suspected pathology. T1-weighted images provide excellent anatomical detail, while T2-weighted sequences highlight fluid collections and edema. Post-contrast T1-weighted images with fat suppression enhance visualization of tumors and inflammatory changes. Advanced MRI protocols such as diffusion-weighted imaging (DWI) and dynamic contrast-enhanced imaging (DCE) are increasingly used in oncology for tumor characterization and therapy response evaluation.

Patient preparation for both modalities includes fasting (in cases of abdominal extension), removal of metal objects (for MRI), and pre-procedure screening for renal function and contrast allergies. Image interpretation requires specialized radiologic expertise and should be integrated into the patient's overall clinical assessment.

12.7 CONCLUSION

CT and MRI are essential adjuncts to the endoscopic and fluoroscopic evaluation of pharyngeal and esophageal disorders. Their complementary strengths in visualizing anatomical structures, soft tissue planes, and pathological changes allow for more accurate diagnosis, staging, and treatment planning, especially in complex or oncologically significant cases. While CT is favored in acute and structural evaluations, MRI provides unparalleled detail in soft tissue characterization and is invaluable in longitudinal patient care. Together, these modalities enhance the diagnostic acumen of the clinician and contribute to safer, more effective management strategies in the care of patients with aerodigestive tract disease.

REFERENCES

1. Curtin HD, Ishwaran H, Mancuso AA. Imaging of the oropharynx and hypopharynx. *Radiol Clin North Am*. 2015;53(1):115–132.
2. Becker M, Zbären P, Läng H, Stoupis C, Vock P, Marchal F. Neoplastic invasion of the laryngeal cartilage: comparison of CT and MR imaging. *Radiology*. 1995;194(2):661–669.
3. Mukherji SK, Castillo M. Head and neck imaging. *Neuroimaging Clin N Am*. 2003;13(3):481–502.
4. Loevner LA, Yousem DM, Montone KT, et al. MR imaging appearance of radiation-induced changes of the head and neck. *Radiographics*. 1997;17(1):141–160.
5. Hermans R. CT and MRI in the assessment of head and neck tumors and tumor recurrence. *Eur J Radiol*. 2000;33(3):239–247.

6. Carroll WR, Lo WW, Coit WE, Bruner JM, Johnson JT. MRI of perineural tumor spread in head and neck cancer. *Laryngoscope*. 1994;104(4):410–415.
7. Abdel Razek AAK, Mukherji SK. State-of-the-art imaging of laryngeal cancer. *AJNR Am J Neuroradiol*. 2018;39(4):642–649.
8. Halpern EJ. Clinical imaging of the esophagus: current practice and future directions. *AJR Am J Roentgenol*. 2007;188(6):1463–1471.
9. Kuehn BM. MRI finds a place in swallowing studies. *JAMA*. 2006;296(5):529–530.
10. American College of Radiology. *ACR–ASNR–SPR practice parameter for the performance of computed tomography (CT) of the neck*. Revised. American College of Radiology; 2021.

Index

Cervicothoracic scoliosis, 82
Chagas disease, 177, 178
Chronic pharyngitis with ulcers, 151
Cleft palate, 8
Collagen disorders, esophageal disorders
    acrosclerosis, 158
    dermatomyositis (polymyositis), 158–159
    lupus erythematous, 159
    rheumatoid arthritis, 159
    scleroderma, 157–158
Cranial base bones, 1
Cricopharyngeal achalasia, 165
Crohn's disease, 182, 192, 194
Curling ulcers, 150
Cushing ulcers, 150

D

Deglutition. *See* Swallowing
Dermatomyositis (polymyositis), 158–159
Diffuse esophageal spasm, 153, 156, 157
Diphtheritis, 148–149
Diverticula
    acquired, 166
    congenital, 166
    epiphrenic diverticula, 171–172
    Killian–Jamieson diverticulum, 166–168
    laryngoceles, 169
    lateral pharyngeal pouches, 169
    of thoracic esophagus, 169–171
    Zenker's diverticula, 29, 42, 51, 52, 57, 165–168
Dynamic barium swallow protocol, 101–103
Dysphagia, 29, 37, 45, 50, 51, 54, 81, 82, 85, 101, 105, 118,
        144, 146, 148, 151, 159, 160, 162, 165, 181–183
    dynamic barium swallow, 101
    dysphagia aortica, 30
    dysphagia lusoria, 30
    esophageal dysphagia, 33, 51
    oropharyngeal dysphagia, 33
    pharyngoesophageal endoscopy of, 57
    solid food dysphagia, 51
    symptoms of, 27

E

Edema, 174
Elevator esophagus, 156
Emphysema, 88
Endochondral bones, 1
Endochondral ossification, 1
Eosinophilic esophagitis, 175
Epidermolysis bullosa, 181
Epiphrenic diverticula, 171–172
Esophageal atresia, 185–186
Esophageal clearance, 137
Esophageal dysmotility, 47
Esophageal leiomyoma, 172
Esophageal melanoma, 174, 175
Esophageal neurofibroma, 191, 192
Esophageal webs, 160–163
Esophagitis
    acute esophagitis, 174
    candidiasis, 176–177

catarrhal acute esophagitis, 176
caustic and chemical esophagitis
    acid agents, 178–179
    alcohol and tobacco use, 179
    alkali substances, 178
    caustic substances, 178
    dust and fumes, 179
    heat esophagitis, 181
    peptic esophagitis, 180–181
Chagas disease, 177, 178
chronic bacterial esophagitis, 176
edema, 174
eosinophilic esophagitis, 175
renal transplant, 176
schistosomiasis, 177–178
thrush, 176
ulcerative esophagitis, 176
Esophagus. *See also* Specific entries
    Auerbach's plexus, 28
    benign and malignant esophageal tumors
        adenocarcinoma, 173, 174
        benign esophageal tumors, 172
        esophageal leiomyoma, 172
        esophageal melanoma, 174, 175
        granular cell tumor, 174
        malignant esophageal tumors, 173
        neurofibromas, 172, 173
        papillomas, 172
        squamous cell carcinoma, 173
    benign strictures
        Barrett's ulcer, 159
        cricopharyngeal (CP) bar, 163, 165–166
        double ring, 163
        hiatal hernia, 159, 160
        reflux esophagitis, 159
        ring-like strictures, 160
        Schatski's ring, 162–164
        webs, 160–163
    cervical esophagus, 29
    clasp and sling fibers of gastroesophageal
            junction, 30
    collagen disorders
        acrosclerosis, 158
        dermatomyositis (polymyositis), 158–159
        lupus erythematous, 159
        rheumatoid arthritis, 159
        scleroderma, 157–158
    computed tomography (CT) imaging, 191–196
    Curling ulcers, 150
    Cushing ulcers, 150
    deficiency disorders
        sideropenic anemia, 182–183
        vitamin deficiency, 183
    detailed structure of, 27–28
    diverticula
        acquired, 166
        congenital, 166
        epiphrenic diverticula, 171–172
        Killian–Jamieson diverticulum, 166–168
        laryngoceles, 169
        lateral pharyngeal pouches, 169
        of thoracic esophagus, 169–171
        Zenker's diverticula, 166–168

For Product Safety Concerns and Information please contact our EU
representative GPSR@taylorandfrancis.com
Taylor & Francis Verlag GmbH, Kaufingerstraße 24, 80331 München, Germany

www.ingramcontent.com/pod-product-compliance
Lightning Source LLC
Chambersburg PA
CBHW061418210326
41598CB00035B/6255

* 9 7 8 1 0 3 2 7 9 1 7 8 4 *